THE STATE OF THE WORLD'S CHILDREN 2009

Acknowledgements

This report was made possible with the advice and contributions of many people, both inside and outside UNICEF. Important contributions were received from the following UNICEF field offices: Afghanistan, Bangladesh, Benin, Brazil, Burundi, Central African Republic, Chad, Côte d'Ivoire, Ghana, Guatemala, Haiti, India, Indonesia, Kenya, Lao People's Democratic Republic, Liberia, Madagascar, Mexico, Morocco, Mozambique, Nepal, Niger, Nigeria, Occupied Palestinian Territory, Pakistan, Peru, Rwanda, Sierra Leone, Sri Lanka, Sudan, Togo, Tunisia and Uganda. Input was also received from UNICEF regional offices and the Innocenti Research Centre.

Special thanks to H. M. Queen Rania Al Abdullah of Jordan, the Honourable Vabah Gayflor, Zulfiqar A. Bhutta, Sarah Brown, Jennifer Harris Requejo, Joy Lawn, Mario Merialdi, Rosa Maria Nuñez-Urquiza and Cesar G. Victora.

EDITORIAL AND RESEARCH

Patricia Moccia, *Editor-in-Chief*; David Anthony, *Editor*; Chris Brazier; Marilia Di Noia; Hirut Gebre-Egziabher; Emily Goodman; Yasmine Hage; Nelly Ingraham; Pamela Knight; Amy Lai; Charlotte Maitre; Meedan Mekonnen; Gabrielle Mitchell-Marell; Kristin Moehlmann; Michelle Risley; Catherine Rutgers; Karin Shankar; Shobana Shankar; Judith Yemane

STATISTICAL TABLES

Tessa Wardlaw, *Chief*, Strategic Information, Division of Policy and Practice; Priscilla Akwara; Danielle Burke; Xiaodong Cai; Claudia Cappa; Ngagne Diakhate; Archana Dwivedi; Friedrich Huebler; Rouslan Karimov; Julia Krasevec; Edilberto Loaiza; Rolf Luyendijk; Nyein Nyein Lwin; Maryanne Neill; Holly Newby; Khin Wityee Oo; Emily White Johansson; Danzhen You

PRODUCTION AND DISTRIBUTION

Jaclyn Tierney, *Chief*, Production and Translation; Edward Ying, Jr.; Germain Ake; Fanuel Endalew; Eki Kairupan; Farid Rashid; Elias Salem

TRANSLATION

French edition: Marc Chalamet
Spanish edition: Carlos Perellón

PROGRAMME AND POLICY GUIDANCE

UNICEF Programme Division, the Division of Policy and Practice and Innocenti Research Centre, with particular thanks to Nicholas Alipui, *Director*, Programme Division; Dan Rohrmann, *Deputy Director*, Programme Division; Maniza Zaman, *Deputy Director*, Programme Division; Peter Salama, *Associate Director*, Health; Jimmy Kolker, *Associate Director*, HIV and AIDS; Clarissa Brocklehurst, *Associate Director*, Water, Sanitation and Hygiene; Werner Schultink, *Associate Director*, Nutrition; Touria Barakat; Linda Bartlett; Wivina Belmonte; Robert Cohen; Robert Gass; Asha George; Christine Jaulmes; Grace Kariwiga; Noreen Khan; Patience Kuruneri; Nuné Mangasaryan; Mariana Muzzi; Robin Nandy; Shirin Nayernouri; Kayode Oyegbite; David Parker; Luwei Pearson; Ian Pett; Bolor Purevdorj; Melanie Renshaw; Daniel Seymour; Fouzia Shafique; Judith Standley; David Stewart; Abdelmajid Tibouti; Mark Young; Alex Yuster

DESIGN AND PRE-PRESS PRODUCTION

Prographics, Inc.

PRINTING

Colorcraft of Virginia, Inc.

DEDICATION

The State of the World's Children 2009 is dedicated to Allan Rosenfield, MD, Dean Emeritus, Mailman School of Public Health, Columbia University, who passed away on 12 October 2008. A pioneer in the field of public health, Dr. Rosenfield worked tirelessly to avert maternal deaths and provide care and treatment for women and children affected by HIV and AIDS in resource-poor settings. He lent his energy and intellect to numerous groundbreaking programmes and institutions, and his passion, dedication, courage and commitment to bringing women's health and human rights to the fore of development remain a source of inspiration.

Foreword

Niger has the highest lifetime risk of maternal mortality of any country in the world, 1 in 7. The comparable risk in the developed world is 1 in 8,000. Since 1990, the base year for the Millennium Development Goals, an estimated 10 million women have died from complications related to pregnancy and childbirth, and some 4 million newborns have died each year within the first 28 days of life. Advances in maternal and neonatal health have not matched those of child survival, which registered a 27 per cent reduction in the global under-five mortality rate between 1990 and 2007.

The State of the World's Children 2009 focuses on maternal and neonatal health and identifies the interventions and actions that must be scaled up to save lives. Most maternal and neonatal deaths can be averted through proven interventions – including adequate nutrition, improved hygiene practices, antenatal care, skilled health workers assisting at births, emergency obstetric and newborn care, and post-natal visits for both mothers and newborns – delivered through a continuum of care linking households and communities to health systems. Research indicates that around 80 per cent of maternal deaths are preventable if women have access to essential maternity and basic health-care services.

A stronger focus on Africa and Asia is imperative to accelerate progress on maternal and newborn health. These two continents present the greatest challenges to the survival and health of women and newborns, accounting for an estimated 95 per cent of maternal deaths and around 90 per cent of neonatal deaths.

Two thirds of all maternal deaths occur in just 10 countries; India and Nigeria together account for one third of maternal deaths worldwide. In 2008, UNICEF, the World Health Organization, the United Nations Population Fund and the World Bank agreed to work together to help accelerate progress on maternal and newborn health in the 25 countries with the highest rates of mortality.

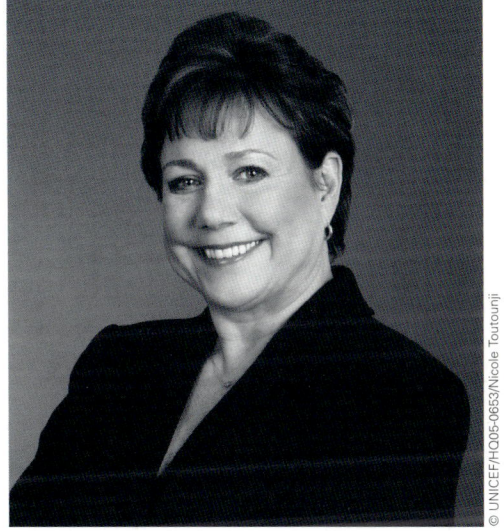

Premature pregnancy and motherhood pose considerable risks to the health of girls. The younger a girl is when she becomes pregnant, the greater the health risks for herself and her baby. Maternal deaths related to pregnancy and childbirth are an important cause of mortality for girls aged 15–19 worldwide, accounting for nearly 70,000 deaths each year.

Early marriage and pregnancy, HIV and AIDS, sexual violence and other gender-related abuses also increase the risk that adolescent girls will drop out of school. This, in turn, entrenches the vicious cycle of gender discrimination, poverty and high rates of maternal and neonatal mortality.

Educating girls and young women is one of the most powerful ways of breaking the poverty trap and creating a supportive environment for maternal and newborn health. Combining efforts to expand coverage of essential services and strengthen health systems with actions to empower and protect girls and women has real potential to accelerate progress.

As the 2015 deadline for the Millennium Development Goals draws closer, the challenge for improving maternal and newborn health goes beyond meeting the goals; it lies in preventing needless human tragedy. Success will be measured in terms of lives saved and lives improved.

Ann M. Veneman
Executive Director
United Nations Children's Fund

CONTENTS

Acknowledgements ii
Dedication ii
Foreword
    Ann M. Veneman
    Executive Director, UNICEF iii

1 Maternal and newborn health: Where we stand 1

Panels
Challenges in measuring maternal deaths 7

Creating a supportive environment for mothers and newborns *by H. M. Queen Rania Al Abdullah of Jordan, UNICEF's Eminent Advocate for Children* 11

Maternal and newborn health in Nigeria: Developing strategies to accelerate progress 19

Expanding Millennium Development Goal 5: Universal access to reproductive health by 2015 20

Prioritizing maternal health in Sri Lanka 21

The centrality of Africa and Asia in the global challenges for children and women 22

The global food crisis and its potential impact on maternal and newborn health 24

Figures
1.1 Millennium Development Goals on maternal and child health 3
1.2 Regional distribution of maternal deaths 6
1.3 Trends, levels and lifetime risk of maternal mortality 8
1.4 Regional rates of neonatal mortality 10
1.5 Direct causes of maternal deaths, 1997–2002 14
1.6 Direct causes of neonatal deaths, 2000 15
1.7 Conceptual framework for maternal and neonatal mortality and morbidity 17
1.8 Food prices have risen sharply across the board 24

2 Creating a supportive environment for maternal and newborn health 25

Panels
Promoting healthy behaviours for mothers, newborns and children: *The Facts for Life* guide 29

Primary health care: 30 years since Alma-Ata 31

Addressing the health worker shortage: A critical action for improving maternal and newborn health 35

Towards greater equity in health for mothers and newborns *by Cesar G. Victora, Professor of Epidemiology, Universidade Federal de Pelotas, Brazil* 38

Adapting maternity services to the cultures of rural Peru 42

Southern Sudan: After the peace, a new battle against maternal mortality 43

Figures
2.1 The continuum of care 27
2.2 Although improving, the educational status of young women is still low in several developing regions 30
2.3 Gender parity in attendance has improved markedly, but there are still slightly more girls than boys out of primary school 33
2.4 Child marriage is highly prevalent in South Asia and sub-Saharan Africa 34
2.5 Female genital mutilation/cutting, though in decline, is still prevalent in many developing countries 37
2.6 Mothers who received skilled attendance at delivery, by wealth quintile and region 38
2.7 Women in Mali receiving three or more antenatal care visits, before and after the implementation of the Accelerated Child Survival and Development (ACSD) initiative 39
2.8 Many women in developing countries have no say in their own health-care needs 40

3 The continuum of care across time and location: Risks and opportunities 45

Panels
Eliminating maternal and neonatal tetanus 49

Hypertensive disorders: Common yet complex 53

The first 28 days of life *by Zulfiqar A. Bhutta, Professor and Chairman, Department of Paediatrics & Child Health, Aga Khan University, Karachi, Pakistan* 57

Midwifery in Afghanistan 60

Kangaroo mother care in Ghana 62

HIV/malaria co-infection in pregnancy 63

The challenges faced by adolescent girls in Liberia *by the Honourable Vabah Gayflor, Minister of Gender and Development, Liberia* 64

Figures
3.1 Protection against neonatal tetanus 48
3.2 Antiretroviral prophylaxis for HIV-positive mothers to prevent mother-to-child transmission of HIV 50
3.3 Antenatal care coverage 51
3.4 Delivery care coverage 52
3.5 Emergency obstetric care: Rural Caesarean section ... 54
3.6 Early and exclusive breastfeeding 59

THE STATE OF THE WORLD'S CHILDREN 2009
Maternal and Newborn Health

4 Strengthening health systems to improve maternal and newborn health 67

Panels

Using critical link methodology in health-care systems to prevent maternal deaths *by Rosa Maria Nuñez-Urquiza, National Institute of Public Health, Mexico* 73

New directions in maternal health *by Mario Merialdi, World Health Organization, and Jennifer Harris Requejo, Partnership for Maternal, Newborn and Child Health* 75

Strengthening the health system in the Lao People's Democratic Republic 76

Saving mothers and newborn lives – the crucial first days after birth *by Joy Lawn, Senior Research and Policy Advisor, Saving Newborn Lives/Save the Children-US, South Africa* 80

Burundi: Government commitment to maternal and child health care 83

Integrating maternal and newborn health care in India 85

Figures

4.1 Emergency obstetric care: United Nations process indicators and recommended levels 70
4.2 Distribution of key data sources used to derive the 2005 maternal mortality estimates 71
4.3 Skilled health workers are in short supply in Africa and South-East Asia in particular 74
4.4 Uptake of key maternal, newborn and child health policies by the 68 Countdown to 2015 priority countries 78
4.5 Asia has among the lowest levels of government spending on health care as a share of overall public expenditure 79
4.6 Post-natal care strategies: Feasibility and implementation challenges 81
4.7 Lower-income countries pay most of their private health-care spending out of pocket 82
4.8 Low-income countries have only 10 hospital beds per 10,000 people 84

5 Working together for maternal and newborn health 91

Panels

Working together for maternal and newborn health *by Sarah Brown, Patron of the White Ribbon Alliance for Safe Motherhood and wife of Gordon Brown, Prime Minister of the Government of the United Kingdom* 94

Key global health partnerships for maternal and newborn health 96

Partnering for mothers and newborns in the Central African Republic 99

UN agencies strengthen their collaboration in support of maternal and newborn health 102

Enhancing health information systems: The Health Metrics Network 105

Figures

5.1 Key global health initiatives aimed at strengthening health systems and scaling up essential interventions 97
5.2 Official development assistance for maternal and neonatal health has risen rapidly since 2004 98
5.3 Nutrition, PMTCT and child health have seen substantial rises in financing 100
5.4 Financing for maternal, newborn and child health from global health initiatives has increased sharply in recent years 101
5.5 Focal and partner agencies for each component of the continuum of maternal and newborn care and related functions 103

References 106

Statistical Tables 113

Under-five mortality rankings 117
Table 1. Basic indicators 118
Table 2. Nutrition 122
Table 3. Health 126
Table 4. HIV/AIDS 130
Table 5. Education 134
Table 6. Demographic indicators 138
Table 7. Economic indicators 142
Table 8. Women 146
Table 9. Child protection 150
Table 10. The rate of progress 154

Acronyms 158

THE STATE OF THE WORLD'S CHILDREN 2009

1 Maternal and newborn health: Where we stand

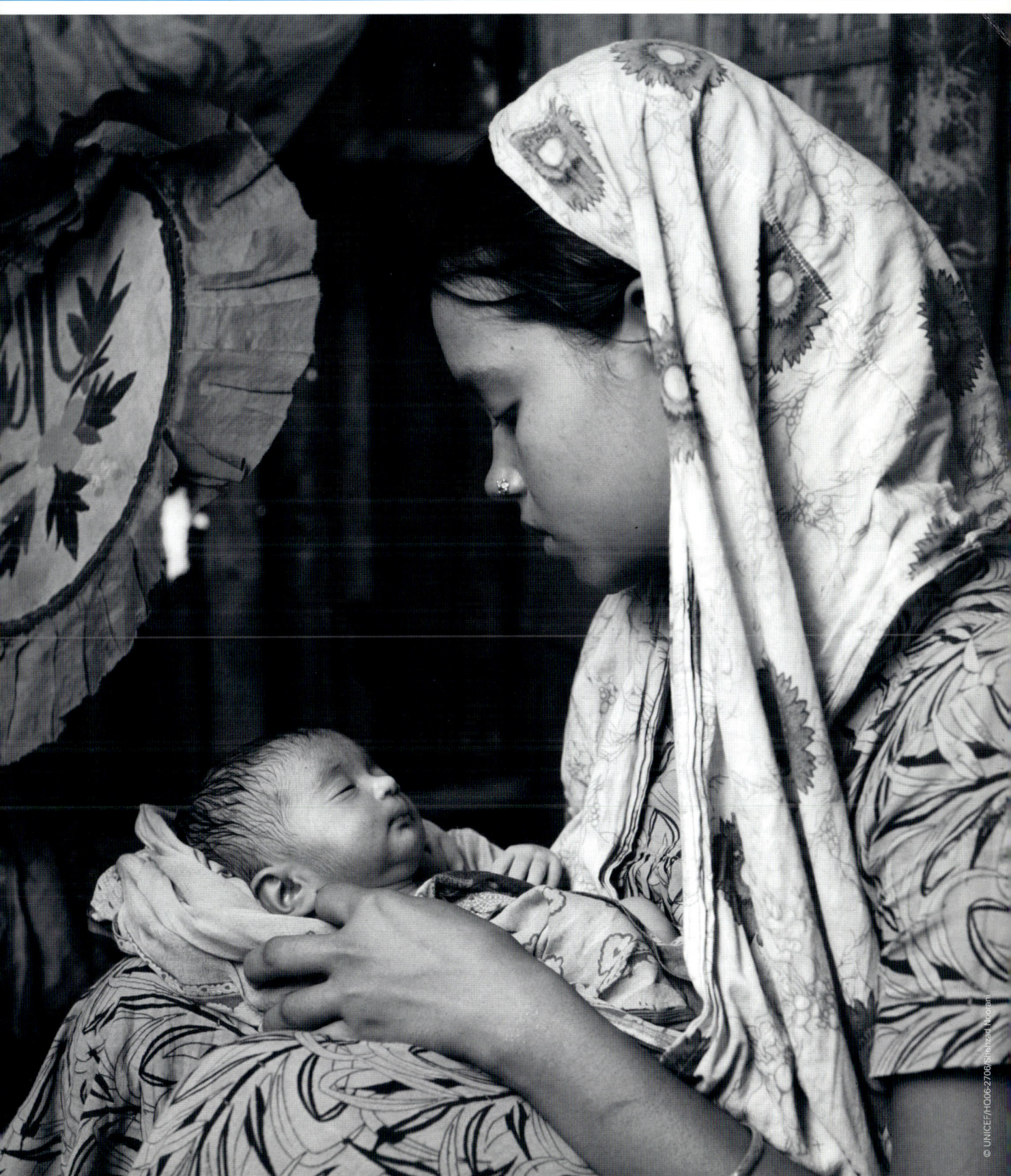

Each year, more than half a million women die from causes related to pregnancy and childbirth, and nearly 4 million newborns die within 28 days of birth. Millions more suffer from disability, disease, infection and injury. Cost-effective solutions are available that could bring rapid improvements, but urgency and commitment are required to implement them and to meet the Millennium Development Goals related to maternal and child health. The first chapter of The State of the World's Children 2009 *examines trends and levels of maternal and neonatal health in each of the major regions, using mortality ratios as benchmark indicators. It briefly explores the main proximal and underlying causes of maternal and neonatal mortality and morbidity, and outlines a framework for accelerating progress.*

Pregnancy and childbirth are generally times of joy for parents and families. Pregnancy, birth and motherhood, in an environment that respects women, can powerfully affirm women's rights and social status without jeopardizing their health.

The enabling environment for safe motherhood and childbirth depends on the care and attention provided to pregnant women and newborns by communities and families, the acumen of skilled health personnel and the availability of adequate health-care facilities, equipment, and medicines and emergency care when needed. Many women in the developing world – and most women in the world's least developed countries – give birth at home without skilled attendants, yet their newborns are usually healthy and survive past their first few weeks of life until their fifth birthday and beyond. Despite the multitude of risks associated with pregnancy and childbirth, the majority of mothers also survive.

But the health risks associated with pregnancy and childbirth are far greater in developing countries than in industrialized ones. They are especially prevalent in the least developed and lowest-income countries, and among less affluent and marginalized families and communities everywhere. Globally, efforts to reduce deaths among women from complications related to pregnancy and childbirth have been less successful than other areas of human development – with the result that having a child remains among the most serious health risks for women. On average, each day around 1,500 women die from complications related to pregnancy and childbirth, most of them in sub-Saharan Africa and South Asia.

The divide between industrialized countries and developing regions – particularly the least developed countries – is perhaps greater on maternal mortality than on almost any other issue. This claim is borne out by the numbers: Based on 2005 data, the average lifetime risk of a woman in a least developed country dying from complications related to pregnancy or childbirth is more than 300 times greater than for a woman living in an industrialized country. No other mortality rate is so unequal.

Millions of women who survive childbirth suffer from pregnancy-related injuries, infections, diseases and disabilities, often with lifelong consequences. The truth is that most of these deaths and conditions are preventable – research has shown that approximately 80 per cent of maternal deaths could be averted if women had access to essential maternity and basic health-care services.[1]

Deaths of newborns in developing countries have also received far too little attention. Almost 40 per cent of under-five deaths – or 3.7 million in 2004, according to the latest World Health Organization estimates – occur in the first 28 days of life. Three quarters of neonatal deaths take place in the first seven days, the early neonatal period; most of these are also preventable.[2]

The gap in risk of maternal death between the industrialized world and many developing countries, particularly the least developed, is often termed the 'greatest health divide in the world'.

The divide in neonatal deaths between the industrialized countries and developing regions is also wide. Based on 2004 data, a child born in a least developed country is almost 14 times more likely to die during the first 28 days of life than one born in an industrialized country.

The health of mothers and newborns is intricately related, so preventing deaths requires, in many cases, implementing the same interventions. These include such essential measures as antenatal care, skilled attendance at birth, access to emergency obstetric care when necessary, adequate nutrition, post-partum care, newborn care and education to improve health, infant feeding and care, and hygiene behaviours. To be truly effective and sustainable, however, these interventions must take place within a development framework that strives to strengthen and integrate programmes with health systems and an environment supportive of women's rights.

A human rights-based approach to improving maternal and neonatal health focuses on enhancing healthcare provision, addressing gender discrimination and inequities in society through cultural, social and behavioural changes, among other means, and targeting those countries and communities most at risk.

The State of the World's Children 2009 examines maternal and newborn health across the world, and in the developing world in particular, complementing last year's report on child survival. While the emphasis of the report remains firmly on health and nutrition, mortality rates are employed as benchmark indicators. Sub-Saharan Africa and South Asia, the regions with the highest numbers and rates of maternal and newborn mortality, are principal focuses. Key threads running through the report are the imperative of creating a supportive environment for maternal and newborn health based on respect for women's rights, and the need to establish a continuum of care for mothers, newborns and children that integrate programmes for reproductive health, safe motherhood, newborn care and child survival, growth and development. The report examines the latest paradigms, policies and programmes and describes key initiatives and partnerships that are striving to accelerate progress. A series of panels, several of which have been contributed by guest collaborators,

Figure 1.1

Millennium Development Goals on maternal and child health

Millennium Development Goal 4: Reduce child mortality	
Targets	**Indicators**
4.A: Reduce by two thirds, between 1990 and 2015, the under-five mortality rate	4.1 Under-five mortality rate
	4.2 Infant mortality rate
	4.3 Proportion of 1-year-old children immunized against measles

Millennium Development Goal 5: Improve maternal health*	
Targets	**Indicators**
5.A: Reduce by three quarters, between 1990 and 2015, the maternal mortality ratio	5.1 Maternal mortality ratio
	5.2 Proportion of births attended by skilled health personnel
5.B: Achieve, by 2015, universal access to reproductive health	5.3 Contraceptive prevalence rate
	5.4 Adolescent birth rate
	5.5 Antenatal care coverage (at least one visit and at least four visits)
	5.6 Unmet need for family planning

* The revised Millennium Development Goals framework agreed by the United Nations General Assembly at the 2005 World Summit, with the new official list of indicators effective as of 15 January 2008, has added a new target (5.B) and four new indicators for monitoring Millennium Development Goal 5.

Source: United Nations, Millennium Development Goals Indicators: The official United Nations site for the MDG indicators, <http://mdgs.un.org/unsd/mdg/Host.aspx?Content=Indicators/OfficialList.htm>, accessed 1 August 2008.

address some of the critical issues in maternal and newborn health and nutrition today.

The current situation of maternal and neonatal health

Since 1990, the estimate of the global annual number of maternal deaths has exceeded 500,000. Although the number of under-five deaths worldwide has fallen consistently – from around 13 million in 1990 to 9.2 million in 2007 – maternal deaths have remained stubbornly intractable. Limited gains have been made worldwide towards the first target of Millennium Development Goal (MDG) 5, which aims to reduce the 1990 maternal mortality ratio by three quarters by 2015; and progress on diminishing maternal mortality ratios has been virtually non-existent in sub-Saharan Africa.[3]

Maternal mortality ratios strongly reflect the overall effectiveness of health systems, which in many low-income developing countries suffer from weak administrative, technical and logistical capacity, inadequate financial investment and a lack of skilled health personnel. Scaling up key interventions – for example, antenatal HIV testing, increasing the number of births attended by skilled health personnel, providing access to emergency obstetric care when necessary and providing post-natal care for mothers and babies – could sharply reduce both maternal and neonatal deaths. Enhancing women's access to family planning, adequate nutrition and affordable basic health care would lower mortality rates further still. These are not impossible, impractical actions, but proven, cost-effective provisions that women of reproductive age have a right to expect.

Maternal health, however, goes beyond the survival of pregnant women and mothers. For every woman who dies from causes related to pregnancy or childbirth, it is estimated that there are 20 others who suffer pregnancy-related illness or experience other severe consequences. The number is striking: An estimated 10 million women annually who survive their pregnancies experience such adverse outcomes.[4]

That maternal health – as epitomized by the risk of death or disability from causes related to pregnancy and childbirth – has scarcely advanced in decades is the result of multiple underlying causes. The root cause may lie in women's disadvantaged position in many countries and cultures, and in the lack of attention to, and accountability for, women's rights.

The 1979 Convention on the Elimination of All Forms of Discrimination against Women (CEDAW), currently ratified by 185 countries, requires signatories to "eliminate discrimination against women in the field of health care in order to ensure, on a basis of equality of men and women, access to health care services, including those related to family planning" (article 12.1). It also stipulates that they "ensure to women appropriate services in connection with pregnancy, confinement and the post-natal period, granting free services where necessary, as well as adequate nutrition during pregnancy and lactation" (article 12.2). Furthermore, the Convention on the Rights of the Child also commits States Parties to "ensure appropriate pre-natal and post-natal health care for mothers" and to "develop preventive health care, guidance for parents and family planning education and services" (article 24). The available evidence suggests that many countries are failing to deliver on these commitments.

Improving women's health is pivotal to fulfilling the rights of girls and women under CEDAW and the Convention on the Rights of the Child and achieving the Millennium Development Goals. In addition to meeting MDG 5, enhancing reproductive and maternal health and services will also directly contribute to attaining MDG 4, which seeks to reduce the under-five mortality rate by two thirds between 1990 and 2015.

Enhancing maternal nutrition will also bring benefits for the achievement of Millennium Development Goal 1, which seeks to eradicate extreme poverty and hunger by 2015. Undernutrition is a process which often starts in utero and may last, particularly for girls and women, throughout the life cycle: A stunted girl is likely to become a stunted adolescent and later a stunted woman. Besides posing threats to

The lifetime risk of maternal death for a woman in a least developed country is more than 300 times greater than for a woman living in an industrialized country.

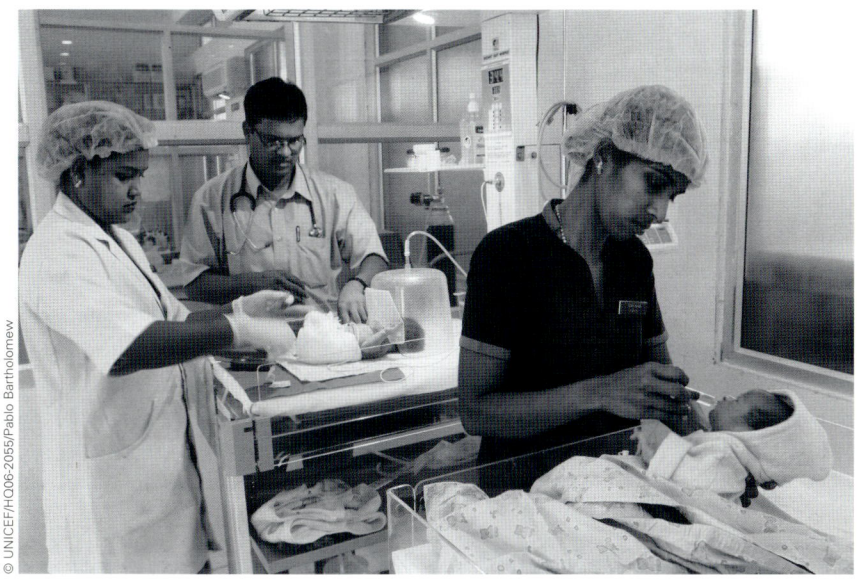

A strong referral system, skilled health workers and well equipped facilities are pivotal to reducing maternal and newborn deaths resulting from complications during childbirth. Health workers treat babies in the Sick Newborn Care Unit, India.

her own health and productivity, poor nutrition that contributes to stunting and underweight increases a woman's likelihood of adverse pregnancy and birth outcomes. Undernourished mothers also have a far higher risk of delivering babies with low birthweight – a condition that gravely heightens the baby's risk of death.[5]

Lowering a mother's risk of mortality and morbidity directly improves a child's prospects for survival. Research has shown that in developing countries, babies whose mothers die during the first six weeks of their lives are far more likely to die in the first two years of life than babies whose mothers survive. In a study conducted in Afghanistan, 74 per cent of infants born alive to mothers who died of maternal causes also subsequently died.[6] Moreover, maternal complications in labour heighten the risk of neonatal deaths, which are rapidly becoming a key focus of child survival efforts as overall rates of under-five mortality decline in most developing countries.

Trends in maternal and newborn health

Maternal mortality

The most recent UN inter-agency estimates suggest that in 2005, 536,000 women died from causes related to pregnancy and childbirth. This figure may be far from precise, however, as measuring maternal mortality is challenging, and in many developing countries the required data are not routinely recorded. Beyond the estimation of maternal mortality, determining and recording the causes of death is a complex process. For a death to be conclusively established as related to pregnancy or childbirth, both the cause of mortality and the pregnancy status and the timing of death in relation to that pregnancy must be accurately noted. This level of detail is sometimes missing in the statistical reporting systems of industrialized countries, and its absence is commonplace in many developing countries, particularly the poorest.[7]

Efforts to improve data collection on maternal mortality have been ongoing for the past two decades, initially involving the World Health Organization (WHO), UNICEF and the United Nations Population Fund (UNFPA), later joined by the World Bank. This inter-agency collaboration pools resources and reviews methodologies to arrive at more precise and comprehensive global estimates of maternal mortality. The figures for 2005 are the most accurate yet and the first to estimate maternal mortality trends by an inter-agency process. (*Further details on the estimation of maternal mortality ratios and levels can be found in the Panel on page 7.*)

In recent years, new methodologies to calculate maternal and neonatal health status, service needs and mortality have been developed by the research community. These efforts are ongoing, enriching the process of arriving at more precise estimates

Africa and Asia account for 95 per cent of the world's maternal deaths, with particularly high burdens in sub-Saharan Africa (50 per cent of the global total) and South Asia (35 per cent).

and causes of mortality and morbidity. In turn, better data and analysis on health status and health services are helping enhance the strategies and frameworks, programmes, policies and partnerships – including those that support gender mainstreaming – that are striving to improve maternal and newborn health.

One issue in the estimation of maternal mortality appears beyond contention: The vast majority of maternal deaths – more than 99 per cent, according to the 2005 UN inter-agency estimates – occurred in developing countries. Half of these (265,000) took place in sub-Saharan Africa and another third (187,000) in South Asia. Between them, these two regions accounted for 85 per cent of the world's pregnancy-related deaths in 2005. India alone had 22 per cent of the global total.

The trend estimates available for maternal mortality indicates the lack of sufficient progress towards Target A of MDG 5, which seeks a 75 per cent reduction in the maternal mortality ratio between 1990 and 2015. Given that the global maternal mortality ratio stood at 430 per 100,000 live births in 1990, and at 400 deaths per 100,000 live births in 2005, meeting the target will require more than a 70 per cent reduction between 2005 and 2015.

Global trends can obscure the wide variations between regions, many of which have made appreciable progress in reducing maternal mortality and are laying the foundations for further improvements by increasing access to basic maternity services. In the industrialized countries, the maternal mortality ratio remained broadly static between 1990 and 2005, at a low rate of 8 per 100,000 live births. Near universal access to skilled care during delivery and emergency obstetric care when necessary have contributed to these diminished levels of maternal mortality; no industrialized countries with data have skilled attendance at birth of less than 98 per cent, and most have universal coverage.

In all of the developing regions outside sub-Saharan Africa, both the absolute numbers of maternal deaths and maternal mortality ratios declined between 1990 and 2005. In sub-Saharan Africa, maternal mortality ratios remained largely unchanged over the same period. Given the region's high fertility rates, this has resulted in higher numbers of maternal deaths over the 15-year period. This lack of progress is particularly worrying, since the region has by far the highest ratios and lifetime risk of maternal mortality and the greatest number of maternal deaths. In West and Central Africa, the regional maternal mortality ratio stands at a staggering 1,100 per 100,000 live births, compared to the average for developing countries and territories of 450 per 100,000 live births. This region includes the country with the highest rate of maternal death in the world: Sierra Leone, with 2,100 maternal deaths per 100,000 live births.

The West and Central Africa region also has the highest total fertility rate, at 5.5 children in 2007. (The total fertility rate measures the number of children who would be born per woman if she lived to the end of her childbearing

Figure 1.2

Regional distribution of maternal deaths*

Maternal deaths, 2005

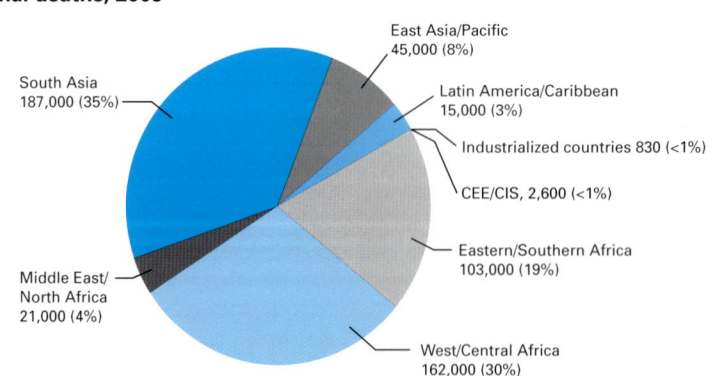

* Percentages may not total 100% because of rounding.

Source: World Health Organization, United Nations Children's Fund, United Nations Population Fund and the World Bank, *Maternal Mortality in 2005: Estimates developed by WHO, UNICEF, UNFPA and the World Bank*, WHO, Geneva, 2007, p. 35.

Challenges in measuring maternal deaths

Maternal mortality is defined as the death of a woman while pregnant or within 42 days of termination of pregnancy, regardless of the site or duration of pregnancy, from any cause related to or aggravated by the pregnancy or its management. Causes of deaths can be divided into direct causes that are related to obstetric complications during pregnancy, labour or the post-partum period, and indirect causes. There are five direct causes: haemorrhage (usually occurring postpartum), sepsis, eclampsia, obstructed labour and complications of abortion. Indirect obstetric deaths occur from either previously existing conditions or from conditions arising in pregnancy which are not related to direct obstetric causes but may be aggravated by the physiological effects of pregnancy. These include such conditions as HIV and AIDS, malaria, anaemia and cardiovascular diseases. Simply because a woman develops a complication does not mean that death is inevitable; inappropriate or incorrect treatment or lack of appropriate, timely interventions underlie most maternal deaths.

Accurate classification of the causes of maternal death, whether direct or indirect, accidental or incidental, is challenging. To accurately categorize a death as maternal, information is needed on the cause of death as well as pregnancy status, or the time of death in relation to the pregnancy. This information may be missing, misclassified or under-reported even in industrialized countries with fully functioning vital registration systems, as well as in developing countries facing high burdens of maternal mortality. There are several reasons for this: First, many deliveries take place at home, particularly in the least developed countries and in rural areas, complicating efforts to establish cause of death. Second, civil registration systems may be incomplete or, even if deemed complete, attribution of causes of death may be inadequate. Third, modern medicine may delay a women's death beyond the 42-day post-partum period. For these reasons, in some cases alternative definitions of maternal mortality are used. One concept refers to any cause of death during pregnancy or the post-partum period. Another concept takes into account deaths from direct or indirect causes that occur after the post-partum period up to one year following pregnancy.

The main measure of mortality risk is the *maternal mortality ratio*, which is identified as the number of maternal deaths during a given period of time per 100,000 live births during the same period, which is generally a year. Another key measure is the *lifetime risk of maternal death*, which reflects the probability of becoming pregnant and the probability of dying from a maternal cause during a women's reproductive lifespan. In other words, the risk of maternal death is related to two main factors: mortality risk associated with a single pregnancy or live birth; and the number of pregnancies that women have during their reproductive years.

Working together to improve estimations of maternal deaths

Several agencies are collaborating to establish more accurate measurements of maternal mortality rates and levels worldwide, and assess progress towards Target A of Millennium Development Goal 5, which seeks to reduce the maternal mortality rate by three quarters between 1990 and 2015. The Maternal Mortality Working Group, which originally comprised the World Health Organization, UNICEF and the United Nations Population Fund, developed internationally comparable global estimates of maternal mortality for 1990, 1995 and 2000.

In 2006, the World Bank, United Nations Population Division and several outside technical experts joined the group, which subsequently developed a new set of globally comparable maternal mortality estimates for 2005, building on previous methodology and new data. The process generated estimates for countries with no national data, and adjusted available country data to correct for under-reporting and misclassification. Of the 171 countries reviewed by the Maternal Mortality Working Group for the 2005 estimations, appropriate national-level data were unavailable for 61 countries, representing one quarter of global births. For these countries, models were used to estimate maternal mortality.

For the 2005 estimates, data were drawn from eight categories of sources: complete civil registration systems with good attribution of data, complete civil registration systems with uncertain or poor attribution of data, direct sisterhood methods, reproductive-age mortality studies, disease surveillance or sample registration, census, special studies and no national data. Estimates for each source were calculated according to a different formula, taking into account factors such as correcting for known bias and determining realistic uncertainty bounds.

Measures of maternal mortality are prepared with a margin of uncertainty, highlighting the fact that while they are the best estimates available, the actual rate may be higher or lower than the average. Although this is true of any statistic, the high degree of uncertainty for maternal mortality ratios indicates that all data points should be interpreted cautiously.

Notwithstanding the challenges of data collection and measurement, the 2005 inter-agency estimates for maternal mortality were sufficiently rigorous to produce trend analysis, assessing progress from the 1990 baseline date of MDG 5 to 2005. The lack of improvement in reducing maternal mortality identified in many developing countries has helped bring greater attention to achieving MDG 5.

The 2005 maternal mortality estimates are far from perfect, and much work is still required to refine the processes of data collection and estimation. But they reflect a strong commitment on the part of the international community to continually strive for greater accuracy and precision. These ongoing efforts will support and guide actions to improve maternal health and ensure that women count.

See References, page 107.

Although the number of under-five deaths worldwide has fallen consistently – from around 13 million in 1990 to 9.2 million in 2007 – the toll of maternal mortality has remained stubbornly intractable above 500,000.

Figure 1.3

Trends, levels and lifetime risk of maternal mortality

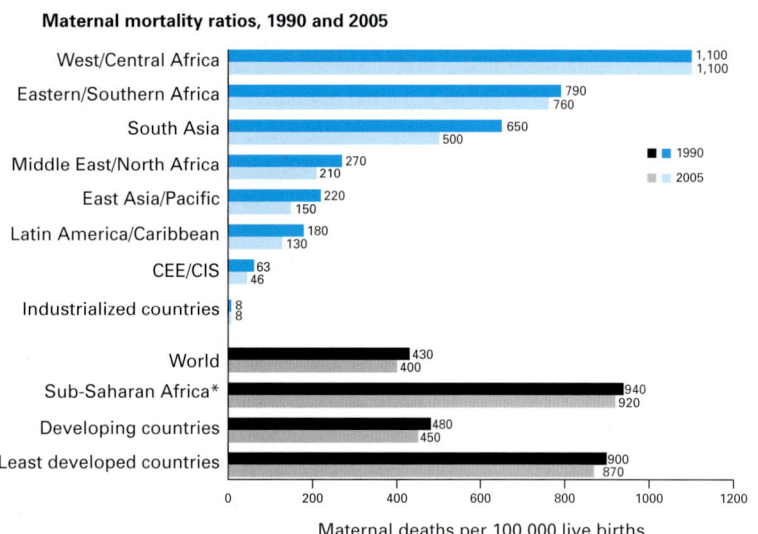

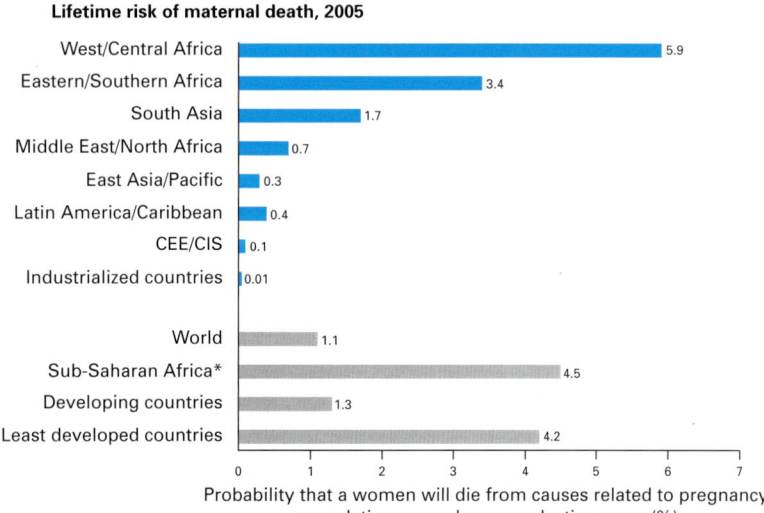

*Sub-Saharan Africa comprises the regions of Eastern/Southern Africa and West/Central Africa.

Source: World Health Organization, United Nations Children's Fund, United Nations Population Fund and the World Bank, *Maternal Mortality in 2005: Estimates developed by WHO, UNICEF, UNFPA and the World Bank*, WHO, Geneva, 2007, p. 35.

years and bore children at each age in accordance with prevailing age-specific fertility rates.) High fertility rates increase the risk that a woman will die from maternal causes. While mortality risks are associated with all pregnancies, these risks rise the more times a woman gives birth.

Elevated fertility rates, combined with weak access to basic health-care and maternity services, can have lifelong implications for women's survival. In the developing world as a whole, a woman has a 1 in 76 lifetime risk of maternal death, compared with a probability of just 1 in 8,000 for women in industrialized countries. By way of comparison, the lifetime risk of maternal mortality ranges from just 1 in 47,600 for a mother in Ireland, to 1 in every 7 in Niger, the country with the highest lifetime risk of maternal death.[8]

Neonatal mortality

Neonatal mortality is the probability of a newborn dying between birth and the first 28 completed days of life. The latest estimates from the World Health Organization, which date from 2004, indicate that around 3.7 million children died within the first 28 days of life in that year. Within the neonatal period, however, there is wide variation in mortality risk. The greatest risk is during the first day after birth, when it is estimated that between 25 and 45 per cent of neonatal deaths occur. Around three quarters of newborn deaths, or 2.8 million in 2004, occur within the first week – the early neonatal period.

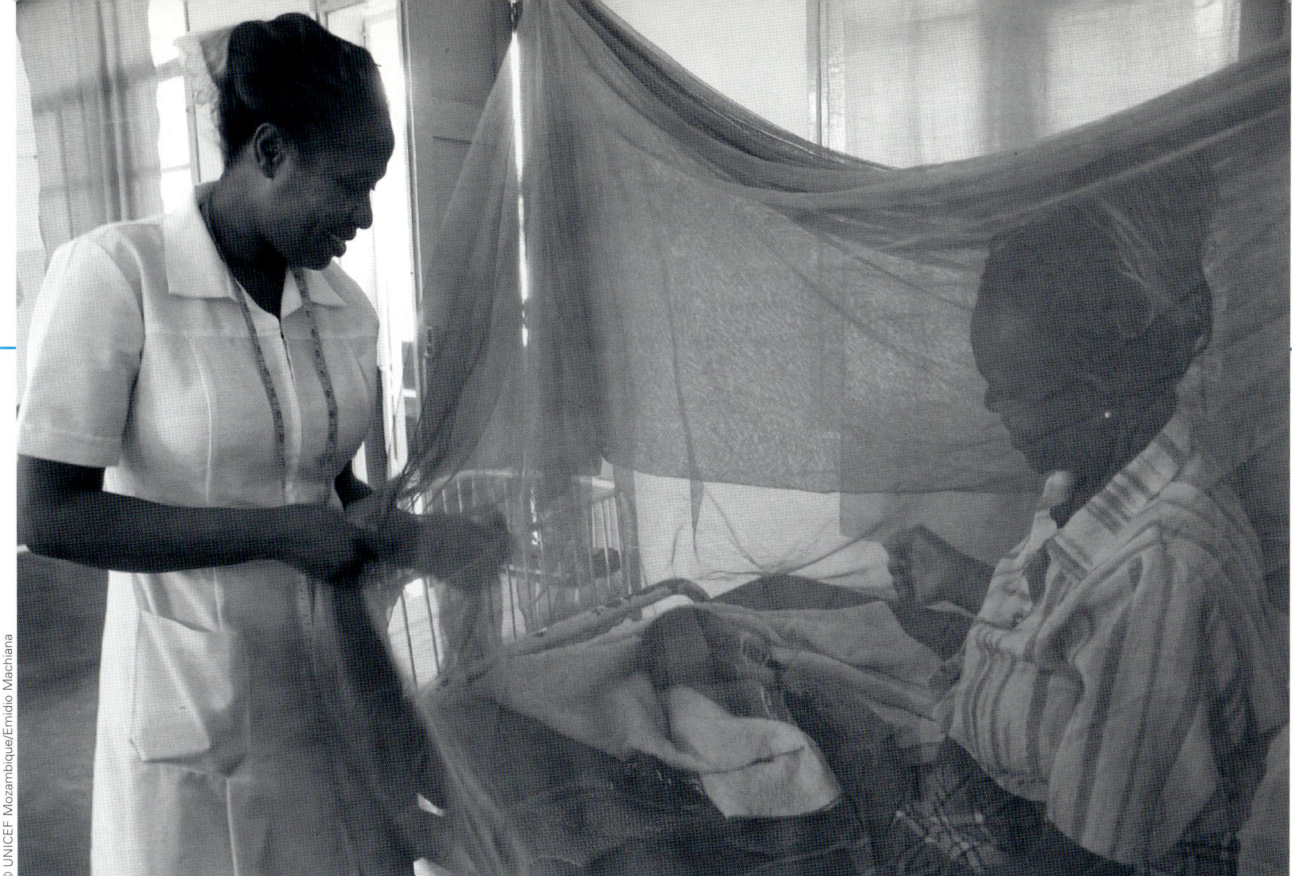

Expanded distribution of insecticide-treated mosquito nets to help prevent malaria and rapid scaling up of programmes to prevent and treat HIV infection are helping to save maternal and newborn lives. *An HIV-positive mother and her newborn son under an insecticide-treated mosquito net are assisted by a nurse in a health centre, Mozambique.*

Like maternal deaths, almost all (98 per cent in 2004) neonatal deaths occur in low- and middle-income countries. The total number of perinatal deaths, which groups stillbirths with early neonatal deaths owing to the fact that they have similar obstetric causes, was 5.9 million deaths in 2004. Stillborns accounted for around 3 million perinatal deaths that year.[9]

Until the mid-to-late 1990s, neonatal mortality figures were estimated from rough historical data. But as more reliable data emerged from household surveys, it became evident that previous estimates had significantly underestimated the incidence of newborn deaths. The global neonatal mortality rate declined by one quarter between 1980 and 2000, but its rate of reduction was much slower than that of the overall under-five mortality rate, which fell by one third. As a consequence, neonatal deaths currently constitute a much higher proportion of under-five deaths than in previous years. In particular, deaths in the first week of life have risen from 23 per cent of under-five deaths in 1980 to 28 per cent in 2000.[10]

In part, the rising proportion of neonatal deaths reflects two key factors: the difficulty of reaching many babies who are born at home with effective and timely neonatal interventions, and the success of many countries in implementing interventions such as immunization that have markedly reduced post-neonatal deaths in the developing world as a whole. This has led in part to a relative neglect of cost-effective, simple neonatal survival interventions. Reducing neonatal deaths therefore has become a major component of new paradigms and strategies for diminishing child mortality and reaching Millennium Development Goal 4.

Regional patterns of neonatal death correlate closely to those for maternal death. The lowest rates, unsurprisingly, are found in industrialized countries, where the neonatal mortality rate in 2004 was just 3 per 1,000 live births. The highest rates of neonatal death in 2004 were found in South Asia (41 per 100,000 live births) and West and Central Africa (44 per 100,000). Owing to a higher number of births, South Asia has the highest number of neonatal deaths among the world's regions.[11]

The main causes of maternal and neonatal mortality and morbidity

Maternal mortality

Direct causes

The timing and causes of maternal and newborn deaths are well known. Maternal deaths mostly occur from the third trimester to the first week after birth (with the exception of deaths due to complications of abortion). Studies show that mortality

The latest inter-agency estimates suggest that 536,000 women died in 2005 from causes related to pregnancy and childbirth.

risks for mothers are particularly elevated within the first two days after birth. Most maternal deaths are related to obstetric complications – including post-partum haemorrhage, infections, eclampsia and prolonged or obstructed labour – and complications of abortion. Most of these direct causes of maternal mortality can be readily addressed if skilled health personnel are on hand and key drugs, equipment and referral facilities are available.[12] (*For further details on birth complications and emergency obstetric care, see Chapter 3.*)

Indirect causes

Many factors contributing to a mother's risk of dying are not unique to pregnancy but may be exacerbated by pregnancy and childbirth. Attributing these causes to pregnancy is difficult owing to the poor diagnostic capacity of many countries' health information systems. Nonetheless, assessing the indirect causes of maternal deaths helps determine the most appropriate intervention strategies for maternal and child health. Collaboration between condition-specific programmes – such as those to address malaria or AIDS – and maternal health initiatives may often be the most effective way to address some of these indirect causes, including those that are highly preventable or treatable, such as anaemia.[13]

Maternal anaemia affects about half of all pregnant women. Pregnant adolescents are more prone to anaemia than older women, and they often receive less care. Infectious diseases such as malaria, which affects around 50 million pregnant women living in malaria-endemic countries every year, and intestinal parasites can exacerbate anaemia, as can poor-quality diets – all of which heighten vulnerability to maternal death. Severe anaemia contributes to the risk of death in cases of haemorrhage.[14]

Anaemia is highly treatable with iron supplements offered through maternal health programmes. This intervention, however, remains limit-

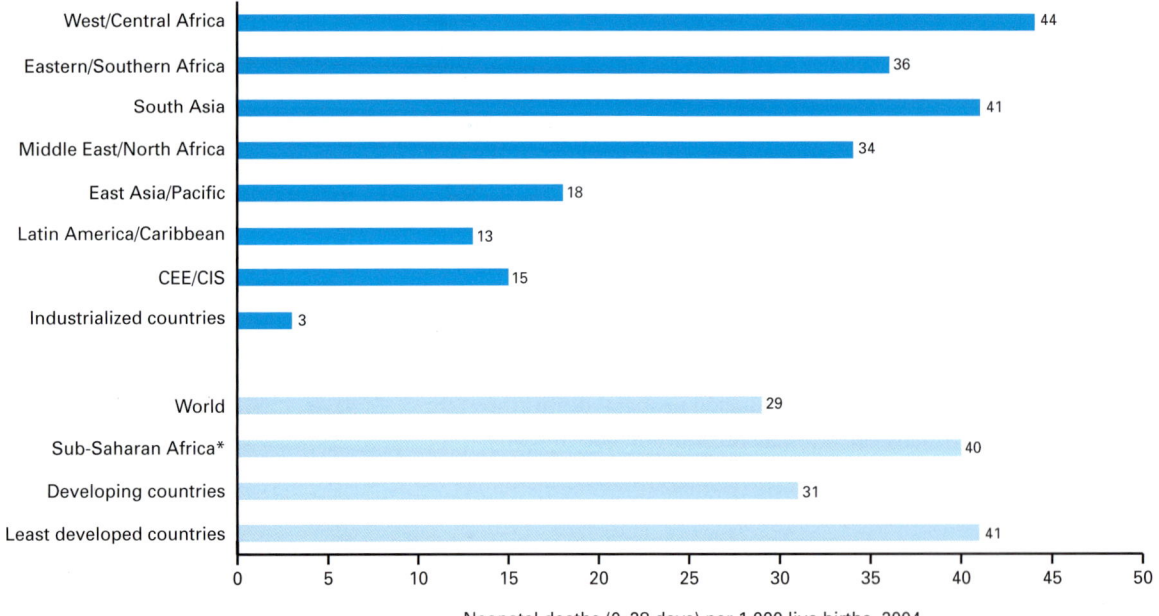

Figure 1.4

Regional rates of neonatal mortality

West/Central Africa: 44
Eastern/Southern Africa: 36
South Asia: 41
Middle East/North Africa: 34
East Asia/Pacific: 18
Latin America/Caribbean: 13
CEE/CIS: 15
Industrialized countries: 3

World: 29
Sub-Saharan Africa*: 40
Developing countries: 31
Least developed countries: 41

Neonatal deaths (0–28 days) per 1,000 live births, 2004

*Sub-Saharan Africa comprises the regions of Eastern/Southern Africa and West/Central Africa.
Source: World Health Organization, using vital registration systems and household surveys.

Creating a supportive environment for mothers and newborns

by H. M. Queen Rania Al Abdullah of Jordan, UNICEF's Eminent Advocate for Children*

In 1631, a beautiful empress, Mumtaz Mahal, died while giving birth to her 14th child. Overwhelmed by grief, her husband constructed a monument in her honour: the Taj Mahal, today one of the best-known buildings in the world.

And yet, while the Taj Mahal's domes and spires are instantly recognizable, there is far less global awareness of the tragedy that inspired its creation.

Nearly 400 years after Mumtaz Mahal lost her life in childbirth, a woman still dies from causes related to pregnancy or childbirth every minute of every day – more than 500,000 women each year, 10 million per generation. How can it be that in our age of modern advances and medical miracles we are still failing to safeguard women as they perpetuate the human race itself?

The answer, of course, is that public health has made breathtaking strides, but those benefits have not been equally shared, either among countries or between the geographical areas and social groups within them. Even though the causes of pregnancy and childbirth complications are the same around the world, their consequences vary dramatically from country to country and region to region. Today, a young woman in Sweden has a 1 in 17,400 lifetime risk of dying of pregnancy-related causes. In Sierra Leone, her risk soars to 1 in 8.

And for every woman who dies, another 20 are afflicted with serious infections or injuries. An estimated 75,000 women each year become victims of obstetric fistula, a physically and psychologically devastating condition that can result in social exclusion.

The toll in women's lives is enormous. But they are not the only ones who suffer. As a group of experts stated during a global conference on women's health in 2007: "In their prime reproductive years, women 'deliver' for their societies in multiple ways: They bear and raise the next generation, and they are critical actors for progress as workers, leaders, and activists." When women's lives are cut short or incapacitated as a result of pregnancy or childbirth, the tragedy cascades. Children lose a parent. Spouses lose a partner. And societies lose productive contributors.

Our world cannot afford to keep sacrificing so many people and so much potential. We know what it takes to prevent and treat the vast majority of pregnancy-related difficulties, from eclampsia and haemorrhage to sepsis, obstructed labour and anaemia. Indeed, the World Bank estimates that such basic interventions as antenatal care, attendance at delivery by skilled health personnel, and accessible emergency treatment for women and newborns could avert almost three quarters of maternal deaths.

But expanding medical interventions is just one part of improving maternal and newborn health. More fundamentally, we need to boost women's empowerment around the world. Consider that in a century increasingly defined by information, we still do not have precise data regarding the numbers of women who die in childbirth each year. Why are maternal deaths only partially enumerated? One possible reason is that, in too many places, women's lives do not fully count.

And as long as women remain disadvantaged in their societies, maternal and newborn health will suffer as well. But if we can empower women with the tools to take control of their lives, we can create a more supportive environment for women and children alike.

Empowerment begins with education, the best development investment we can make – from ensuring that girls as well as boys are able to attend primary school to teaching women to read and write, and providing public health education. Although much remains to be done, many countries are beginning to make strides in this direction. In Jordan, for example, nursing students from the University of Jordan are volunteering to educate girls in public schools about women's health issues.

Study after study shows that educated women are better equipped to earn income to support their families, more likely to invest in their children's health care, nutrition and education, and more inclined to participate in civic life and to advocate for community improvements.

Educated mothers are also more likely to seek proper health care for themselves; according to the 2007 *Millennium Development Goals Report*, "84 per cent of women who have completed secondary or higher education are attended by skilled personnel during childbirth, more than twice the rate of mothers with no formal education."

Children of educated mothers are 50 per cent more likely to survive until the age of five and beyond than those whose mothers did not receive or complete schooling. For girls in particular, education can make the difference between hope and despair. Research shows that young people who complete primary school are less likely to be infected by HIV than those who never managed to graduate from primary school.

Educated girls are also more likely to delay marriage and less likely to get pregnant while very young, reducing the risk of dying in childbirth while they are still children themselves. As girls continue their education, their earning potential increases, enabling them to break the bonds of poverty too often passed down through the generations.

Put simply, changing the trajectory for girls can change the course of the future. And if these girls grow into women who choose to become mothers themselves, they will view pregnancy and childbirth as something to celebrate, not fear.

See References, page 107.

*Her Majesty Queen Rania Al Abdullah of Jordan is UNICEF's Eminent Advocate for Children and a tireless global advocate for child protection, early childhood development, gender parity in education and women's empowerment.

ed in both coverage and effectiveness in some developing countries, mostly as a result of low access to basic health care and, more specifically, to quality antenatal care and support. Encouragingly, there are signs that efforts to address anaemia by fortifying staple foods like flour are beginning to accelerate at the national level in a number of developing countries.[15]

Maternal iodine deficiency during pregnancy is associated with a higher incidence of stillbirths, miscarriage and congenital abnormalities. These risks can be reduced and prevented by ensuring optimal maternal iodine status before or during pregnancy. Universal salt iodization and, in some cases, iodine supplementation are essential to ensure optimum iodine intake during pregnancy and childhood.[16]

Malaria is another deadly risk for mothers and babies. In malaria-endemic areas, the disease contributes to around one quarter of severe maternal anaemia cases, heightens the risk of stillbirth and miscarriage, and contributes to low birthweight and neonatal deaths. Prevention of malaria through the use of insecticide-treated mosquito nets is therefore vital to reduce its impact on pregnant women and newborns. In addition, intermittent preventive treatment of malaria for pregnant women in the second and third trimesters is increasingly used in sub-Saharan Africa to avert anaemia and placental malaria.[17]

The precise contribution of HIV and AIDS to maternal deaths is difficult to assess since, despite the expansion of programmes to prevent mother-to-child transmission of HIV, the HIV status of many pregnant women is still unknown. HIV and pregnancy might interact in several ways. The virus may heighten the risk of such obstetric complications as haemorrhage, sepsis and complications of Caesarean section. Pregnancy, in turn, may raise the risk of HIV-related illnesses such as anaemia and tuberculosis, or accelerate HIV progression. Current research findings are indicative rather than conclusive, and more research is needed to clarify the degree of causality in both directions. It is believed that in countries with high prevalence of HIV, the AIDS epidemic may have reversed previous advances in maternal mortality. What can be assessed with greater certainty, at least partially, is the number of women identified as living with HIV who gave birth – around 1.5 million in 108 low- and middle-income countries in 2006.

Efforts to address the AIDS epidemic and its impact on maternal and newborn health are intensifying in four key areas: prevention of infection among adolescents and young people; antiretroviral treatment for HIV-positive women and mothers who require antiretroviral therapy; prevention of mother-to-child transmission; and paediatric treatment of HIV. Advances are being made in all four areas and encouraging results are ensuing. For example, coverage of antiretroviral prophylaxis for HIV-positive mothers to prevent mother-to-child transmission rose from 10 per cent of HIV-infected pregnant women in low- and middle-income countries in 2004 to 33 per cent in 2007. Despite this appreciable progress, much more needs to be done to provide women with interventions for HIV prevention, care and therapy – including testing and counselling, and quality sexual and reproductive health services in addition to medicines.[18]

Although the consequences of co-infection with HIV and malaria parasites are not fully understood, available evidence suggests that the infections act synergistically and result in adverse outcomes. Recent evidence suggests that HIV-positive women with placental malaria are more likely to give birth to low-birthweight infants. Research also suggests that low-birthweight infants are more susceptible to HIV infection as a result of mother-to-child transmission of the virus than infants of normal birthweight. Antiretroviral treatment for HIV-positive women and children and the use of insecticide-treated mosquito nets can reduce the risk of malaria still further.[19] (*For further details on HIV and malaria co-infection, see the Panel in Chapter 3, page 63.*)

For every woman who dies from pregnancy-related complications, around 20 more incur injuries, infections and disabilities – approximately

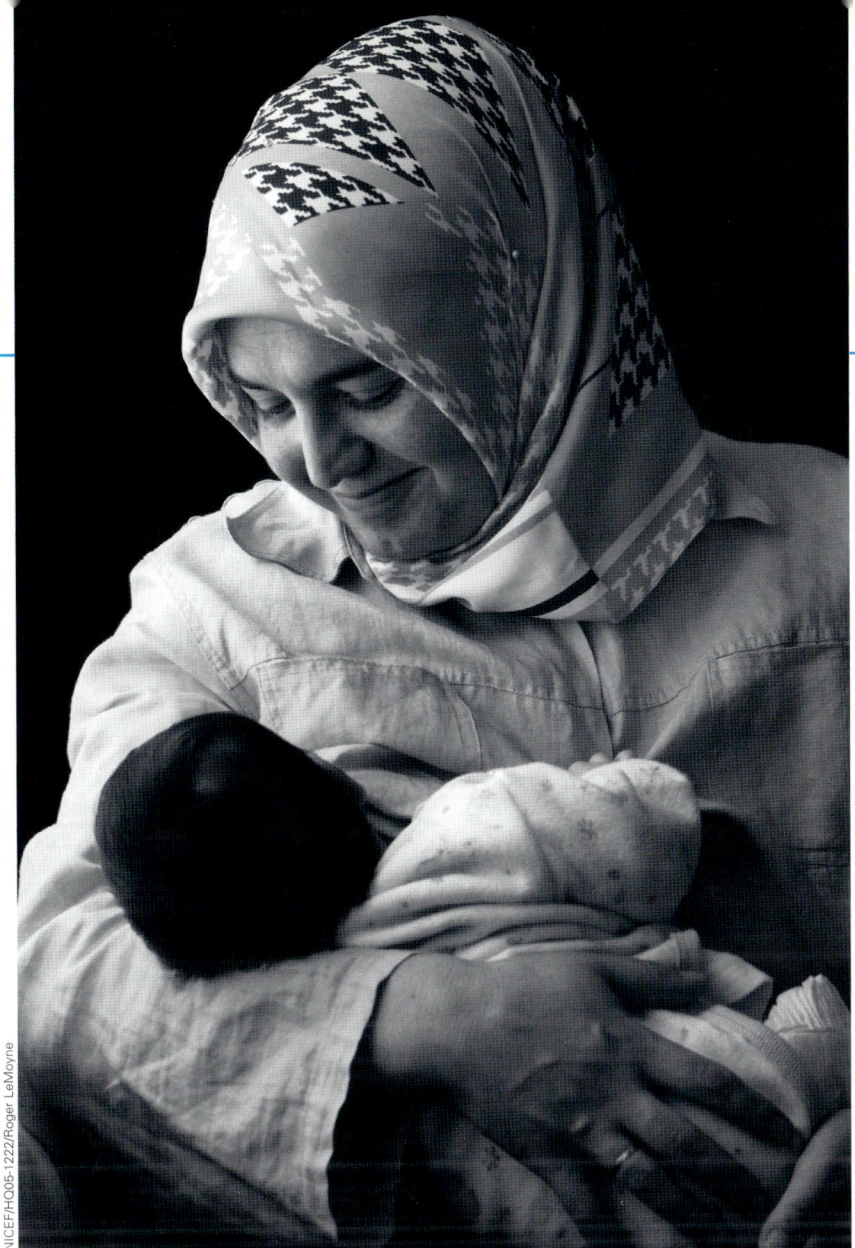

Exclusive breastfeeding for the first six months of life helps protect newborns and infants from disease, reduces the risk of mortality and encourages healthy child development. *A woman breastfeeds her newborn at the Uskudar Ana ve Cocuk Sagligi Klinigi, a clinic operated by the Ministry of Health in Istanbul, Turkey.*

10 million women each year. Among the most distressing conditions is obstetric fistula, which occurs when prolonged pressure from the baby's head during extended, problematic labour causes tissue damage in the birth canal. In the period following the birth, holes open up and there is leakage from the bladder and/or the rectum into the vagina. Fistula can be easily treated by health workers with appropriate surgical skills, but many of the estimated 75,000 women afflicted by this condition each year never receive treatment. Instead, they not only have to cope with the physical discomfort and emotional distress of the condition, they also may risk being shunned by their husbands and families.

Another debilitating condition is uterine prolapse, which occurs when the muscles, ligaments and tissue supporting the pelvic structure give way, causing the uterus to fall into the vaginal canal. Limited mobility, chronic back pains and urinary incontinence are three consequences of prolapse, which, if severe, can also make it impossible for women to undertake household and other routine tasks. A number of factors can cause uterine prolapse, including prolonged labour, difficult delivery, frequent pregnancies, inadequate obstetric care and heavy manual labour.

Other forms of maternal morbidity include anaemia, infertility, chronic infection, depression and incontinence – all of which may result in domestic problems including physical and psychological abuse, household dissolution and social exclusion.[20]

Neonatal mortality

Some 86 per cent of newborn deaths globally are the direct result of three main causes: severe infections – including sepsis/pneumonia, tetanus and diarrhoea – asphyxia and preterm births. Severe infections are estimated to account for 36 per cent of all newborn deaths. They can occur at any point during the first month of life but are the main cause of neonatal death after the first week. Clean delivery practices are clearly important in preventing infection, but maternal infections also need to be identified and treated during pregnancy. Infections in newborns require rapid identification and treatment as soon as possible following childbirth.

Asphyxia (difficulty in breathing after birth) causes 23 per cent of newborn deaths and can largely be prevented by improved care during labour and delivery. The condition can be alleviated by a trained health worker who is able to detect its signs and resuscitate the newborn. Preterm birth (deliv-

Pregnancy- and childbirth-related complications are an important cause of mortality for girls aged 15–19 years worldwide, accounting for 70,000 deaths every year.

ery at less than 37 weeks of completed gestation) directly causes 27 per cent of newborn deaths. Infants born prematurely find it more difficult than full-term babies to feed, maintain normal body temperature and withstand infection. Preventing malaria in pregnant women can have a positive impact on the incidence of premature births in malaria-endemic areas.[21]

According to the latest international estimates, which cover the period 2000–2007, 15 per cent of all newborns are born with low birthweight (defined as infants weighing less than 2,500 grams at birth). Low birthweight, which is caused by preterm birth or intrauterine growth restriction, is an underlying factor in 60–80 per cent of neonatal deaths. The majority of such cases occur in South Asia in particular, and also in sub-Saharan Africa, the regions with the highest rates of undernutrition among girls and women. Maternal undernutrition is correlated with a higher incidence of low birthweight in infants.[22]

Intrauterine growth restriction, which refers to restricted growth of the fetus during pregnancy, is a leading risk for perinatal deaths. Like low birthweight, it is also associated with maternal undernutrition and ill health, among other factors. With correct identification and proper management, including early treatment of maternal diseases and good nutrition, the condition can be contained and need not result in lifelong consequences.[23]

The intergenerational nature of the solution to intrauterine growth restriction underlines the fact that improving maternal and newborn health is not simply a practical matter of making available better and more extensive maternal health services. It also involves tackling head on the neglect of women's basic rights in many societies.

In addition to adequate nutrition for women, birth spacing is also central to avoiding preterm births, low birthweight in infants and neonatal deaths; studies show that birth intervals of less than 24 months significantly increase these risks. It is also imperative to secure girls' access to proper nutrition and health care from birth through childhood and into adolescence, womanhood and their potential childbearing years.[24]

For every newborn baby who dies, another 20 suffer birth injury, com-

Figure 1.5
Direct causes of maternal deaths, 1997–2002*

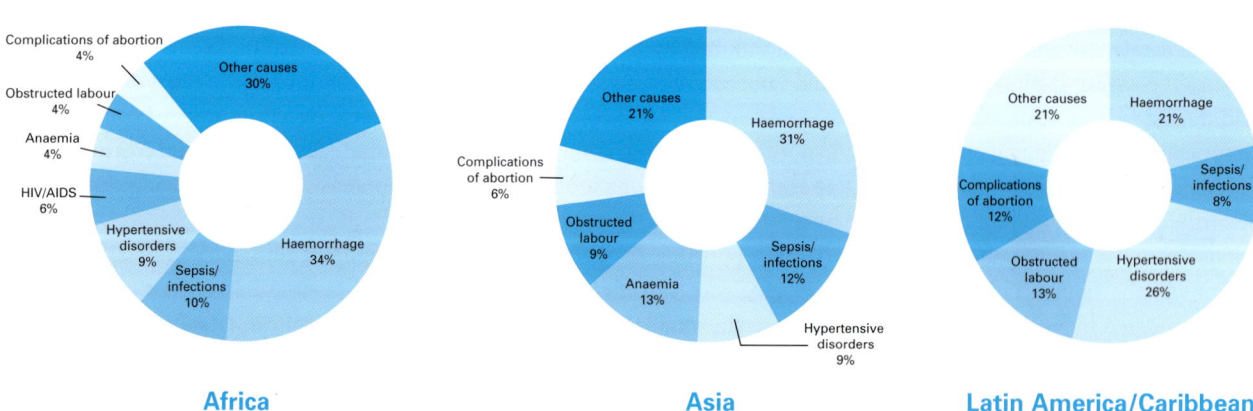

Africa   Asia   Latin America/Caribbean

* Data refer to the most recent year available during the period specified. Percentages may not total 100% because of rounding.
Source: Khan, Khalid S., et al., 'WHO Analysis of Causes of Maternal Death: A systematic review', *The Lancet*, vol. 367, no. 9516, 1 April 2006, p.1069.

For every woman who dies from a pregnancy-related cause, another 20 more incur injuries, infections and disabilities – around 10 million women each year.

plications arising from preterm birth or other neonatal conditions. More than 1 million children who survive birth asphyxia each year, for example, end up suffering disabilities such as cerebral palsy or learning difficulties.[25]

Underlying and basic causes of maternal and neonatal mortality and morbidity

In addition to the direct causes of maternal and newborn mortality and morbidity, there are a number of underlying factors at the household, community and district levels that also serve to undermine the health and survival of mothers and newborns. They include lack of education and knowledge, inadequate maternal and newborn health practices and care seeking, insufficient access to nutritious food and essential micronutrients, poor environmental health facilities and inadequate basic health-care services and limited access to maternity services – including emergency obstetric and newborn care. There are also basic factors, such as poverty, social exclusion and gender discrimination that underpin both the direct and underlying causes of maternal and newborn mortality and morbidity. (*For a fuller outline of how these factors interact, see Figure 1.7 on page 17.*)

Of particular importance is the restricted access to quality health care services that many women face. Maternal health and access to quality contraception and reproductive health services save women's lives and are also important factors underlying newborn health and survival. Studies show that women's health throughout the life cycle, from childhood through adolescence and into adulthood, is critical in determining maternal and neonatal health outcomes. Access to institutional facilities and skilled health personnel at birth are also important factors; it should come as no surprise that the countries with the highest rates of neonatal mortality have among the lowest rates of skilled attendants at birth and institutional deliveries.[26]

Poverty undermines maternal and neonatal health in several ways. It can heighten the incidence of direct causes of mortality, such as maternal infections and undernutrition, and discourage care seeking or reduce access to health-care services. It can also undermine the quality of the

Figure 1.6

Direct causes of neonatal deaths, 2000*

Low birthweight, which is related to maternal malnutrition, is a causal factor in 60–80 per cent of neonatal deaths.

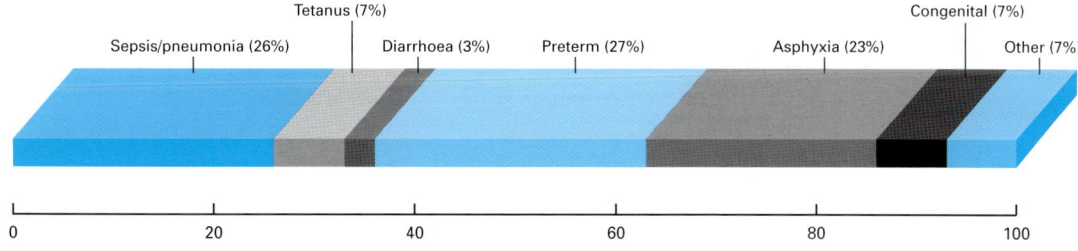

* Percentages may not total 100% because of rounding.

Source: Lawn, Joy E., Simon Cousens and Jelka Zupan, '4 million neonatal deaths; When? Where? Why?', *The Lancet*, vol. 365, no. 9462, 5 March 2005, p. 895.

services provided even when they are available. Information from 50 Demographic and Health Surveys from 1995 to 2002 reveals that within regions, neonatal mortality rates are around 20–50 per cent higher for the poorest 20 per cent of households than for the richest quintile. Similar inequities are also prevalent for maternal mortality.[27]

Providing a supportive social context for the rights of women and girls is also critical to reducing maternal and neonatal mortality and morbidity. Efforts to increase health interventions to address the proximate causes of maternal and neonatal deaths and ill health, and to ameliorate maternal undernutrition, curb infectious diseases and improve hygiene facilities and practices will be only partly successful unless the social context in which women and girls reside respects their rights. As Chapter 2 shows, expanding service delivery may prove insufficient if women and girls are denied access to essential commodities or services because of cultural, social, or familial impediments.

Accelerating progress on maternal and newborn health

Many of the causal factors responsible for maternal and neonatal morbidity and mortality are well known and interrelated, as illustrated in the conceptual framework in Figure 1.7. While there are still many gaps in our knowledge of the extent and causes of maternal and newborn deaths, we

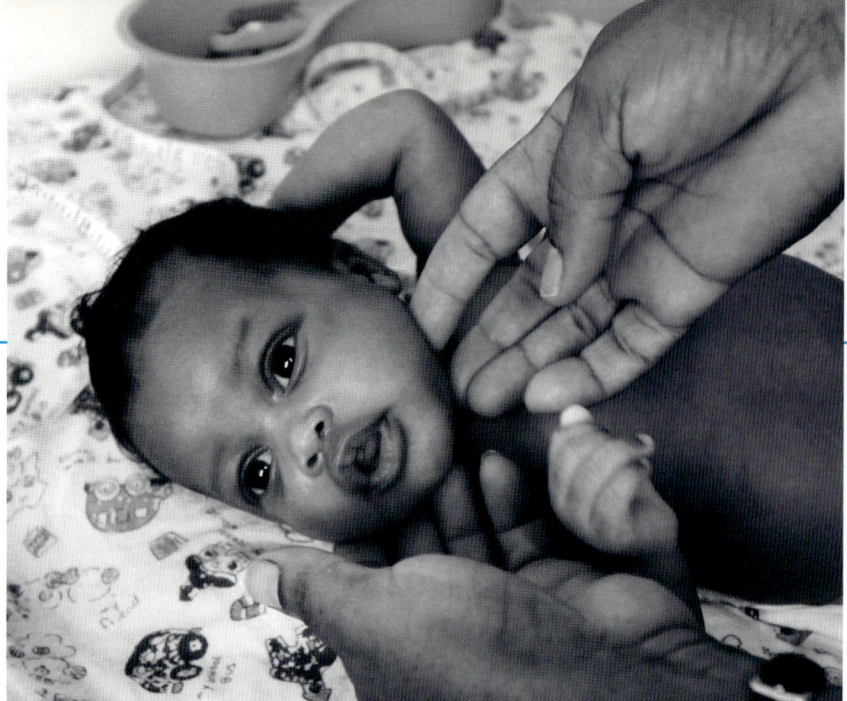

Improving maternity services is essential to enhancing maternal and newborn health and survival. A nurse examines a six-week-old baby during a check-up at a community health centre, Jamaica.

certainly know enough to implement interventions that could save millions of lives. The main methods of reducing maternal and newborn mortality and morbidity are well established and understood. These include:

- Promoting access to family planning services, based on individual country policies.

- Quality antenatal care providing a comprehensive package of health and nutrition services.

- Preventing mother-to-child transmission of HIV and offering antiretroviral treatment for women in need.

- Basic preventive and curative interventions, including immunization against neonatal tetanus for pregnant women, routine immunization, distribution of insecticide-treated mosquito nets and oral rehydration salts, among others.

- Access to improved water and sanitation, and adoption of improved hygiene practices, especially at delivery. Clean water for hygiene and drinking is essential for safe delivery.

- Access to skilled health personnel – a doctor, nurse or midwife – at delivery.

- Basic emergency obstetric care at a minimum of four facilities per 500,000 population – adapted to each country's circumstances – for women who experience some complication.

- Comprehensive emergency obstetric care at a minimum of one facility in every district or one per 500,000 population.

- A post-natal visit for every mother and newborn as soon as possible after delivery, ideally within 24 hours, with additional visits towards the end of the first week and at four to six weeks.

- Knowledge and life skills for pregnant women and families on the danger signs of maternal and newborn health and about referral systems.

- Maternal nutrition counselling and supplementation as needed as part of

The burden of neonatal deaths is also high, as each year almost 4 million newborns die within the first 28 days of life.

Figure 1.7

Conceptual framework for maternal and neonatal mortality and morbidity

This conceptual framework on the causes of maternal and newborn deaths illustrates that health outcomes are determined by interrelated factors, encompassing nutrition, water, sanitation and hygiene, health-care services and healthy behaviours, and disease control, among others. These factors are defined as proximate (individual), underlying (household, community and district) and basic (societal). Factors at one level influence other levels. The framework is devised to be useful in assessing and analysing the causes of maternal and newborn mortality and morbidity, and in planning effective actions to enhance maternal and neonatal health.

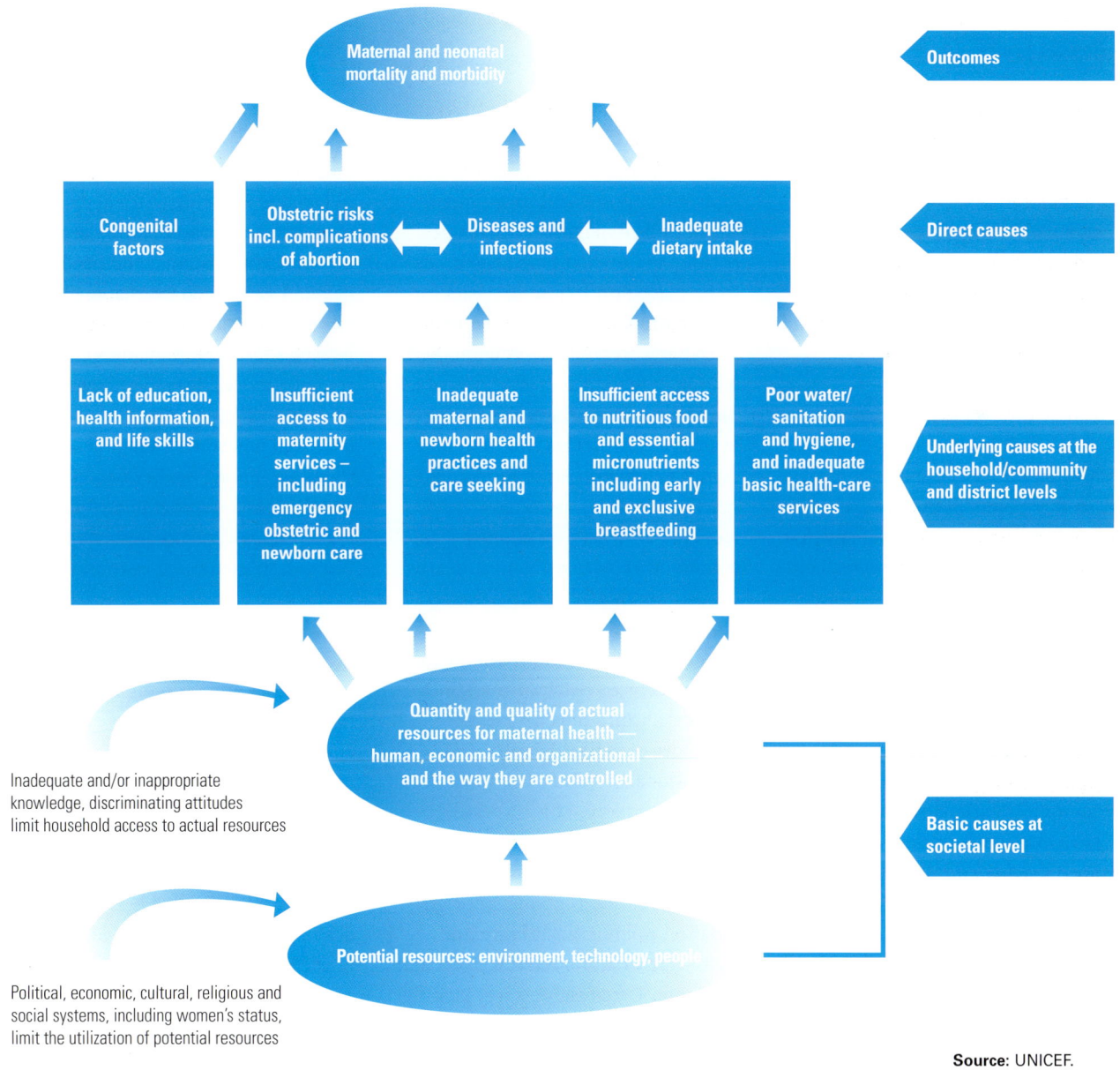

Source: UNICEF.

MATERNAL AND NEWBORN HEALTH: WHERE WE STAND

A child born in a least developed country is almost 14 times more likely to die during the first 28 days of life than one born in an industrialized country.

routine antenatal, post-natal and neonatal care.

- Essential care for all newborns, including initiation of breastfeeding within the first hour of birth, exclusive breastfeeding, infection control, warmth provision and avoidance of bathing during the first 24 hours.

- Extra care for small babies, multiple births and severe congenital abnormalities.

- Integrated Management of Neonatal and Childhood Illness, or the equivalent, in health facilities that provide care to women and children.[28]

For these interventions to work, however, it is increasingly recognized that essential services must be provided, at key points in the life cycle, through dynamic health systems that integrate a continuum of home, community, outreach and facility-based care. This concept of a continuum of care for maternal, neonatal and child health has arisen in recent years from the recognition that an integrated approach reaps more dividends than myriad separate initiatives. The continuum must exist, however, in a supportive environment that safeguards women's rights and prioritizes maternal and newborn health. Chapter 2 explores the elements required to create and sustain such an environment.

Among the most vital elements in the continuum of care is the presence of skilled professionals throughout pregnancy, birth, post-partum and neonatal care, supported by referrals to adequately staffed facilities equipped to manage emergencies. The emerging role of mid-level providers such as nurses and midwives in broadening access to emergency obstetric care is also showing promising potential in the developing world.

In particular, given that the risks of maternal and newborn death are greatest during the first 24–48 hours after birth, post-natal care urgently needs to be expanded during this period, and greater emphasis needs to be placed on follow-up visits for babies and mothers. Visits shortly after birth are vital for new mothers, who may remain at higher risk of mortality and morbidity for up to a year after birth. This is usually not possible, however, as maternal and newborn services are often sorely lacking in the poorest countries and communities where the most deaths occur. Particularly in sub-Saharan Africa, factors such as distance, migration, urbanization, armed conflict, disease and lack of investment in public health have left severe shortages of skilled health professionals.

Women and newborns in fragile states – countries that experience weak institutional policy, poor governance, political instability and weak rule of law – require particular attention. Often these states lack the institutional capacity and adequate resources to deliver basic social and infrastructure services and offer security to citizens. Fragile states hold around 8 per cent of the world's population, but they account for 35 per cent of global maternal deaths and comprise 8 of the 10 countries with the highest maternal mortality ratios. These countries also account for 21 per cent of global neonatal deaths, and comprise 9 of the 10 countries with the most elevated rates of neonatal mortality.[29]

Strengthening governance and the rule of law and restoring peace and security are requisites for accelerating progress on improving maternal and newborn health. Donors and international agencies also face the challenge of moving beyond short-term humanitarian response to long-term development assistance, and ensuring that maternal, child and newborn health and women's rights are among the key issues in negotiations and programmes aimed at improving governance, resolving conflict and strengthening institutions.[30]

In the least developed countries, insufficient resources have been dedicated to maternal and neonatal health, with the result that the poor have been effectively denied access to clinics and hospitals, especially in rural areas. This may be due to the absence of such a facility, the poor quality and condition of health centres and hospitals, the lack of skilled health personnel or personnel with low skills levels, or the existence of user fees and other costs that the poor cannot afford. The continuum of care concept refers not only to the needs of mothers and

Focus On: Maternal and newborn health in Nigeria: Developing strategies to accelerate progress

Nigeria is Africa's most populous country, with 148 million inhabitants in 2007, 25 million of them under age five. With almost 6 million births in 2007 – the third highest number in the world behind India and China – and a total fertility rate of 5.4, Nigeria's population growth continues to be rapid in absolute terms.

In addition to its sizeable population, Nigeria is known for its vast oil wealth. Nonetheless, poverty is widespread; according to the latest *World Development Indicators 2007*, published by the World Bank, more than 70 per cent of Nigerians live on less than US$1 per day, impairing their ability to afford health care.

Poverty, demographic pressures and insufficient investment in public health care, to name but three factors, inflate levels and ratios of maternal and neonatal mortality. The latest United Nations inter-agency estimates place the 2005 average national maternal mortality ratio at 1,100 deaths per 100,000 live births and the lifetime risk of maternal death at 1 in 18. When viewed in global terms, the burden of maternal death is brought into stark relief: Approximately 1 in every 9 maternal deaths occurs in Nigeria alone.

The women who survive pregnancy and childbirth may face compromised health; studies suggest that between 100,000 and 1 million women in Nigeria may be suffering from obstetric fistula. Neonatal deaths in 2004 stood at 249,000, according to the latest World Health Organization figures, with 76 per cent taking place in the early neonatal period (first week of life). Inadequate health facilities, lack of transportation to institutional care, inability to pay for services and resistance among some populations to modern health care are key factors behind the country's high rates of maternal, newborn and child mortality and morbidity.

Disparities in poverty and health among Nigeria's numerous ethnolinguistic groups and between its states are marked. Poverty rates in rural areas, estimated at 64 per cent in 2004, are roughly 1.5 times higher than the urban-area rate of 43 per cent. Moreover, the poverty rate in the north-east region, which stands at 67 per cent, is almost twice the level of 34 per cent in the more prosperous south-east.

Low levels of education, especially among women, and discriminatory cultural attitudes and practices are barriers to reducing high maternal mortality rates. A study at the Jos University Teaching Hospital in the north-central region shows that nearly three quarters of maternal deaths in 2005 occurred among illiterate women. The mortality rate among women who did not receive antenatal care was about 20 times higher than among those who did. Of the several ethnic groups represented among the patients, Hausa-Fulani women accounted for 22 per cent of all deliveries and 44 per cent of all deaths. The Hausa-Fulani represent the largest ethnic group in northern Nigeria and are therefore critically affected by this region's higher poverty rates.

Cultural attitudes and practices that discriminate against women and girls contribute to maternal mortality and morbidity. Child marriage and high rates of adolescent births are commonplace across Nigeria, exposing girls and women of reproductive age to numerous health risks.

Given these complex realities, developing strategies to accelerate progress on maternal and newborn health remains a considerable challenge. But the Government of Nigeria, together with international partners, is attempting to meet the challenge. In 2007, it began to implement a national Integrated Maternal, Newborn and Child Health (IMNCH) Strategy to fast-track high-impact intervention packages that include nutritional supplements, immunization, insecticide-treated mosquito nets and prevention of mother-to-child transmission of HIV.

The strategy is to be rolled out in three phases, each lasting three years, and has been designed along the continuum of care model to strengthen Nigeria's decentralized health system, which operates at the federal, state and local levels. In the initial phase, covering 2007–2009, the key focus will be identifying and removing bottlenecks, while delivering a basic package of services using community-based and family-care strategies. A sizeable proportion of expenditure will go towards artemisinin-based combination therapy to combat malaria in women, children and newly recruited and trained health workers, particularly in rural areas. As basic healthcare improves, it is anticipated that the demand for clinical services will increase.

The second and third phases of the IMNCH will place greater emphasis on building health infrastructure. Over nine years, the strategy aims to revitalize existing facilities, construct clinics and hospitals, and create incentives – such as dependable salaries, hardship allowances and performance-based bonuses – that will help retain skilled health professionals in Nigeria's health system.

The IMNCH strategy, if implemented in full and on time, can markedly improve maternal and newborn health. Together with this package, the country has recently passed the National Health Insurance Scheme, which integrates the public and private health sectors to make health care more affordable for Nigerians. If the government passes the National Health Bill, which is currently before the legislature, a direct funding line for primary health care will become available. These health-system improvements have the potential to set a new course for meeting Millennium Development Goals 4 and 5 in Africa's largest nation.

See References, page 107.

For every newborn baby who dies, another 20 suffer birth injury, complications arising from preterm birth or other neonatal conditions.

children across time, but also to increasing access to health services by linking households and communities, clinics and hospitals. Chapter 3 looks in more depth at how to integrate and strengthen the services available to mothers and newborns and deliver them at key points in the life cycle and at key locations.

Implementing and extending continua of care for mothers, newborns and children will require both integrating and scaling up a range of actions. Chapter 4 examines the key paradigms, policies, and programmes that are driving the process forward.

The final chapter of *The State of the World's Children 2009* calls for concerted action and strong, cohesive partnerships to improve maternal and neonatal survival and health. The goals are already clear – and it is also evident that the world as a whole has fallen behind on the Millennium Development Goal to reduce child mortality (MDG 4) and even further behind on the goal to improve maternal health (MDG 5). It is clear that progress has to be significantly accelerated. The experiences of several developing countries, explored in depth in subsequent chapters, have proved that rapid progress is possible when sound strategies, political commitment, adequate resources and collaborative efforts are applied in support of the health of both mothers and newborns.

Expanding Millennium Development Goal 5: Universal access to reproductive health by 2015

In 2005, Heads of State meeting at the United Nations to review commitments made in the Millennium Declaration – the outcome document of the Millennium Summit of 2000 – not only reaffirmed the development goals elaborated in 2000 and ever since known as the Millennium Development Goals (MDGs), they also added four new targets to support them.

One of the major changes to the MDG configuration is the inclusion of a specific target on reproductive health: Millennium Development Goal 5, Target B, which seeks to "Achieve, by 2015, universal access to reproductive health." This new target falls within the goal's overarching objective of improving maternal health and complements its original target and associated indicators. The indicators selected to monitor progress towards MDG 5, Target B, are shown below:

Contraceptive prevalence rate – Percentage of women aged 15–49 in union currently using contraception.

Adolescent birth rate – Annual number of births to women aged 15–19 per 1,000 women in that age group. Alternatively, it is referred to as the age-specific fertility rate for women aged 15–19.

Antenatal care coverage – Percentage of women aged 15–49 attended at least once during pregnancy by skilled health personnel (doctors, nurses or midwives) and the percentage attended by any provider at least four times.

Unmet need for family planning – Refers to women who are fecund and sexually active but are not using any method of contraception and report not wanting any more children or wanting to delay the birth of the next child.

The addition of the reproductive health target to the MDGs reflects a long process linking reproductive health issues to development, human rights and gender equity, whose landmark event was the International Conference on Population and Development (ICPD) held in Cairo in 1994. Since then, other important events, notably the Fourth World Conference on Women (Beijing, 1995) and ICPD+5 – the UN General Assembly Special Session on the International Conference on Population and Development held in 1999 – have confirmed and extended the recommendations of the original ICPD gathering, including the goal of universal access to reproductive health services by 2015.

See References, page 107.

Focus On: Prioritizing maternal health in Sri Lanka

Sri Lanka is a story of success against the odds. A lower-middle-income country – in 2006, Sri Lanka's annual gross national income per capita was less than US$1,500 – it has also experienced a protracted civil conflict and the devastation of the 2004 Indian Ocean tsunami. Yet the country's progress in human development, particularly in maternal and child health and education, has been one of the key success stories among developing countries in recent decades. Sri Lanka's maternal mortality ratio declined from 340 per 100,000 live births in 1960 to 43 per 100,000 live births in 2005, and 98 per cent of births now take place in hospitals. Rates of antenatal care (at least one visit) and skilled attendance at birth stand at 99 per cent. In 2007, the country had an overall fertility rate of 1.9 – compared to 3.0 for the South Asia region. These results have also had positive effects on child survival: The under-five mortality rate has fallen from 32 per 1,000 live births in 1990 to 21 per 1,000 live births in 2007. The latest available data suggest that the neonatal mortality rate has also fallen, to around 8 per 100,000 births in 2004.

In basic education, too, Sri Lanka's performance has been outstanding. According to the latest international estimates, net primary school enrolment stands at more than 97 per cent for both girls and boys, while literacy rates among young people aged 15–24 are 97 per cent for males and 98 per cent for females. Administrative data suggest that the completion rate for primary school is 100 per cent. Given the positive correlation between education and maternal and child survival, these are the results of sustained investment in all three areas.

The key to Sri Lanka's outstanding improvements in maternal health was the expansion of a synergistic package of health and social services to reach the poor. The country's health system, which dates back to the late 19th century, first targeted universal provision of improved health care, sanitation and disease management. It subsequently added specific interventions to improve the health of women and children. Over the years, successive governments have followed a prudent approach of prioritizing health-care services to mothers and the poor while spending economic and human resources judiciously. The resulting improvements in women's health are supported and strengthened by measures to empower women socially and politically through education, employment and social engagement.

Sri Lanka's early written records and colonial past give a unique perspective of the evolution of maternal health in the country, starting with 9th- and 10th-century medical texts. Formal midwifery training was established under the British colonial government in 1879, and the Registrar General has recorded maternal mortality since 1902. This wealth of information and knowledge makes it possible to evaluate results of differing approaches to maternal health over time. Clear mandatory competencies helped professionalize midwives, and a no-blame policy helped make inquiries into maternal deaths routine.

The results were dramatic – maternal mortality was halved between 1947 and 1950. Thirteen years later, maternal mortality rates were cut in half again. Once health structures and networks were in place, increasingly better organization and clinical management have allowed Sri Lanka to cut the maternal mortality ratio by 50 per cent every 6 to 11 years. In addition, women's literacy rose from 44 to 71 per cent between 1946 and 1971. The rates of skilled attendance at birth and institutional delivery also grew. The public health midwife's role became more that of an institutional delivery assistant, as home midwife-assisted deliveries declined from 9 per cent in 1970 to just 2 per cent in 1995. Beginning in 1965, midwives also played a role in expanding government family planning services.

Sri Lanka's development of its health system has long been a model for other developing countries, demonstrating the degree of success that can be achieved in maternal and child health when sound strategies, sufficient resources and political commitment are judiciously applied. Despite its noteworthy advances in maternal and child health, challenges remain. In recent years, the country has faced a shortage of health workers; according to the *World Health Statistics 2008*, in the 2000–2006 period the country had only 6 doctors and 17 nurses and midwives per 10,000 inhabitants. In addition, services have deteriorated as financial resources have been squeezed, with health spending at around 4 per cent of GDP in 2005. Private spending on health, most of which is out-of-pocket, accounts for more than half of total health expenditure.

A further challenge for Sri Lanka will be to ensure food security, particularly if global food prices remain high. The country still has marked levels of undernutrition among newborns and children under five. According to the latest international estimates, more than 1 in every 5 newborns are born with low birthweight, and 23 per cent of children under five are moderately or severely underweight. Improving the level of exclusive breastfeeding for children less than six months old from its current level of 53 per cent will be vital to sustaining Sri Lanka's gains in neonatal and child mortality.

See References, page 107.

The centrality of Africa and Asia in the global challenges for children and women

The continents of Africa and Asia* present the largest global challenges to the survival of children and women. Their progress in such critical areas as child and maternal health, nutrition and education, among others, is pivotal to achievement of the Millennium Development Goals.

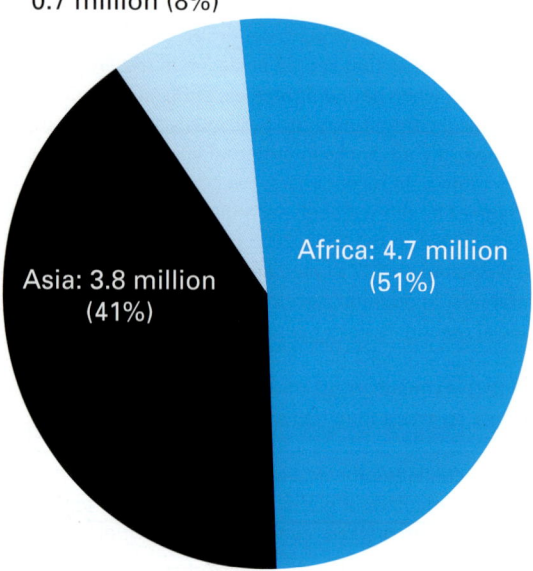

Source: UNICEF global databases.

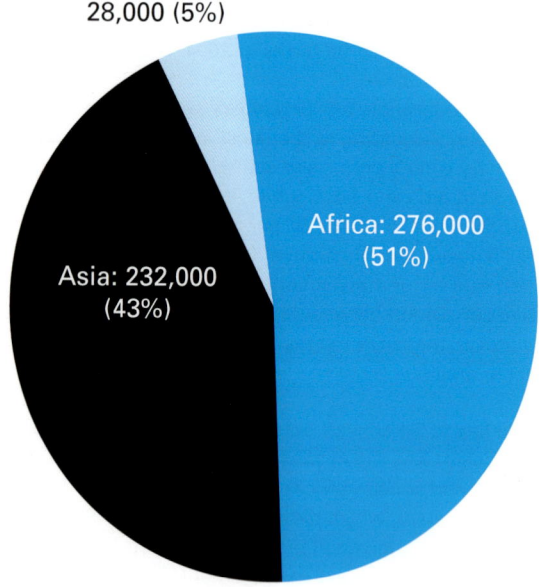

Source: UNICEF global databases.

Deaths among children under five

- In 2007, 9.2 million children died before age five. Africa and Asia together accounted for 92 per cent of these deaths.

- Half of the world's under-five deaths occurred in Africa, which remains the most difficult place in the world for a child to survive until age five.

- Although Asia has seen a remarkable reduction in the annual number of child deaths since 1970, it still accounted for 41 per cent of global under-five deaths in 2007.

Maternal deaths

- In 2005, the latest year for which firm estimates are available, an estimated 536,000 women died from causes related to pregnancy and childbirth. Almost all – 95 per cent – of these maternal deaths occurred in Africa and Asia.

- Africa is the continent with the highest rate of maternal mortality, estimated at 820 maternal deaths per 100,000 live births in 2005. Asia's rate of maternal death is 350 per 100,000 live births.

- In Africa, the lifetime risk of maternal death is 1 in 26, four times higher than in Asia and more than 300 times higher than in the industrialized countries.

The full burden of maternal and child deaths in Africa and Asia – for each continent and for the two combined – is frequently understated due to the lack of continent-wide estimates for key Millennium Development Goal indicators. This panel presents a snapshot of key child and maternal indicators for Africa and Asia, and in their totality provides a complementary perspective to the regional breakdown presented in the Statistical Tables, pages 113-157 of this report.

Aggregating the data on children from these two vast continents provides a stark reminder of the overwhelming importance of making rapid progress across both Africa and Asia if global development goals are to be realized. In the push to accelerate progress at the continental level, however, the often startling disparities in the status of women and children and in rates of progress within countries and continents must not be forgotten. The issue of disparities and inequalities affecting children will be examined in greater detail in future editions of *The State of the World's Children*.

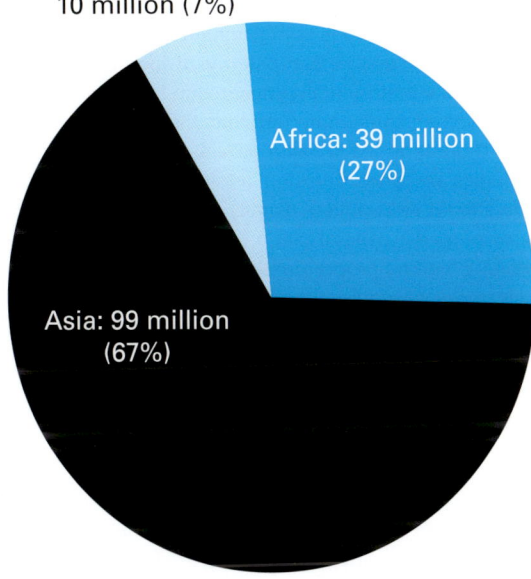

Underweight children under five, 2007
Rest of the world: 10 million (7%)
Africa: 39 million (27%)
Asia: 99 million (67%)

Source: UNICEF global databases.

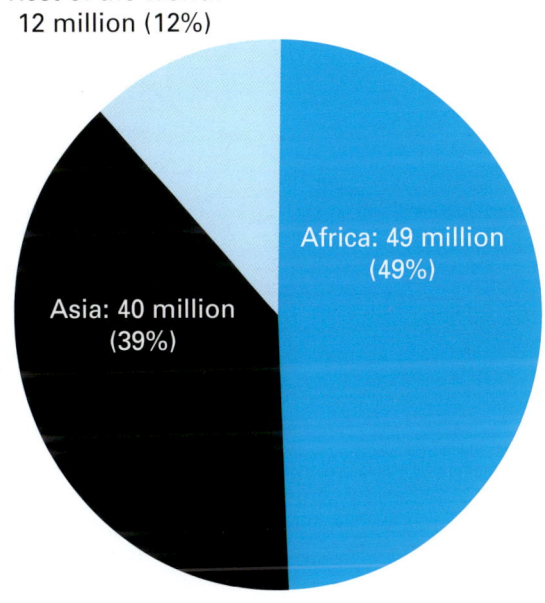

Primary-school-age children out of school, 2007
Rest of the world: 12 million (12%)
Africa: 49 million (49%)
Asia: 40 million (39%)

Source: UNICEF global databases.

Nutritional status of young children

- In 2007, 148 million children under age five in the developing world were underweight for their age.

- Two thirds of these children live in Asia, and just over one quarter live in Africa.

- Together, Africa and Asia account for 93 per cent of all underweight children under age five in the developing world.

Primary education

- In 2007, 101 million children of primary school age were not in school.

- Almost half of these children live in Africa, and 39 per cent live in Asia.

- Across the two regions, approximately 20 per cent of girls and 16 per cent of boys of primary school age are either not enrolled or are not attending primary school.

* Africa includes all member states of the African Union. Asia includes the countries in the UNICEF regions of East Asia and the Pacific and South Asia. Numbers may not always add up due to rounding.

The global food crisis and its potential impact on maternal and newborn health

The recent, precipitous rise in global prices that began in 2006 and continued in 2007–2008 has illustrated the vulnerability of millions to hunger and undernutrition, particularly those in countries where food security is still a major concern. The sharp increases involved such basic foodstuffs as vegetable oils, grains, dairy products and rice. Although fluctuations in the prices of commodities are common, what distinguished the situation in 2008 was that the hike in world prices affects not just a selected few products but nearly all major food and feed commodities.

Figure 1.8

Food prices have risen sharply across the board*

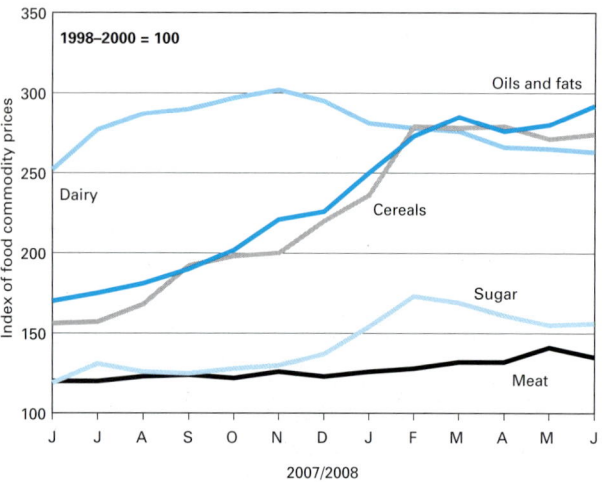

* The food commodity price indices displayed above are the weighted averages of price indices from a basket of basic goods under each commodity group. The weights are the average export trade shares for 1998–2000. For examples, the Oils and Fats Price Index consists of the price indices of 11 different oils (including animal and fish oils) weighted with average export trade shares of each oil product for 1998–2000. For a fuller explanation of the composition of each food commodity group index, see Source.

Source: Food and Agriculture Organization of the United Nations, Food Price Indices, <http://www.fao.org/worldfoodsituation/FoodPricesIndex/en>, accessed 1 August 2008.

By June 2008, the Food and Agriculture Organization of the United Nations (FAO) had identified 22 developing countries as being particularly vulnerable to the food crisis. Its assessment was based on a combination of three risk factors:

- An underweight prevalence rate of 30 per cent or more in the population.
- A high degree of dependence on imports of food staples such as rice, wheat and maize.
- A high degree of dependence on imported petroleum products.

Comoros, Eritrea, Haiti, Liberia and Niger are among the countries that demonstrate worrisome levels of all three of these identified risk factors. It comes as little surprise that most of these nations are among the least developed and lowest-income countries. Even within these countries, however, it is the poorest sections of society – who spend the largest proportion of their disposable income on food – that are likely to be hardest hit by the food crisis.

Addressing the special nutritional needs of mothers and newborns

During an emergency such as a food crisis, pregnant and lactating mothers, together with infants, are among those considered most at risk of undernutrition, owing to their higher nutritional requirements. For example, pregnant women require almost 285 additional calories per day, and lactating women require an additional 500 calories per day. Their micronutrient needs are also higher, and they require adequate intake of iron, folate, vitamin A and iodine to ensure the health of both mother and infant.

In the face of the food crisis, FAO has urged a rapid supply response to restore a better balance between food supply and demand, especially in the countries worst affected. In addition, while food aid is being supplied to countries, policies must be applied to offset patterns of food distribution between family members that may result in pregnant and lactating women consuming less than their minimum requirements. Where food aid is being provided to those most at risk of shortages and undernutrition, additional food for pregnant women should be supplied, usually as a take-home ration, either through the general ration distribution or through supplementary feeding programmes. Pregnant and lactating women may also require other complementary, nutrition-related interventions, including food fortification, micronutrient supplementation, additional safe drinking water, malaria management during pregnancy, prophylaxis for management of internal parasites, and nutrition education counselling.

Communication and advocacy campaigns concerning food aid should highlight the special nutritional needs of pregnant and lactating women and include messages to families and communities explaining why these women are being provided extra food. The information should stress the importance of exclusive breastfeeding for the first six months of a child's life, with complementary feeding for older infants. For HIV-positive mothers, breastfeeding practices may differ, since the virus can be transmitted through breast milk, depending on the availability and safety of replacement feeding.

Information and early warning continue to have a crucial role in ensuring that timely and appropriate action can be taken to avoid suffering. FAO's Global Information and Early Warning System is demonstrating its capacity to alert the world to emerging food shortages. More needs to be done, however, to create strong response mechanisms to food crises and to develop national and international policies that prioritize and safeguard food and nutrition security – and take into account the special nutritional needs of women and young children.

See References, page 107.

THE STATE OF THE WORLD'S CHILDREN 2009

2 Creating a supportive environment for maternal and newborn health

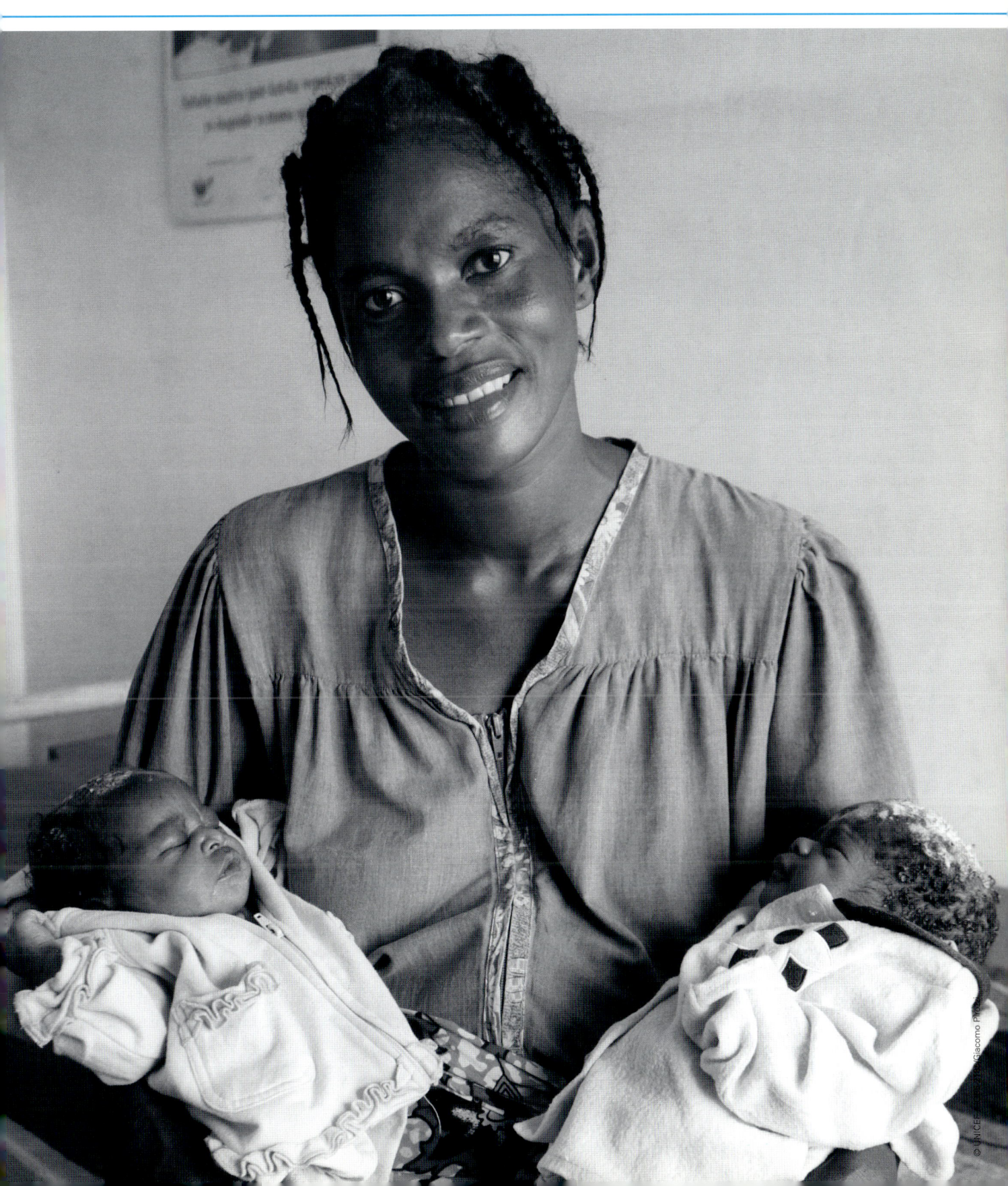

Improving maternal and newborn health requires delivering essential services at critical times and in key locations where they can be readily accessed by women and children. Establishing and consolidating these continua of care necessitate more than just enhanced primary-health-care interventions; it also demands a supportive environment for mothers and children that safeguards and promotes their rights. The second chapter of The State of the World's Children 2009 *explores the fundamentals of the supportive environment and the ways in which it strengthens efforts to enhance primary health care.*

In October 2008, more than 500 health leaders from 65 countries met in Almaty, Kazakhstan, at an international conference marking the 30th anniversary of the Alma-Ata Declaration on primary health care. The participants exchanged experiences from the past three decades and renewed their commitment to the principles of primary health care as a way of strengthening health systems. The World Health Organization launched the *World Health Report 2008*, which also addressed the theme of primary health care, on the eve of the conference.

The Alma-Ata Declaration, which emerged from a similar meeting convened by UNICEF and WHO in 1978 in the same city, in effect charted a new course for public health. It advocated that countries broaden the remit of health care beyond medical interventions to address the social, cultural and infrastructure constraints on providing quality health services to all their citizens. A principal focus of the primary-health-care approach that emerged from Alma-Ata is the same as the subject of this report: care for mothers and children. Other core priorities included disease control, access to family planning, safe water supplies and sanitation. Citizens were to be encouraged to participate in their own health care, particularly in the provision of preventive care and adoption of healthy behaviours and practices.[1] *(See Panel on page 29)*

Considerable progress has been achieved across the developing world in the 30 years that have ensued, in controlling several major diseases, including polio and measles, and in reducing child mortality – particularly in the post-neonatal period (between 29 days and five years of age). Yet given the widening inequities in healthcare provision between and within countries across the developing world, the Alma-Ata agenda of comprehensive primary health care – which emphasizes the importance of a supportive environment and preventive and curative interventions in determining health outcomes – is perhaps as pertinent today as it was in 1978.

There is a growing recognition among health policymakers and practitioners that the interrelated health needs of women, newborns and children require the type of integrated solutions championed in the Alma-Ata Declaration. This recognition has resulted in renewed interest in and support for integrated frameworks of health-service delivery. Regular refinement of such frameworks as the Integrated Management of Childhood Illness, introduced by UNICEF and the World Health Organization in 1992, and collaboration between national and international partners over the past two decades have recently consolidated into a comprehensive paradigm that integrates the hitherto often disparate programmes for maternal and child health: *the continuum of care for mothers, newborns and children.*

The continuum of care

The continuum of care aims to integrate maternal, newborn and child health care. Its central premise can be summarized as follows: essential services for mothers, newborns and children are most effective when they are

The interrelated health needs of women and newborns require integrated primary-health-care solutions.

delivered in integrated packages at critical points in the life cycle of mothers and children, in a dynamic health system that spans key locations, underpinned by an environment supportive of the rights of women and children.

The *critical points* for service delivery are adolescence, pre-pregnancy, pregnancy, birth, post-partum, neonatal, infancy and childhood.

The *essential services for mothers, newborns and children* include basic health care, quality maternal, newborn and child health care, adequate nutrition and improved water and sanitation facilities, and hygiene practices.

The *key delivery modes for services* are household and community, outreach and outpatient, and health facilities.[2]

The *supportive environment* requires respect for the rights of women and children; quality education; a decent standard of living; protection from abuse, exploitation, discrimination and violence; equal participation in home, community, social and political life; empowerment of women; and greater involvement of men in maternal and child care.

The continuum of care broadly reflects a set of strategic principles based on lessons learned from a century of evolving health-care systems and practices. These principles were explored in depth in *The State of*

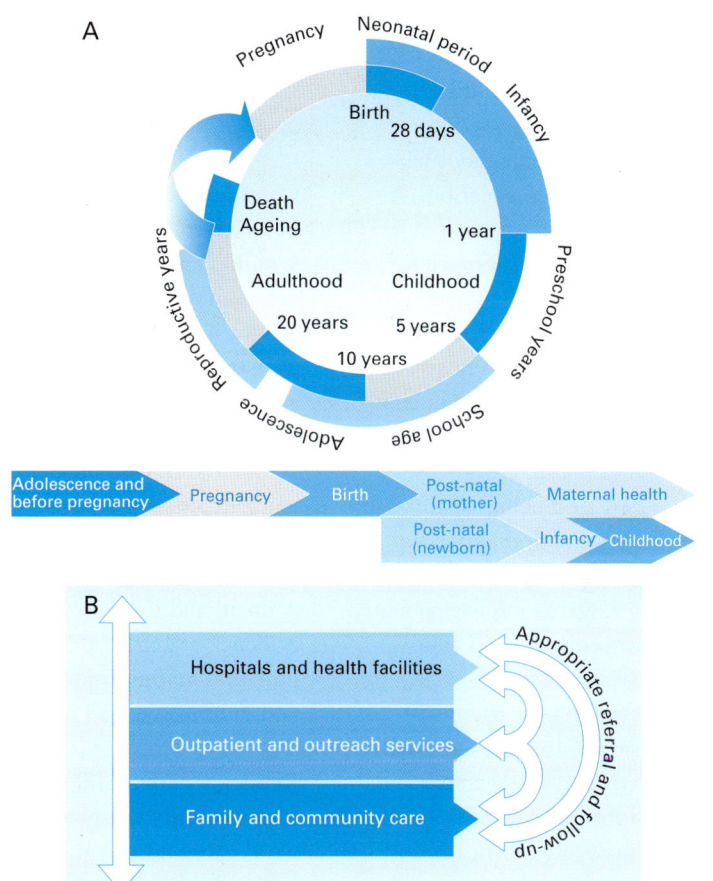

Figure 2.1

The continuum of care

Connecting care during the lifecycle (A) and at places of caregiving (B). Adapted from Partnership for Maternal, Newborn and Child Health, with permission.

Source: Kevbes, Kate J., et. al., 'Continuum of Care for Maternal, Newborn and Child Health: From slogan to service delivery', *The Lancet*, vol. 370, no. 9595, 13 October 2007, p.1360.

the World's Children 2008 and are summarized here.

- Actions to improve the health of women, newborns and children are most effective and sustainable when they are integrated and delivered in convenient, cost-effective packages to communities and families.

- Health systems are most useful when they integrate dynamically the different modes of care – facility-based, outreach and outpatient services, and community and family care.

- Strengthening health systems to improve health outcomes for mothers and children requires combining and integrating the

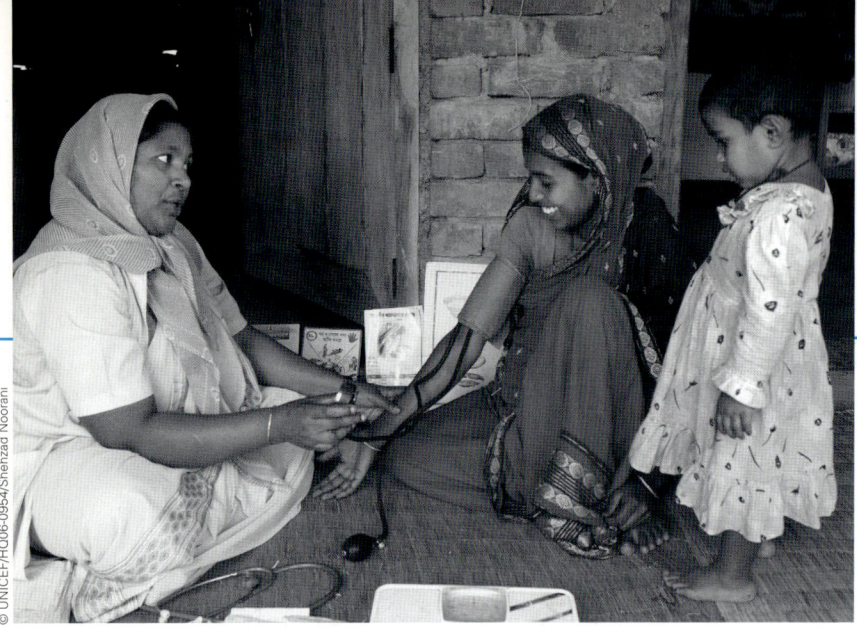

Much ill health among women during pregnancy is preventable, detectable or treatable through antenatal visits. *A health worker prepares to measure a pregnant woman's blood pressure at a clinic, Bangladesh.*

strengths of vertical and horizontal approaches to health-service delivery, rather than choosing either approach in isolation.

- A results-oriented approach to health-systems development, centred on effective and evidence-based interventions, is useful in setting agendas and policies and in monitoring and evaluating progress.

- Results are best achieved through collaborative action between programmes, policies and partnerships working towards improving maternal, newborn and child care.[3]

These precepts form the basis of programmes, policies and partnerships seeking to establish and extend continua of quality health care for mothers, newborns and children. To be truly effective, however, and to move closer to meeting the Alma-Ata challenge of delivering primary health care for all, essential services for mothers and children require a supportive environment that safeguards and promotes their rights. Without actions to address gender discrimination, inequities and abuses that are perpetuated against women and girls in particular, actions in support of enhanced primary health care risk being much less effective, sustainable or even possible.

Consider, for example, the problem of low birthweight, which is a background factor in 70 per cent of neonatal deaths. Most low birthweight babies suffered intrauterine growth restriction in the womb, usually as a result of the poor nutritional and health status of the mother before and during pregnancy. The majority of such cases occur in South Asia, the region with highest rates of undernutrition among girls and women, and the only one with clear evidence of gender discrimination in nutrition among children under five and in adolescence.[4]

Reducing neonatal deaths necessitates not only the provision of antenatal care and the attendance of skilled health personnel at delivery; it also requires that girls and women receive adequate nutrition and health care from birth through childhood and into adolescence, womanhood and their potential childbearing years.

This is but one example – more are given in the remainder of this chapter – of how the survival and health of newborns and children depend critically on the fulfilment of women's rights. For this reason, the exploration of the continuum of care for mothers and newborns begins by examining the various constituents of a supportive environment for the rights of women and girls.

Creating a supportive environment for women and children

Improving maternal and newborn health is not simply a practical matter of making available better and more extensive maternity services. It also involves addressing and reversing the neglect of women's rights and the structural discrimination and maltreatment often suffered by girls and women.

Discrimination on the basis of gender – often passed on from generation to generation by cultural tradition and economic, social and political norms – has numerous pernicious effects. It can deny girls and women access to education, which research shows could lower their exposure to the risks of maternal and infant deaths.[5] It may prevent them from receiving, or from seeking, adequate health care and vital life skills to protect them against sexually transmitted infections – including HIV – inadequate birth spacing, violence, abuse and exploitation. It can constrain their income-earning capacity when they become women and can force them into a life of servitude and subservience when they marry – often when they are still children under 18 years of age.

Promoting healthy behaviours for mothers, newborns and children: The *Facts for Life* guide

Creating a supportive environment for maternal and newborn health requires altering behaviours that discriminate against women and girls and adopting healthy practices that safeguard them from disease and injury. Healthy practices, such as exclusively breastfeeding an infant for the first six months of its life or washing hands with soap, must be evidence-based and established by medical experts.

Describing these practices to parents and other caregivers in non-technical language is critical to empowering women and girls and supporting maternal and newborn health. Twenty years ago, eight UN agencies – UNICEF, WHO, UNFPA, the United Nations Educational, Scientific and Cultural Organization, the United Nations Development Programme, the Joint United Nations Programme on HIV/AIDS, the World Food Programme and the World Bank – jointly published a guide to make such life-saving knowledge available to everyone. The guide, entitled *Facts for Life*, was addressed to communicators – health workers, the media, government officials, non-governmental organizations, teachers, religious leaders, employers, trade unions, women's groups, community organizations and others. Its third edition, published in 2002, addressed a broad range of topics:

- Timing of births
- Safe motherhood
- Child development and early learning
- Breastfeeding
- Nutrition and growth
- Immunization
- Diarrhoea
- Coughs, colds and more serious illnesses
- Hygiene
- Malaria
- HIV and AIDS
- Injury prevention
- Disasters and emergencies

Clear, brief and practical key messages explained recommended actions and offered supplementary information.

One underlying principle of the guide is that communication involves more than simply providing information. It also requires presenting the information in an interesting and accessible way and helping people understand its relevance. The guide also discusses ways to take action and overcome bottlenecks and barriers.

Facts for Life has been widely disseminated, with more than 15 million copies in circulation in 215 languages by 2002. A new edition of the guide is being prepared.

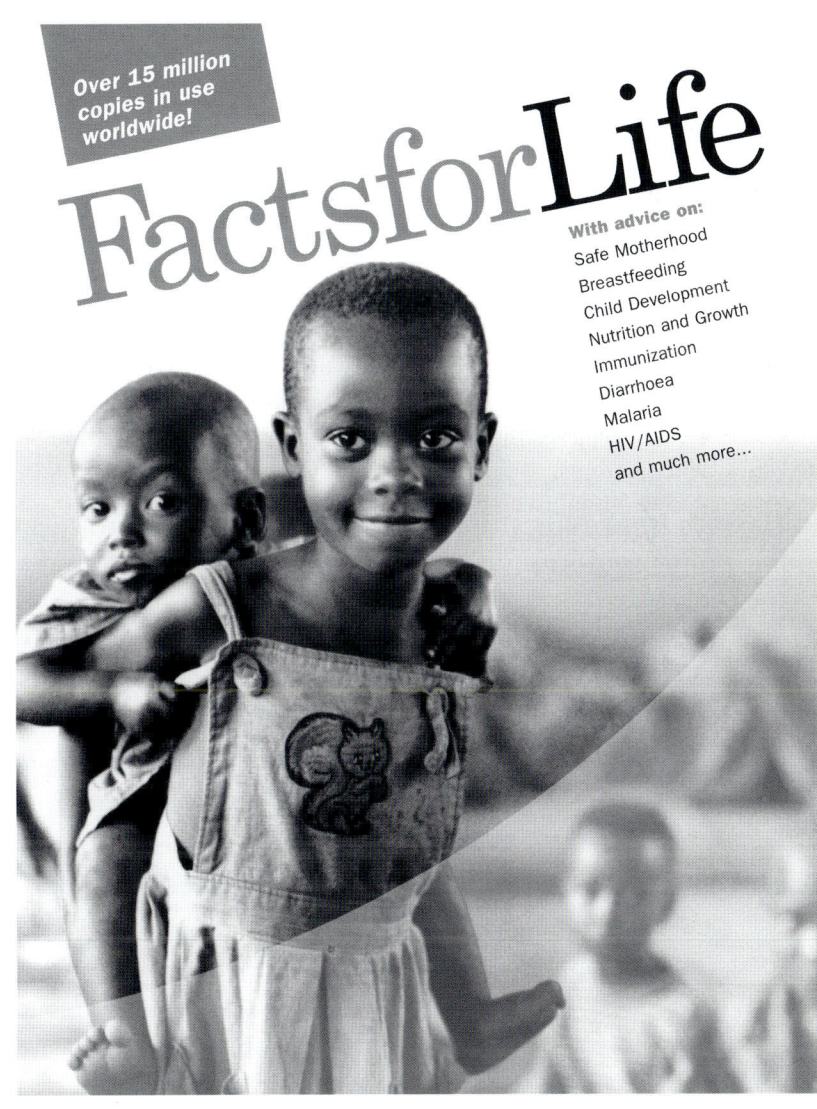

Gender equality produces a double dividend, enhancing the lives of both women and children.

In addition, the heavy workloads of women – who in general work longer hours than men – can deny them the time for leisure and rest.

Creating a supportive environment for maternal and newborn health requires challenging the social, economic and cultural barriers that perpetuate gender inequality and discrimination. This will involve several key actions: educating girls and women, and reducing the poverty they experience; protecting girls and women from abuse, exploitation, discrimination and violence; fostering their participation and their involvement in household decision-making and economic and political life; and empowering them to claim their rights and essential services for themselves and their children. Greater involvement of men in maternal and newborn health care and in addressing gender discrimination and inequalities is also critical to establishing a supportive environment. The remainder of this chapter will briefly examine each of these challenges in turn.

Quality education and a decent standard of living

Securing a quality education

Education is a right for children and adolescents under the 1948 Universal Declaration of Human Rights, the 1989 Convention on the Rights of the Child and other human rights instruments.[6] It is also pivotal to improving maternal and neonatal health, reducing the incidence of child marriage – with its largely inevitable consequences of premature pregnancy and motherhood, eliminating extreme poverty and hunger, and enhancing knowledge of health risks and life skills. Since discrimination against girls and women is known to begin early, promoting gender equality and respect for the rights of women and encouraging fathers to play active roles in child care, should begin with early childhood education programmes.

Figure 2.2

Although improving, the educational status of young women is still low in several developing regions

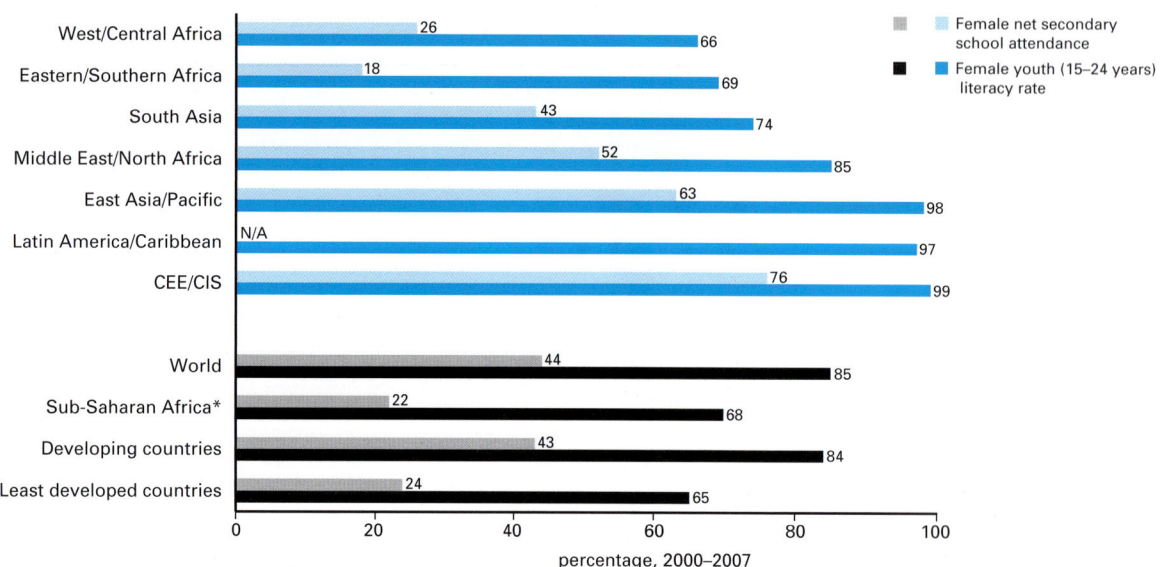

* Sub-Saharan Africa comprises the regions of Eastern/Southern Africa and West/Central Africa.

Sources: *Female youth literacy rate*—UNESCO Institute of Statistics. *Female net secondary school attendance*—Demographic and Health Surveys and Multiple Indicator Cluster Surveys.

30   THE STATE OF THE WORLD'S CHILDREN 2009

Primary health care: 30 years since Alma-Ata

The 1978 Declaration of Alma-Ata was groundbreaking because it linked the rights-based approach to health to a viable strategy for attaining it. The outcome document of the International Conference on Primary Health Care, the declaration identified primary health care as the key to reducing health inequalities between and within countries and thereby to achieving the ambitious but unrealized goal of "Health for All" by 2000. Primary health care was defined by the document as "essential health care" services, based on scientifically proven interventions. These services were to be universally accessible to individuals and families at a cost that communities and nations as a whole could afford. At a minimum, primary health care comprised eight elements: health education, adequate nutrition, maternal and child health care, basic sanitation and safe water, control of major infectious diseases through immunization, prevention and control of locally endemic diseases, treatment of common diseases and injuries, and the provision of essential drugs.

The declaration urged governments to formulate national policies to incorporate primary health care into their national health systems. It argued that attention be given to the importance of community-based care that reflects a country's political and economic realities. This model would bring "health care as close as possible to where people live and work" by enabling them to seek treatment, as appropriate, from trained community health workers, nurses and doctors. It would also foster a spirit of self-reliance among individuals within a community and encourage their participation in the planning and execution of health-care programmes. Referral systems would complete the spectrum of care by providing more comprehensive services to those who needed them most – the poorest and the most marginalized.

Alma-Ata grew out of the same movement for social justice that led to the 1974 Declaration on the Establishment of a New International Economic Order. Both stressed the interdependence of the global economy and encouraged transfers of aid and knowledge to reverse the widening economic and technological divides between industrialized countries and developing countries, whose growth had, in many cases, been stymied by colonization. Examples of community-based innovations in poorer countries after World War II also provided inspiration. Nigeria's under-five clinics, China's barefoot doctors and the Cuban and Vietnamese health systems demonstrated that advances in health could occur without the infrastructure available in industrialized countries.

The International Conference on Primary Health Care was itself a milestone. At the time, it was the largest conference ever held devoted to a single topic in international health and development, with 134 countries and 67 non-governmental organizations in attendance. Yet there were obstacles to fulfilling its promise. For one thing, the declaration was non-binding. Furthermore, conceptual disagreements over how to define fundamental terms such as 'universal access', which persist today, were present from the beginning. In the context of the cold war, these terms revealed the sharp ideological differences between the capitalist and communist worlds, discord perhaps heightened by the fact that the Alma-Ata conference took place in what was then the Union of Soviet Socialist Republics.

As the 1970s gave way to a new decade, a tumultuous economic environment contributed to a diversion away from primary health care in favour of the more affordable model of selective health care, which targeted specific diseases and conditions. Nonetheless, despite the mixed success of primary health care in the countries where it has been implemented, advances in improving public health illustrate the community-based model's flexibility and applicability.

Insufficient progress towards the Millennium Development Goals, coupled with the threats posed to global health and human security by climate change, pandemic influenza and the global food crisis, have led to renewed interest in comprehensive primary health care. Yet the many challenges that prevented Alma-Ata's implementation have evolved and must be confronted to achieve its goals now. Drawing on the growing body of evidence about cost-effective initiatives that integrate household and community care with outreach and facility-based services – such as those for maternal and child health described in Chapter 3 – will enable governments, international partners and civil society organizations to revitalize primary health care.

See References, page 108.

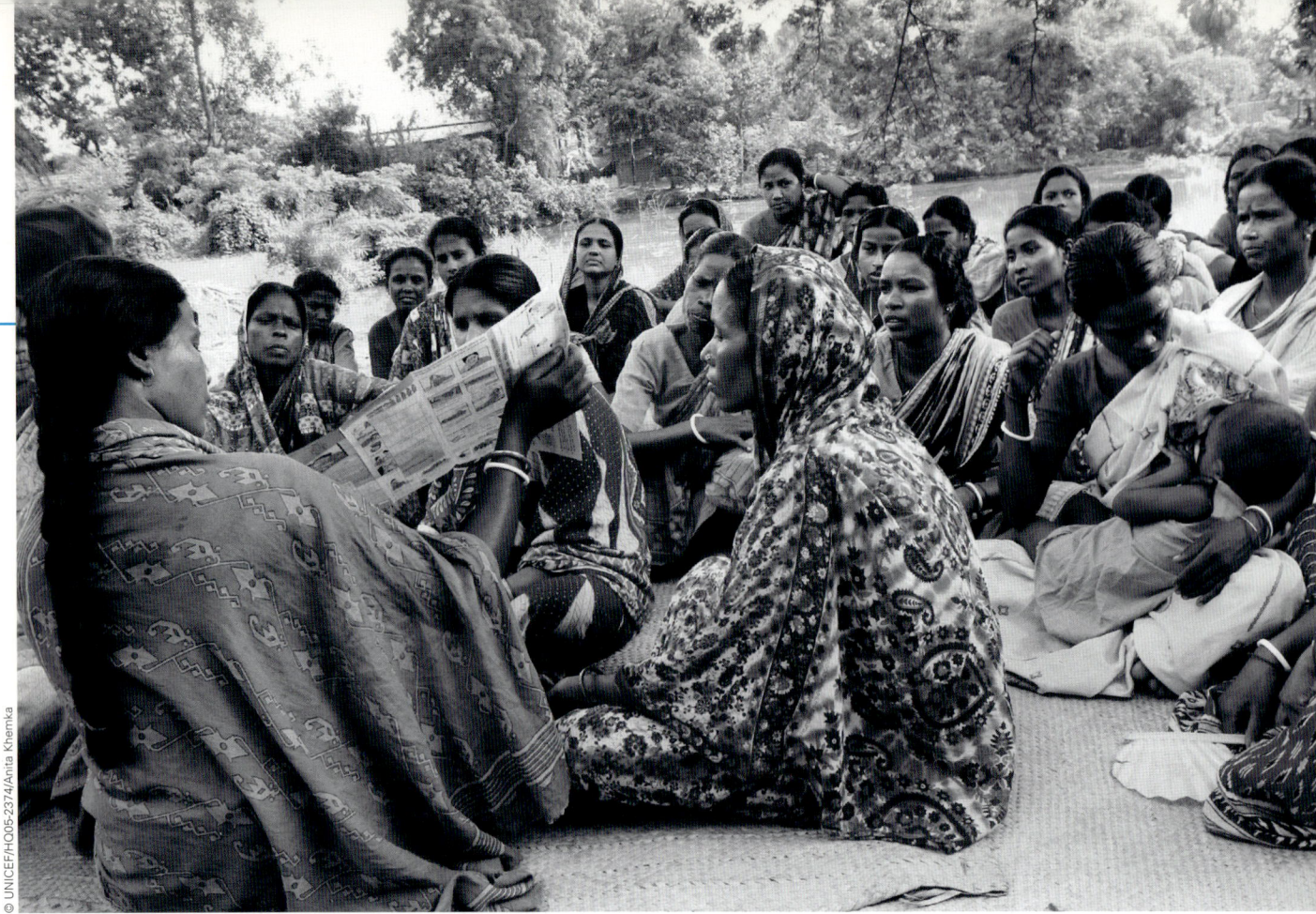

Outreach health providers bring vital services to communities and households. *A community health worker holds up an infant growth chart during an education session for young mothers, India.*

Securing quality education for girls and young women is a key challenge of the Millennium Development Goals, which aim to achieve universal primary education (MDG 2) and to eliminate gender disparity at all levels of education by 2015 as part of efforts to promote gender equality and empower women (MDG 3).

Although considerable progress has been made in reaching gender parity in primary education – all regions are currently deemed to be on track to meet this target – there are sizeable gaps in several countries and in West and Central Africa in particular. Furthermore, gaps have closed less rapidly in secondary education.[7]

Research has long confirmed the merits of education not only for women and girls, but also for families and societies. Studies show that educated adolescents are more likely to wait until they are out of their teenage years – when pregnancy risks are highest – before starting a family, and are also likely to have healthier babies.[8] The benefits of delaying pregnancy until after adolescence are high. Consider the following facts:

- Maternal deaths related to pregnancy and childbirth are an important cause of mortality for girls aged 15–19 worldwide, accounting for 70,000 deaths each year.[9]

- The younger a girl is when she becomes pregnant, the greater the health risks. Girls who give birth before the age of 15 are five times more likely to die in childbirth than women in their twenties.[10]

- If a mother is under the age of 18, her infant's risk of dying in its first year of life is 60 per cent greater than that of an infant born to a mother older than 19.[11]

- Even if the child survives, he or she is more likely to suffer from low birthweight, undernutrition and late physical and cognitive development.[12]

The gains from education go beyond reducing the risk of maternal and newborn deaths and ill health. Research shows that educated women are more likely to delay marriage, ensure their children are immunized, be better informed about nutrition for themselves and their children, and undertake improved birth spacing practices. In turn, their children have higher survival rates than those of uneducated women and tend to be better nourished.[13]

Education is also essential to the fulfilment of women's rights. It

32   THE STATE OF THE WORLD'S CHILDREN 2009

Creating a supportive environment for maternal and newborn health requires challenging the social, cultural and economic barriers that perpetuate gender inequity.

enhances women's influence in household decision-making and opens up opportunities for women's economic and political participation.

Protection from abuse, exploitation, discrimination and violence

Preventing child marriage

Child marriage is a violation of child rights, compromising the development of girls and often resulting in premature pregnancy and social isolation. Although child marriage is not directly addressed in the Convention on the Rights of the Child, it is linked to other rights and is recognized in the Universal Declaration of Human Rights as the "right to free and full consent to marriage" (article 16). The Convention on the Elimination of All Forms of Discrimination against Women states that "the betrothal and the marriage of a child shall have no legal effect" and calls upon states to set legal minimum ages for marriage and to make marriage registration compulsory (article 16). Despite international commitment to change, many societies and communities continue the marriage of their young daughters and sons due to strong social pressures at the community level. Worldwide, more than 60 million women aged 20–24 were married before they reached the age of 18.[14] In the developing world excluding China, the latest international estimates indicate that 36 per cent of women aged 20–24 were married or in union before the age of 18. In some regions, the incidence of child marriage is particularly high, at 49 per cent in South Asia, and 44 per cent in West and Central Africa, according to the latest estimates.[15]

In addition to an increased risk of maternal death from pregnancy and childbirth, adolescent wives are also susceptible to violence, abuse and exploitation. Child marriage also increases the risk that adolescent girls will drop out of school – with attendant negative implications for maternal and newborn health and for income-earning capacity, described previously. This, in turn, contributes to the vicious cycle of gender discrimination, with poorer families being more willing to permit the premature marriage of daughters out of economic necessity.[16]

Given the health risks associated with adolescent pregnancy and birth (*see page 32*), the greater likelihood of adolescent pregnancy for girl wives, and the high incidence of this practice across several developing regions, it is evident that improving maternal health requires ending child marriage. This will require, among other actions,

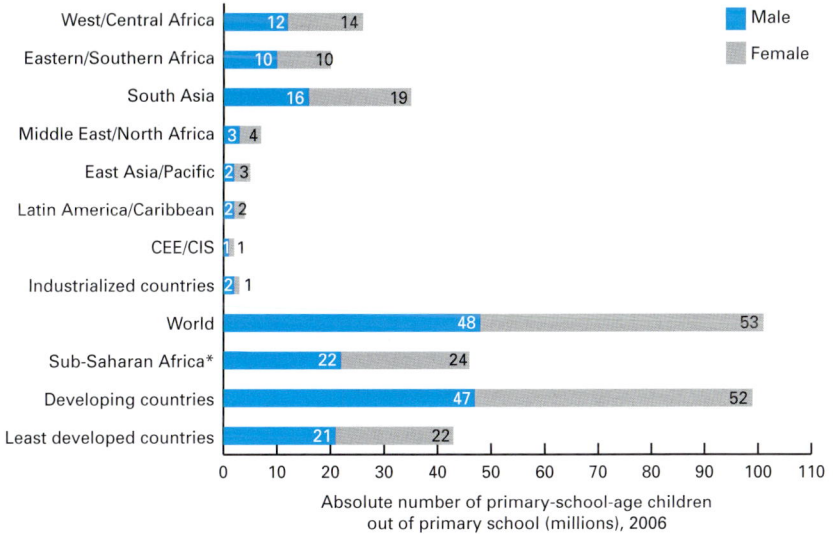

Figure 2.3

Gender parity in attendance has improved markedly, but there are still slightly more girls than boys out of primary school

* Sub-Saharan Africa comprises the regions of Eastern/Southern Africa and West/Central Africa.

Source: Estimates derived by the Statistical Information Section, United Nations Children's Fund, using attendance data from household surveys (Demographic and Health Surveys and Multiple Indicator Cluster Surveys) and UNESCO Institute of Statistics.

stronger government legislation to set and enforce the age of 18 as the minimum legal age of marriage, and to promote both birth and marriage registration; the former is required to establish the age of the child.

While child marriage is becoming less common overall, the pace of change is slow. Challenging prevailing attitudes towards child marriage will also require addressing gender inequality. Action by parties other than governments is crucial, including religious and community leaders, as is the promotion of education, particularly at the secondary level. For their part, civil society and the media can help foster an open dialogue to address and challenge the economic pressures and societal traditions that perpetuate child marriage.

Abandoning female genital mutilation/cutting

Female genital mutilation and cutting violates girls' and women's human rights, denying them their physical and mental integrity, their right to freedom from violence and discrimination and, in the most extreme cases, their lives.

Around 70 million girls and women aged 15–49 in 27 countries of Africa and the Middle East are estimated to have undergone this practice. Though the practice has declined, its prevalence is still strong in several countries and communities.[17]

In addition to being a rights violation, female genital mutilation and cutting pose serious risks for childbirth, heightening the possibility of such complications as obstructed labour and post-partum haemorrhage in contexts outside the hospital setting.

A study by the World Health Organization showed that not only does female genital mutilation/cutting (FGM/C) affect the reproductive health of women and cause severe

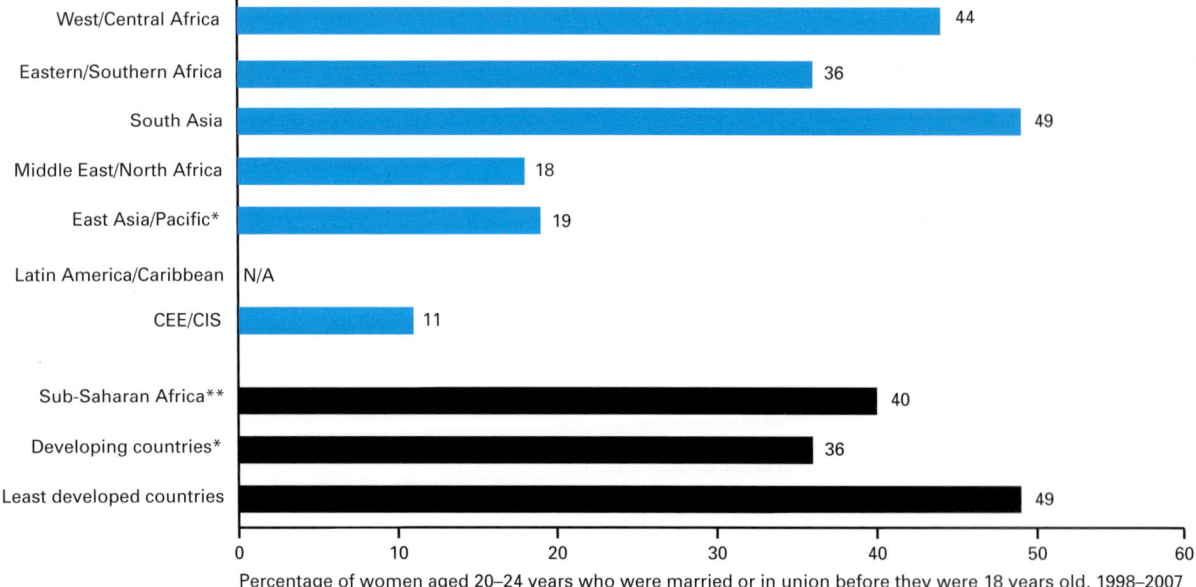

Figure 2.4

Child marriage is highly prevalent in South Asia and sub-Saharan Africa

Percentage of women aged 20–24 years who were married or in union before they were 18 years old, 1998–2007

- West/Central Africa: 44
- Eastern/Southern Africa: 36
- South Asia: 49
- Middle East/North Africa: 18
- East Asia/Pacific*: 19
- Latin America/Caribbean: N/A
- CEE/CIS: 11
- Sub-Saharan Africa**: 40
- Developing countries*: 36
- Least developed countries: 49

* Excludes China. ** Sub-Saharan Africa comprises the regions of Eastern/Southern Africa and West/Central Africa.

Source: Demographic and Health Surveys, Multiple Indicator Cluster Surveys and other national surveys.

Addressing the health worker shortage: A critical action for improving maternal and newborn health

One of the biggest challenges for maternal and neonatal health is the shortage of skilled health personnel. A 2006 World Health Organization survey reveals that while Africa accounts for more than 24 per cent of the global disease burden, it has only 3 per cent of the world's health workers and spends less than 1 per cent of total global resources dedicated to health, even after loans and grants from abroad are taken into account. In contrast, the Americas region, which covers Latin America and the Caribbean along with North America, has only 10 per cent of the global burden of disease but commands 37 per cent of the world's health workers and spends more than 50 per cent of global resources allocated to health.

According to the World Health Organization, the world is facing a shortage of 4.3 million health workers, with every region except Europe showing a shortfall. More specifically, there are not enough skilled health workers – doctors, nurses or midwives – to attend all the world's births. A study by the Joint Learning Initiative found that countries needed an average of 2.28 health-care professionals per 1,000 people to achieve the minimum desired level of coverage for skilled attendance at delivery. Of the 57 countries that fall below this threshold, 36 are in sub-Saharan Africa. Although the countries with the largest shortages of health workers in absolute terms are found in Asia – notably in Bangladesh, India and Indonesia – the largest relative need is in sub-Saharan Africa. This region would need to increase its numbers of health workers by 140 per cent to reach the requisite density. An earlier WHO estimate calculated that 334,000 skilled birth attendants would need to be trained worldwide in the coming years to cover 73 per cent of births.

Shortages of skilled health workers arise from many factors, including underinvestment in training and recruitment, weak incentives for health-care workers, low remuneration and high levels of stress. Heavy migration of skilled health workers from developing countries to industrialized nations – spurred by the burgeoning demand for health workers in industrialized countries with ageing populations – has also taken its toll. A survey of 10 African countries showed that the number of locally trained doctors now working in eight Organisation for Economic Co-operation and Development countries was equivalent to 23 per cent of the doctors still domestically employed in those countries.

Demographic trends within countries are also strong influences on the health worker shortage. Rapid urbanization in developing countries is exacerbating the shortage of health workers in rural areas, as trained professionals seek work in more affluent urban conurbations. Health workers, who usually qualify in urban settings, are often reluctant to base themselves in a rural location on the grounds that it involves greater hardship, more basic living conditions and less access to urban amenities and entertainment. One survey in South and South-east Asia found, for example, that rural postings were shunned because of lower income, low prestige and social isolation.

AIDS, too, is having a deleterious effect on health systems in the countries where it has reached epidemic proportions. Health workers in these countries face the same risks in their private lives as other people in high-prevalence countries, but are also exposed to significant risks at work in circumstances where protective equipment and practices are often deficient. A 2004 study in South Africa indicated that younger health workers there had an HIV-prevalence rate of 20 per cent. Such workers deserve much greater protection and care, including better supplies of protective equipment, safety schemes to prevent needle-stick injuries, prophylaxis in the event of possible exposure to the virus, and antiretroviral treatment if they become infected with HIV.

Establishing continua of quality health care to reduce maternal and neonatal mortality and morbidity will require strategies to reduce the shortfalls in health-care personnel. While part of this gap will be filled by the recruitment and training of community health workers – whose resourcefulness has been shown to have great potential to provide basic services – much more needs to be done to train and retain skilled health-care workers, particularly in sub-Saharan Africa and South Asia.

See References, page 108.

---

pain, it can also result in prolonged bleeding, infection, a variety of reproductive health problems including infertility, and even death. It also affects newborns of women who have been subjected to the practice. The study provides clear evidence that complications in deliveries are significantly more likely among women with FGM/C. It also found that FGM/C is harmful to babies and leads to an extra one to two perinatal deaths per 100 deliveries.[18]

The risks to both mothers and babies increase according to the severity of the mutilation, but can include shock, haemorrhaging, infection and ulceration of the genital area – all of which increase the risks of maternal and neonatal mortality and distress.[19]

Abandoning female genital mutilation and cutting is critical to ensuring safe motherhood and reducing neonatal deaths. Successful initiatives in Senegal and other countries where female genital mutilation and cutting is widespread are based on the collective abandonment of this practice through community empowerment, open dialogue and a collective consensus.[20]

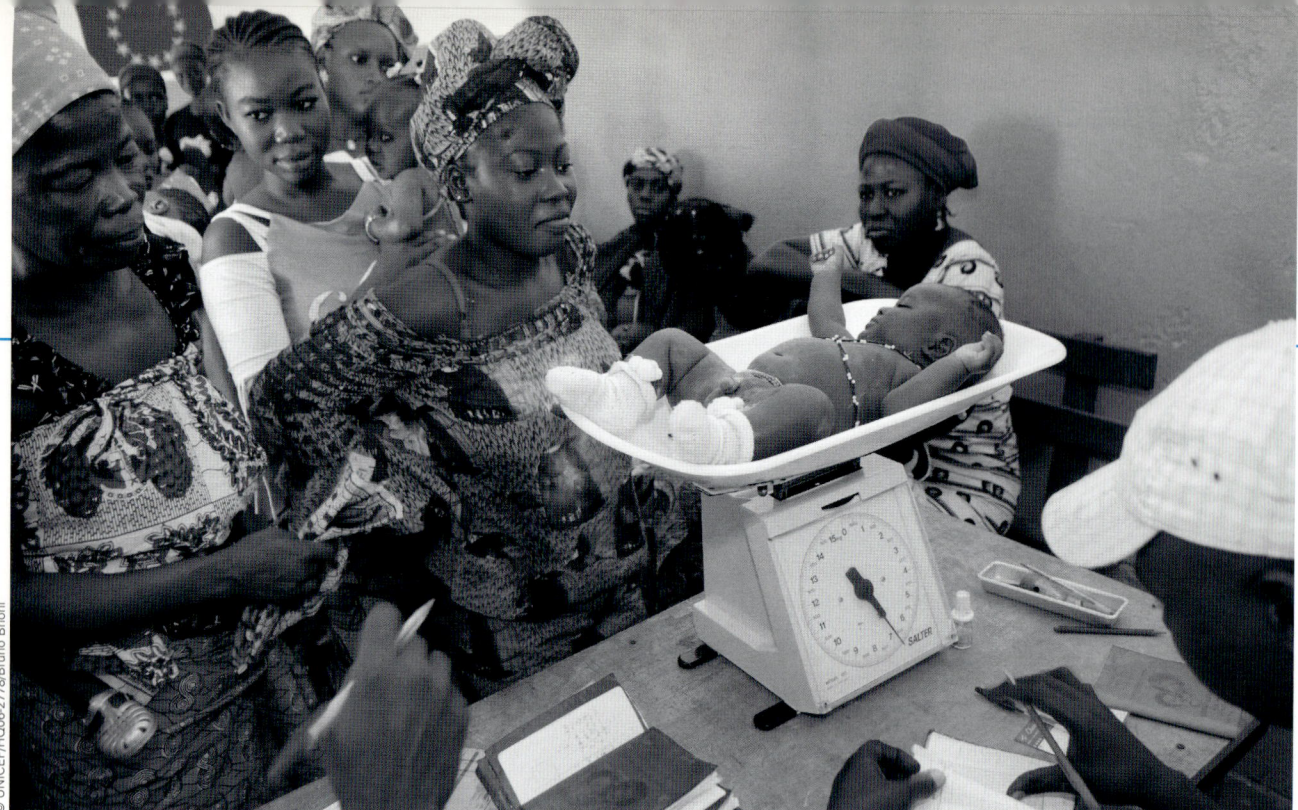

Enhancing health facilities and strengthening referral systems are effective ways of improving maternal and newborn health. *A mother watches as her infant is weighed by a health care worker at a maternal and child health centre, Côte d'Ivoire.*

Eliminating violence, abuse and exploitation of women and girls

Violence is prevalent in all societies. It undermines the physical health and emotional and psychological well-being of its victims. Gender inequities within households, workplaces and societies can foster a permissive context for violence.

The extent of violence against women and girls and its impact on them has long been acknowledged. Until relatively recently, however, its measurement was largely restricted to specific studies. Large-scale studies by the World Health Organization and the recent United Nations studies on violence against women and children have revealed astounding levels of violence against women and children, but also sharp disparities in levels within countries and regions.[21] The health consequences of violence increase the risk of poor physical and reproductive outcomes. Although many of the studies are indicative rather than conclusive, they show a correlation between violence against women and girls and increased risk of maternal mortality and morbidity.

- A study of 400 villages in rural India revealed that 16 per cent of all deaths among pregnant women were due to partner violence.[22]

- Sexual violence, especially rape, can result in involuntary pregnancies, particularly when used as a weapon of war in such conflicts as those in Bosnia and Herzegovina and in Rwanda, when women were raped repeatedly until they conceived.[23]

- Data suggest that involuntary pregnancies carry a greater risk than those that are wanted and that women with unwanted pregnancies are less likely to receive early antenatal care or give birth under medical supervision. Such pregnancies may also carry a greater risk of unsafe abortion – a significant cause of maternal death – depression, suicide and adverse family reactions to the pregnancy.[24]

- Violence before or during pregnancy can lead to multiple health risks for the mother and child, including miscarriage, preterm labour and fetal distress. It can also prevent them from seeking medical care. A study from Nicaragua has shown that around 16 per cent of low birthweight in infants was related to physical abuse of a partner during pregnancy.[25]

- There are also reproductive implications of violence against women, including chronic pain, genital bruising and scarring, and unhealthy weight loss.[26]

- The psychological consequences of violence against women can also be devastating: depression, stress and anxiety disorders, post-traumatic stress and suicide.[27]

- Violence against mothers can create difficulties for the care and feeding of newborns. In addition, increasing evidence suggests that infants and young children are also at risk from

Combating violence against women and children is critical to improving maternal and newborn health.

violence, and that deaths from physical violence are underestimated.[28]

Combating violence and abuse against women and girls is a multifaceted process that will require strong action from governments, civil societies, international partners and communities to confront and address both the direct and underlying causes and consequences. Comprehensive mechanisms, covering legislation and its enforcement, research, programmes and budgets, increasing women's voices in the debate and sustaining attention on the issue, will be imperative to reduce violence from its current level.

Participation in family, community, economic, social and political life

Discrimination on the basis of gender can prevent women – the primary caregivers for children in all societies – from fully participating in the critical decisions and actions taken in households and communities that can affect maternal and child health. This issue was examined extensively in *The State of the World's Children 2007: The double dividend of gender equality*, which showed that in a number of countries across sub-Saharan Africa, South Asia and the Middle East and North Africa, more than one third of women surveyed said that their husbands alone made the decisions regarding their health care. A considerable percentage of women surveyed in 30 countries across six regions reported that they were not fully involved in household decision-making.[29]

Enabling women to participate more equally in the critical and routine decision-making processes that affect their lives, and those of their children, is pivotal to creating a supportive environment for maternal and newborn health. When women are able to participate in key decisions, studies have shown that they are more likely to ensure that their children are well nourished and to seek appropriate medical care for themselves and their children.[30]

Enhancing women's ability to participate in household decisions is only

Figure 2.5

Female genital mutilation/cutting, though in decline, is still prevalent in many developing countries

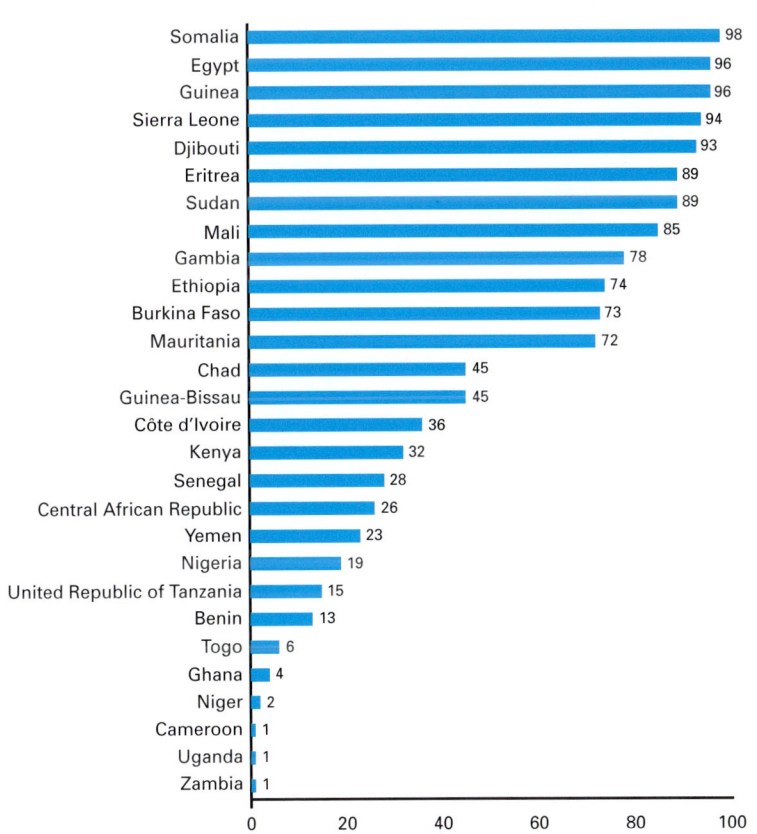

Percentage of girls and women aged 15–49 who have been mutilated/cut, 2002–2007*

* Data refer to the most recent year available during the period specified.

Source: Demographic and Health Surveys, Multiple Indicator Cluster Surveys and other national surveys.

Towards greater equity in health for mothers and newborns

by Cesar G. Victora, Professor of Epidemiology, Universidade Federal de Pelotas, Brazil

The issue of equity in health outcomes, and in access to essential primary-health-care services, is receiving greater attention in the field of maternal, newborn and child health. This focus is increasingly supported by emerging evidence and research on the extent of disparities in health and other development areas. Inequities are defined as systematic differences between population groups that are unfair and avoidable, and generally include disparities related to socio-economic position, gender, ethnic group and place of residence, among other factors.

Having a skilled attendant at delivery – a key intervention for improving maternal and neonatal health and survival – is among the most inequitably distributed health interventions. Figure 2.6 shows the average share of births attended by skilled health personnel, based on results from recent national surveys of low- and middle-income countries. There are marked inequalities between the regions of the world, with Europe and Central Asia showing the highest coverage levels for all income groups, and sub-Saharan Africa and South Asia in particular trailing well behind.

In addition to variations between regions, within each region there are important disparities by socio-economic position – as observed by comparing skilled attendance at delivery across income quintiles. Among the poorest 20 per cent of South Asian mothers, fewer than 10 per cent of births are delivered by a skilled attendant, compared to 56 per cent of births for mothers from the richest income quintile in that region. The other developing regions exhibit similar disparities; even in Europe and Central Asia – where most countries with survey information are former socialist republics – the proportion of deliveries attended by skilled health personnel is significantly lower for the poorest women than for the most affluent.

Other measures of disparity in health-care provision are also pronounced. Urban mothers and children in developing countries tend to have greater access to health care and better health status than their rural counterparts. Socio-economic inequities are similarly marked within urban areas, where health conditions among slum dwellers are particularly adverse. Within countries, state and provincial differentials in maternal and child health are also often wide, as exemplified by the sharp variations in health indicators between Brazil's more prosperous southern states and its more impoverished north-eastern regions.

Poor mothers and children are underserved along the whole continuum of care. Data from several sub-Saharan African countries were used to document the proportion of mothers and children who received a package of four essential interventions: antenatal care, skilled attendance at delivery, postnatal care and childhood immunization. Coverage with all four interventions was two to six times higher – depending on the country – among the richest groups than it was in the poorest groups. This inequitable pattern of health-care

Figure 2.6

Mothers who received skilled attendance at delivery, by wealth quintile and region

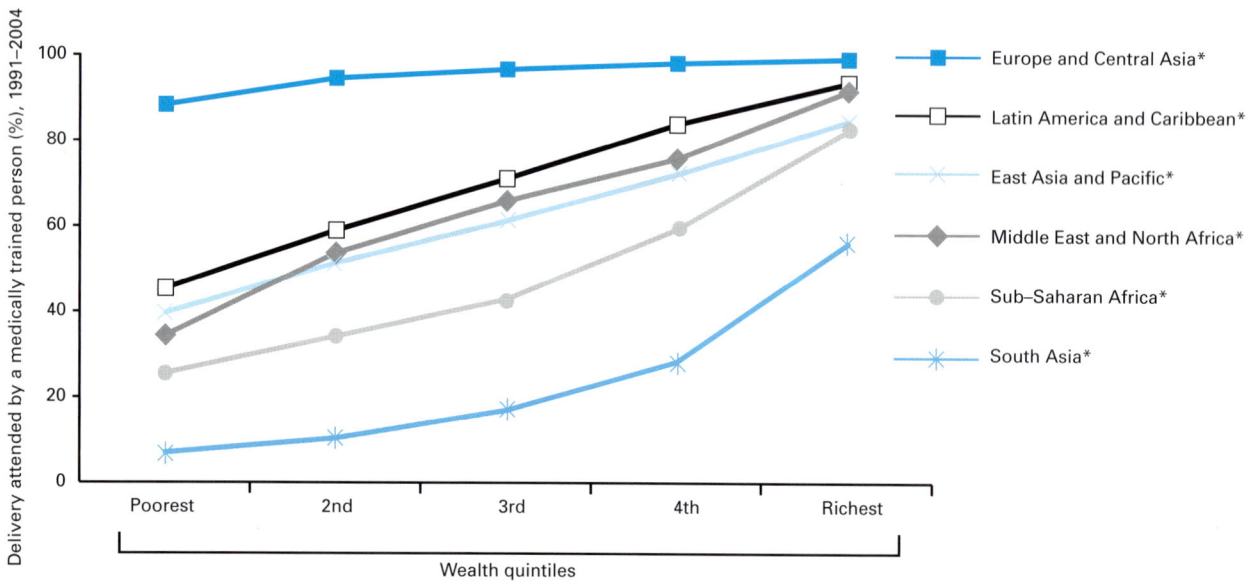

* See References on page 108.

Source: Gwatkin, D. R., et al., *Socio-economic differences in health, nutrition, and population within developing countries: An overview*, Health, Nutrition and Population, World Bank, Washington, D.C., September 2007, pp. 123–124.

provision both reflects and entrenches the social exclusion faced by the poorest and the most marginalized groups and helps explain why maternal, neonatal and child mortality show such marked socio-economic variations.

Health systems have an important role in overcoming these disparities. Examples from across the developing world show that much can be, and is being, done to address and reduce disparities in access to essential services.

- In the *United Republic of Tanzania*, prioritizing interventions to combat diseases that affect poor mothers and children, and allocating district health budgets preferentially to these conditions, led to marked reductions in mortality.

- In *Peru*, the poorest departments (provinces) in the country are earmarked as the first to receive new vaccines; only after high coverage levels are reached in these districts are vaccines rolled out to the rest of the country.

- In *Bangladesh*, the Integrated Management of Childhood Illness (IMCI) strategy was systematically deployed in the poorest areas of the country; a similar strategy is employed by *Brazil's* Family Health Programme.

Because the poor are more likely to live in rural and remote areas, use of appropriate channels for reaching them with essential services should be a primary concern of the health sector. Figure 2.7 shows how implementation of the Accelerated Child Survival and Development (ACSD) strategy has reduced inequities in access to antenatal care in Mali. Whereas both ACSD and control districts showed marked social disparities before the programme was deployed in 2001, five years later access to antenatal care was significantly more equitable in districts with ACSD than in the control areas. The ACSD strategy relied heavily on outreach initiatives aimed at improving access for rural mothers living in remote areas. This finding, however, was not replicated in other ACSD countries where outreach activities were not strongly implemented.

The reduction of inequalities in health is essential for the full achievement of human rights. Gaps in health-care provision contribute to the generation of these inequalities; consequently, health systems also play a role in their elimination. This is particularly true because the greatest gains in maternal, neonatal and child survival depend on effectively reaching the poorest and the most marginalized, who suffer the greatest burden of disease. There are many examples of successful initiatives that, when implemented with sufficient political support and adequate resources, have led to substantial reductions in health inequities. The main challenge for countries and societies is to disseminate these success stories, adopt best practices, and generate and sustain the political will to put equity at the top of the health agenda.

See References, page 108.

Figure 2.7

Women in Mali receiving three or more antenatal care visits, before and after the implementation of the Accelerated Child Survival and Development (ACSD) initiative

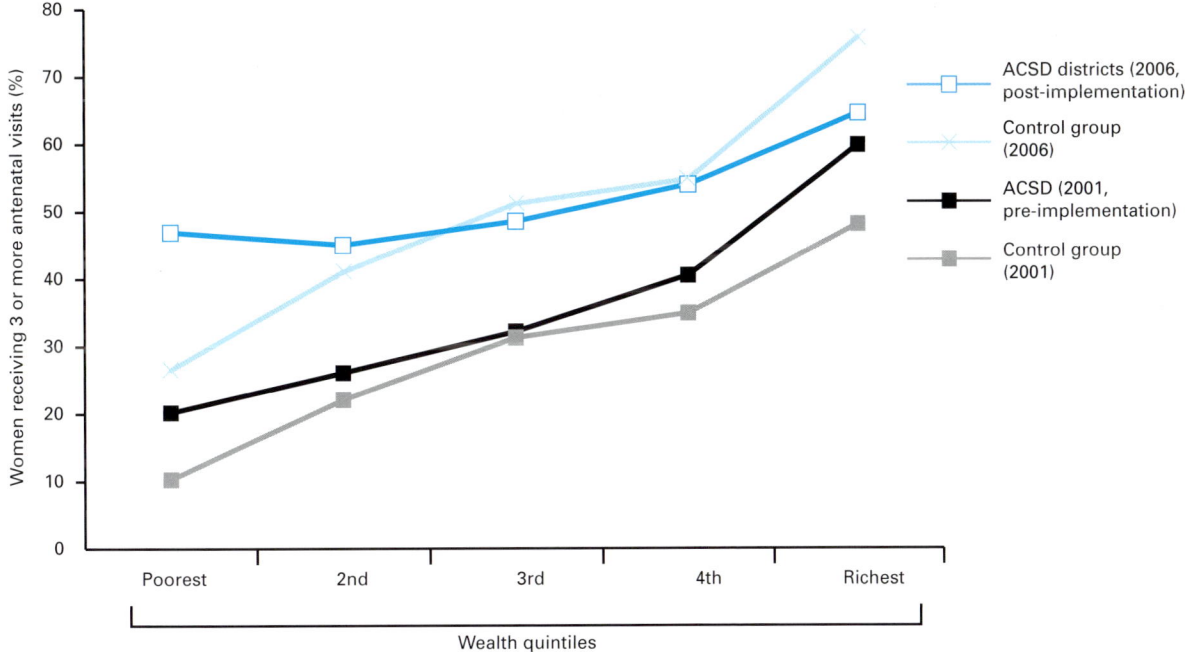

Source: Johns Hopkins University 2008.

Figure 2.8

Many women in developing countries have no say in their own health-care needs

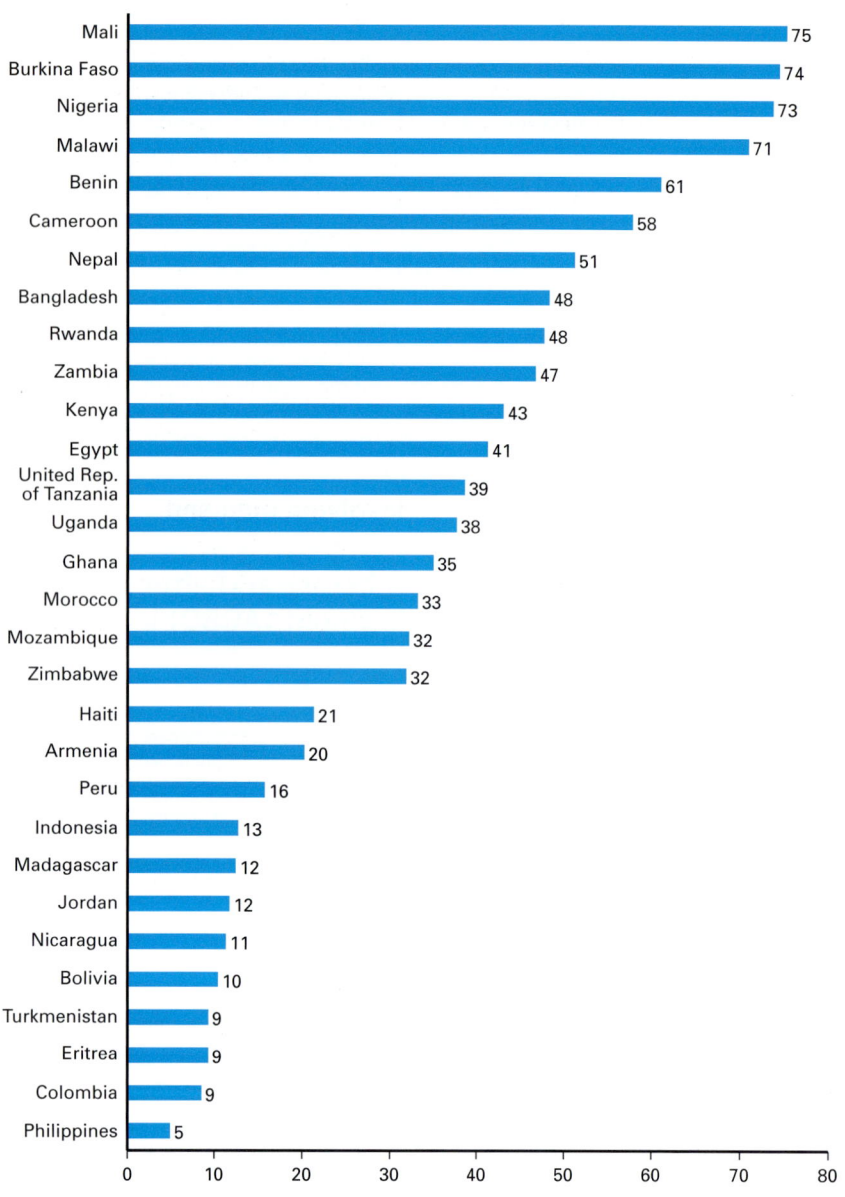

Percentage of women who say their husbands alone made the decisions regarding their health care, 2000–2004*

* Data refer to the most recent year available during the period specified.

Source: UNICEF calculations based on data derived from Demographic and Health Surveys.

part of the solution. Evidence from Demographic and Health Surveys indicates that much of women's decision-making power is exerted at the community level.[31] When women are empowered to participate in their communities, they can challenge the attitudes and practices that entrench gender discrimination, share work, pool resources and collectively devise and sustain initiatives to improve maternal and newborn health. It is the acumen of women acting collectively that is among the strongest reasons why most newborns and mothers survive pregnancy and childbirth.

Increasing women's participation in key decision-making processes in employment and political life is also critical to improving maternal and newborn outcomes. Improving economic status can be vital to enhancing women's participation in decision-making, with attendant implications for the health of their children. When women have greater influence in the management of household decisions, they are more likely than men to ensure that children eat well and receive medical care.[32] Owning assets can also enhance women's influence in household decision-making; a study in rural Bangladesh showed that women who have a greater share of assets than their husbands before their own wedding have a stronger influence on household decision-making.[33]

Despite some progress at increasing their representation in national legisla-

Encouraging women to participate more fully in decision-making is key to creating a supportive environment for mothers and newborns.

tures, women still accounted for less than 19 per cent of parliamentarians worldwide as of May 2008.[34] According to United Cities and Local Governments, an organization that has been publishing data on women in local decision-making since 2003, they are also underrepresented in municipal governments, accounting for just 9 per cent of mayors in 60 countries surveyed and 21 per cent of local councillors in 67 countries surveyed.[35] Given their limited, and relatively recent, engagement in parliamentary politics, the influence of women parliamentarians in determining maternal and newborn health outcomes is still unclear. The evidence suggests, however, that women parliamentarians are likely to strongly support and promote measures to assist women and children – prioritizing initiatives to provide improved child care and strengthen women's rights.[36]

Women's groups can also make a difference at the local level. In 2004, the advocacy by women's rights activists persuaded the Government of Morocco to support a landmark family law countering gender inequality and protecting children's rights. In the same year, women's groups in Mozambique successfully campaigned to raise the legal age of marriage by two years to 16 with parental consent and to 18 without.[37]

Empowering women to participate more fully in household decisions, the economy and political life is key to creating a supportive environment for mothers and newborns. But the benefits of women's participation go well beyond their impact on health outcomes. They enable communities and societies to focus attention on the critical issues that affect two thirds of their citizens – women and children – and to arrive at decisions from a richer base of influences and considerations.

Empowering women and girls

There is a considerable body of evidence testifying to the multiplier effects of investing in gender equality and women's empowerment. Targeted investments in the education, reproductive health, and economic and political rights of women can bring about progress in poverty reduction, sustainable development and peace.

The focus on wider economic and social benefits in international reports is understandable – they are often making a case for investment that competes with other development priorities for limited funds. But it is easy to lose sight of the benefits of women's empowerment in and of itself. Women who are empowered are more able to take control of their own lives, act as change agents in their communities and actively pursue the best interests of their children and families. This may take the form of ensuring that income entering the household is spent on the things that matter most, such as nutritious food, education and health care. It may also mean demanding the services that will afford women the best possible care during pregnancy and delivery and will safeguard the health of their babies.

Cooperation between women at a local level is often a vital encouragement for women's empowerment. Informal women's groups generally gather for a practical purpose, such as organizing a vegetable garden to provide a source of income independent of their husbands – though the sense of solidarity and the problems shared in such groups can add to the sense of empowerment and to the demand for better maternal, neonatal and child health services.

Involving men and adolescent boys in maternal and newborn health and care

Men are often conspicuously absent from reports advocating gender equality – except in so far as they represent the problem. They may appear in the guise of abusers or domestic tyrants, as wasters frittering away precious family income on inessentials or as irresponsible sexual partners taking no responsibility for contraception.

In the field of maternal and newborn health, men are generally missing from the literature. The hundreds of millions of fathers and partners who are actively involved in seeking the best possible maternity care and who take full parental responsibility for their children's well-being could be forgiven for feeling disregarded.

Focus On: Adapting maternity services to the cultures of rural Peru

Peru, a lower-middle-income country where 73 per cent of the population lives in urban areas, has made enormous progress in reducing child deaths from 1 in every 6 children in 1970 to 1 in 50 by 2006. Between 1990 and 2007, the country's under-five mortality rate dropped by 74 per cent – the fastest rate of decline in the entire Latin American and Caribbean region for that period. It has had less success, however, in the area of maternal health. Its maternal mortality ratio, estimated at 240 maternal deaths per 100,000 live births in 2005, is among the highest in the region. Moreover, Peruvian women face a lifetime risk of maternal mortality estimated in 2005 at 1 in 140, twice the regional average of 1 in 280.

The country's relative lack of progress in reducing maternal deaths has resulted in its inclusion on the expanded list of priority countries for the Countdown to 2015 initiative, whose criteria have now been broadened to include maternal mortality thresholds in addition to those for child mortality set out in 2005. According to the Ministry of Health, women in rural areas are twice as likely as those in urban areas to die from causes related to pregnancy. A skilled attendant was present at just 20 per cent of deliveries in rural communities in 2000, compared to 69 per cent in urban areas.

Like other Latin American and Caribbean countries, Peru's challenge for improving maternal and newborn health – and greatest potential for progress – is to address disparities due to ethnicity, geography and extreme poverty. This will require delivering quality services to women and infants in or near their places of residence and providing integrated routine and emergency maternity and newborn care.

Part of the challenge is to adapt current health services, often facility-based or outreach, to the customs of the communities currently underserved by the health system. For example, following tradition and cultural practice, rural women may prefer to give birth at home in an upright position, under the guidance of traditional birth attendants, rather than in a health centre delivery room. Moreover, even if these mothers did decide to seek formal care, distance to a health facility, cost of services, language barriers and other impediments might deter them.

Ensuring that mothers have the option of delivering in their homes, with the assistance of skilled birth attendants and a strong referral system to emergency obstetric care, if it is needed, may be an appropriate way to integrate formal health services with traditional practices. Towards this end, the Ministry of Health, in conjunction with UNICEF Peru, has developed a maternal health project that includes four key strategies:

- Establishing maternal waiting houses to resolve the difficulty posed by geographic distance from health services.

- Fostering family and community support to make maternity and the mother's condition a priority.

- Increasing access to the Integral Health Service, which covers the cost of antenatal, intrapartum and post-partum care for poor families.

- Adapting maternity services to eliminate barriers between the staff at health facilities and mothers who have deeply rooted cultural traditions for childbirth.

The maternal waiting houses, dubbed 'Mamawasi', are constructed to encourage women in rural areas to choose the option of giving birth in health centres instead of at home. Currently, there are almost 400 houses located on grounds belonging to health centres or hospitals; others are in rented buildings in the regions of Apurímac, Ayacucho and Cuzco. Pregnant women from near and distant communities can stay in the waiting rooms until they deliver. Women from remote villages may stay for weeks or months. The Mamawasi is designed to resemble a typical indigenous family home in a farming village. Expectant mothers are allowed to bring family members with them to the houses, which increases their confidence and comfort level in using the service.

Health centres have also changed their practices. For instance, the vertical birth position is accommodated, a family member or traditional midwife is allowed to accompany women during birth, and the centres are kept at a warmer temperature.

This programme has transformed everyday health services by promoting cultural sensitivity in health care. Huancarani district, located in the Andean province of Paucartambo, in the Cuzco region, has been the most successful in implementing the new strategy. Overall, almost 3 out of every 4 pregnant women now visit health-care centres in the regions served, especially for childbirth, whereas previously the ratio was 1 in 4. The programme has been integrated into district and provincial health policies and was adopted in 2004 by the Ministry of Health as a national standard to be implemented throughout the country. The Ministry of Health has also created training modules to teach health personnel how to make services culturally appropriate.

See References, page 108.

Focus On: Southern Sudan: After the peace, a new battle against maternal mortality

After 21 years of conflict, civil war between the north and south of the Sudan came to an end in 2005. While the fighting has mostly ceased, Southern Sudan is facing another struggle – against maternal and neonatal mortality. According to the 2006 Sudan Household Health Survey, the maternal mortality ratio for Western Equatoria, a province in Southern Sudan, stood at 2,327 deaths per 100,000 live births, one of the highest in the world. The 2006 neonatal mortality rate was 51 deaths per 1,000 live births, significantly above the Sudan's national ratio of 41 per 1,000 live births.

Overall health-care coverage, mostly managed through a small number of non-governmental organizations, is estimated at just 25 per cent. Even when health care is available, maternal health services are limited and not often used. Part of the reason may be a lack of education. The United Nations Population Fund (UNFPA) estimates that in 2006 the literacy rate for Southern Sudanese women was just 12 per cent, compared to 37 per cent for men; women therefore have limited access to health information.

Another possible reason is that pregnant women must travel long distances on foot to reach antenatal centres; consequently, attendance rates vary sharply depending on location, from 17.4 per cent in Unity State in 2006 to nearly 80 per cent in Western Equatoria. Fewer than 15 per cent of births in Southern Sudan are attended by skilled health personnel, and 80 per cent take place at home under the supervision of relatives, traditional birth attendants or village midwives (a female birth attendant who has typically received around nine months of training). Yet most of the causes of maternal death – including prolonged obstructed labour, haemorrhage, sepsis and eclampsia – could be managed by better-trained attendants.

The quality of available antenatal and delivery services is low due to a lack of technically skilled service providers. In all 10 states of Southern Sudan, midwives, traditional birth attendants and other maternal and neonatal care providers lack the necessary training required to perform simple lifesaving or nursing procedures. Lack of equipment and supplies, poor referral systems and inadequate physical infrastructure and transportation also impede health-care delivery. Post-natal care services are virtually non-existent, despite the fact that most of the maternal and newborn deaths in Southern Sudan occur during the post-natal period.

Against this background, the Government of Southern Sudan and its partners are making efforts to strengthen maternal health services. The Interim Health Policy for 2006–2011 outlines an integrated approach that recognizes the need to improve health services while protecting women's rights. The Ministry of Health has committed to establishing more primary, reproductive and maternal health facilities, while supporting the use of mass media and counselling services to disseminate information on nutrition, harmful traditional practices and sexual health. To meet immediate health-care needs, community midwives who hold basic qualifications are being 'fast-tracked', with support from UNFPA. In June 2006, the first fistula repair centre in Southern Sudan was established at the Juba Teaching Hospital.

To accelerate implementation of this strategy, the Government has already established a Reproductive Health Directorate and is recruiting state coordinators to facilitate, monitor and coordinate maternal and neonatal health activities in each state. UNICEF is supporting the expansion of antenatal and emergency obstetric services in several states and the dissemination of key health messages over the radio and through community outreach.

There are challenges ahead. The return of refugees and the movements of many displaced populations, Southern Sudan's high fertility rate (6.7) and increasing rates of HIV infection among some populations necessitate a systematic health programme. The struggle may be a long one, but those committed to winning it are already at work.

See References, page 108.

The other side of the coin is that in removing men from the picture, they may somehow be let off the hook, validated in their lack of responsibility for this most essential aspect of family life.

The birth of a child, particularly a first child, is often a landmark moment in a man's life. It can crystallize his sense of himself as a caring, responsible human being on whom other people depend. More generally, involving men in the care of their pregnant partners and newborn children can be a significant opportunity to establish a positive, supportive relationship that will last a lifetime.

Evidence has shown that men are more likely to be engaged, participatory fathers when they feel positive about themselves and their relationships, and when families and friends support their involvement in their children's lives. A man who shares the responsibility for parenthood is also more likely to share the household decision-making with his female partner, thereby contributing to her own empowerment.[38]

Programmes that encourage the participation of both men and women can help this process by increasing communication between the sexes and encouraging a more equal division of childcare duties. In addition, workplaces need to recognize the role played by both parents in child rearing, so that men as well as women are encouraged to reconcile their work and family responsibilities.

Linking the supportive environment to the continuum of care

Creating a supportive environment for maternal and neonatal health will provide a strong foundation for upscaling essential interventions within a dynamic continuum of care, which is the focus of Chapter 3.

THE STATE OF THE WORLD'S CHILDREN 2009

3 The continuum of care across time and location: Risks and opportunities

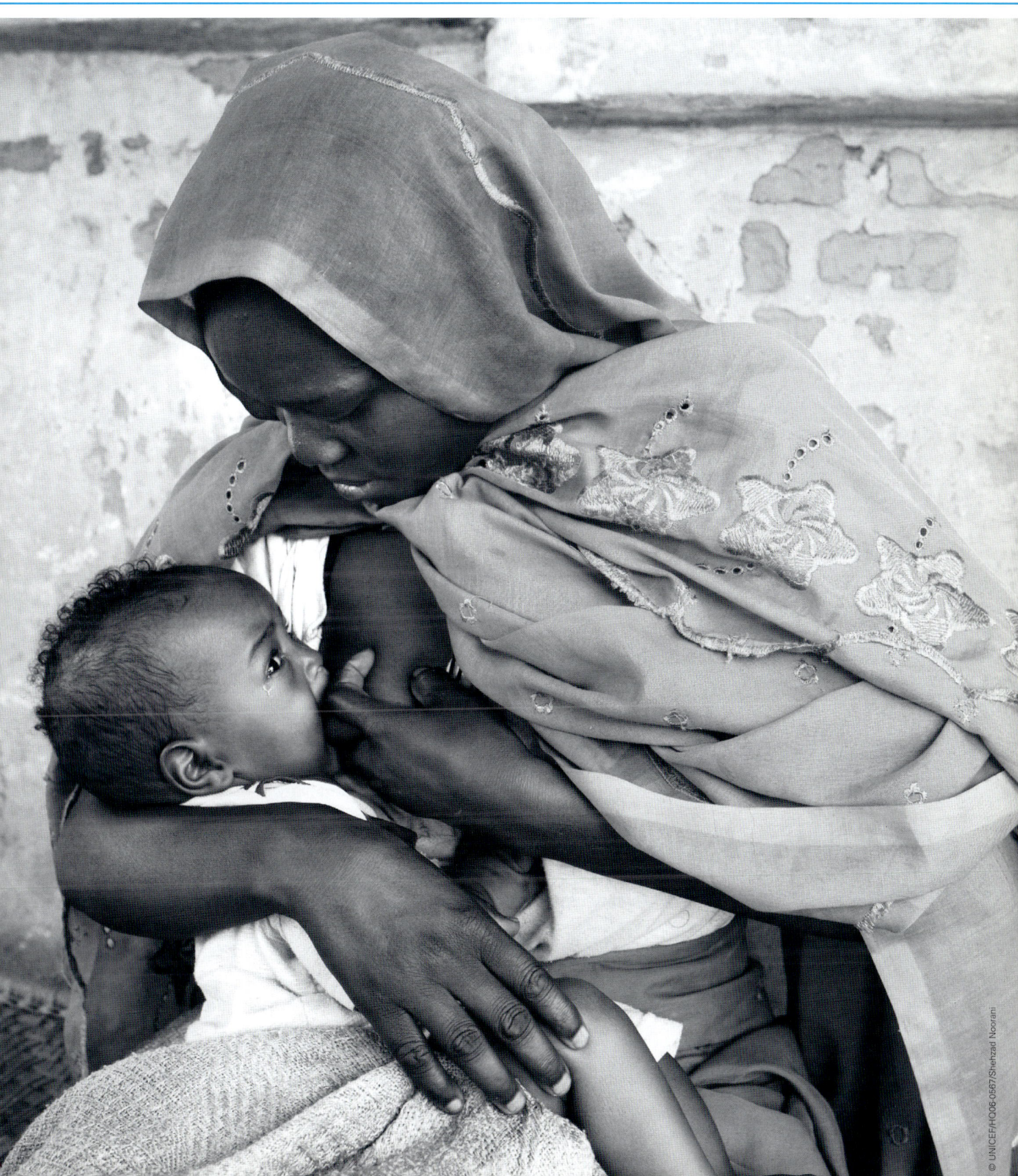

An effective continuum of care delivers essential services for mothers and children at critical points in adolescence, pre-pregnancy, pregnancy, birth, post-natal and neonatal periods and at key locations of the household and community, through outreach/outpatient interventions and in health facilities where they can be readily accessed by women and children. Community partnerships in health are essential components of a continuum of care. Perhaps most vital to reducing maternal and newborn mortality, however, are quality antenatal care, skilled health personnel attending deliveries and post-natal care for mothers and newborns. Ensuring that emergency obstetric and newborn care is available to address birth complications could save many lives currently lost during childbirth and the early neonatal period. The third chapter of The State of the World's Children 2009 *examines the key services underpinning the continuum of care and how these interventions can be expanded and improved.*

The continuum of care: Delivering services at critical points

At every stage of life, from childbirth to old age, there are pressing health demands. The services that aim to respond to the interrelated health needs of mothers and newborns require high levels of continuity and integration – characteristics that have not always been evident in national and international health policies, programmes and partnerships seeking to improve maternal and newborn health.

The continuum of care framework aims to transcend the traditional emphasis on single, disease-specific interventions. It advocates a model of primary health care that embraces every stage of maternal, newborn and child health. The success of this framework, however, depends on delivering essential services and implementing improved practices at key points in the life cycle, linking mothers, newborns and their households and communities with quality basic health care and maternity services.[1]

Chapter 3 outlines the essential services required to support a continuum of maternal and neonatal care, including enhanced nutrition; safe water, sanitation and hygiene facilities and practices; disease prevention and treatment; quality reproductive health services; adequate antenatal care; skilled assistance at delivery; basic and comprehensive emergency obstetric and newborn care; post-natal care; neonatal care; and Integrated Management of Neonatal and Childhood Illness.

This chapter also briefly examines the points of delivery for health services: at the household and community level, outreach and outpatient services, and facility-based care.

Quality reproductive health services

While targets for reproductive health were not initially included in the Millennium Development Goals (MDGs), at the World Summit in September 2005 the decision was taken to achieve universal access to reproductive health by 2015.

Subsequently, a new MDG framework was adopted and the revised goals of January 2008 include a reproductive health target (*see Panel, page 24, for details of the new target and indicators*).

The new target reflects, in part, a growing consensus on the need to improve reproductive health. Another goal is to curb the growing incidence of reproductive tract and sexually transmitted infections, including HIV. The World Health Organization (WHO) has identified unsafe sex as the second most important risk factor for death and disability in the poorest countries and the ninth most important in developed countries.[2] Almost half of all new HIV infections occur in young people, particularly women, with around double the number of women as men infected with HIV in sub-Saharan Africa.[3]

Building reproductive health capacity at the national level will necessitate identifying problems, setting priorities and formulating strategies with the participation of all stake-

Adequate nutrition for women, including increased food intake and micronutrient supplementation, is critical to the health and survival of mothers and newborns.

holders. WHO has identified five key priorities for action on reproductive health-care services. These include strengthening health systems capacity; improving information for setting priorities; mobilizing political will; creating supportive legislative and regulatory frameworks; and strengthening monitoring, evaluation and accountability.[4]

Enhancing nutrition for mothers and newborns

Adequate nutrition for adolescent girls and pregnant women is critical for the health and survival prospects of both mothers and newborns. The undernutrition of young mothers increases the health risks for both them and their babies. A low body mass index (less than 18.5 kg/m²) for pregnant women increases the risk of both maternal and neonatal mortality; the same applies if a mother is stunted. Low body mass can restrict the growth of the fetus, which is a risk factor for neonatal conditions such as low birthweight.[5]

Programmes targeted towards improving maternal health are increasingly focusing on enhancing the nutrition of girls and women across the life cycle. Along with increased food intake, folic acid and iron supplementation are being encouraged during pre-pregnancy and pregnancy, and vitamin A supplementation during the postpartum period. In addition, dietary diversification, the use of iodized salt and deworming are key interventions to strengthen the nutritional status of pregnant women and mothers.

Folic acid supplementation to prevent neural tube defects has proved successful, and in general, antenatal programmes should also offer other micronutrients, such as zinc. There are proven links between zinc deficiency and stunting, diarrhoea and malaria.[6]

Gaining the confidence of pregnant women through such programmes of micronutrient supplementation can be a useful way to encourage their continued attendance for other forms of professional antenatal care. Increased use of clinics and hospitals will also help in collecting data on the health of pregnant women and mothers, which is

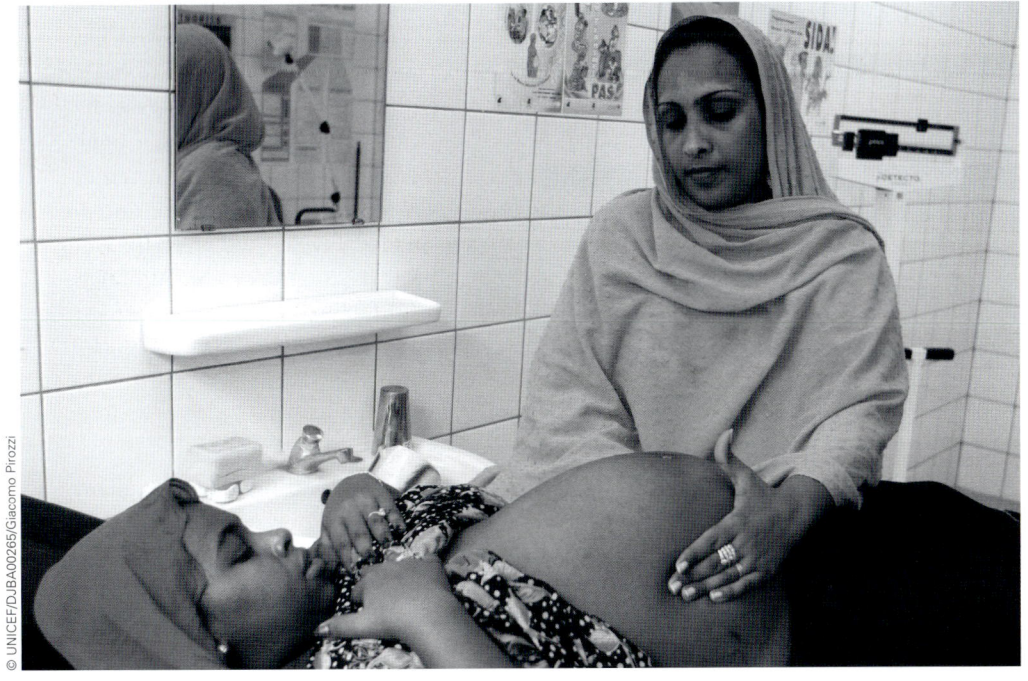

More skilled health workers are needed to provide vital services to women at critical points during pregnancy. *A pregnant woman lies on a table as a nurse performs an antenatal consultation at the Engueila Health Centre, Djibouti.*

Reducing the incidence of infectious conditions and preventing and treating HIV and malaria are vital to improving maternal and newborn health.

particularly scarce in the least developed regions and poorest countries and communities.

Addressing infectious diseases, HIV and malaria

As Chapter 1 underscored, severe infections are among the leading direct causes of maternal and neonatal deaths. They accounted for roughly 36 per cent of neonatal deaths in 2000, the latest year for which firm estimates of cause of death are available. Reducing the incidence of infectious conditions such as sepsis/pneumonia, tetanus and sexually transmitted infections, and preventing and treating HIV and malaria, are therefore critical to improving maternal and newborn health (see Panel on Eliminating maternal and neonatal tetanus, page 49).

Preventing HIV infection in women of childbearing age and treating infected pregnant women with available drug combinations can greatly reduce the transmission of the virus to children. Raising levels of comprehensive knowledge of HIV among young women and men aged 15–24 is vital to averting infection. In 14 of the 17 countries with sufficient data, HIV prevalence rates among pregnant women aged 15–24 have declined since 2000/2001.[7] This positive development is encouraging, but much more needs to be done to boost HIV prevention activities and to address the social, economic and political drivers of the AIDS epidemic.

In line with the new MDG focus on reproductive health, programmes aimed at improving maternal survival should include interventions to help reduce the incidence of, and treat, sexually transmitted infections.

The distribution of insecticide-treated mosquito nets to pregnant women in malaria-endemic areas can reduce the incidence of malaria infection, improving the health of both the pregnant woman and her unborn child. Intermittent preventive treatment of malaria during pregnancy is being used to both prevent and treat the disease. It consists of administering a single dose of a combined antimalarial medicine at least twice during pregnancy whether the pregnant woman has the disease or not. Although considered efficacious, coverage of this treatment remains limited in malaria-endemic areas.[8]

Expanding antenatal care

Much ill health among pregnant women is preventable, detectable or treatable through antenatal visits. Antenatal care provides an opportunity to reach pregnant women with multiple interventions that could be

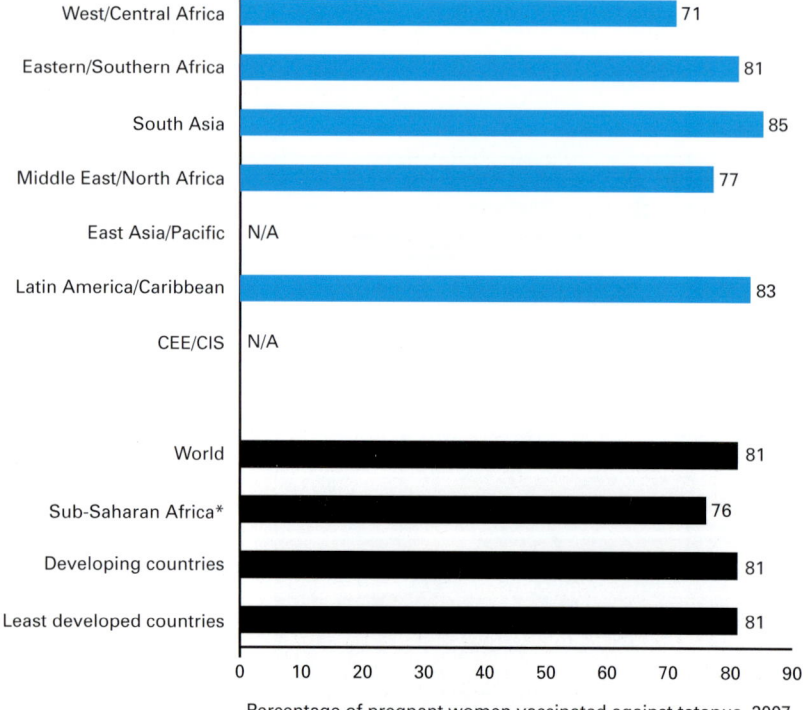

Figure 3.1

Protection against neonatal tetanus

Percentage of pregnant women vaccinated against tetanus, 2007

* Sub-Saharan Africa comprises the regions of Eastern/Southern Africa and West/Central Africa.

Source: UNICEF and the World Health Organization.

Eliminating maternal and neonatal tetanus

Tetanus remains a significant cause of maternal and neonatal deaths, taking the lives of more than 180,000 newborns and between 15,000 and 30,000 mothers in 2002. The condition develops when a bacterium, *Clostridium tetani*, infects a cut or wound. Unclean delivery or abortion practices can result in maternal tetanus, while neonatal tetanus is caused by the unhygienic care of the umbilical cord or umbilical stump in babies. In the absence of intensive hospital care, neonatal tetanus is nearly always fatal. As with other causes of maternal and neonatal deaths, most of the fatalities from tetanus take place in sub-Saharan Africa and Asia, especially in poor and marginalized communities where women have limited or no access to quality health care and little knowledge of safe delivery practices.

Tetanus is readily preventable through the vaccination of adult women and through hygienic delivery practices. Increasing implementation of both measures, particularly immunization of pregnant women, has significantly reduced the number of cases and deaths from maternal and neonatal tetanus since 1980, the earliest year for which comprehensive data are available. In 1988, tetanus was responsible for causing around 800,000 neonatal deaths, and more than 90 countries reported one or more cases of neonatal tetanus per 1,000 live births at the district level. By mid-2008, the number of countries reporting one or more cases of maternal and neonatal tetanus at the district level had dropped to 46.

Immunization has been among the most significant counteractions against maternal and neonatal tetanus. Tetanus toxoid has proved efficacious against the disease, with two doses providing protective concentrations of antitoxins in the majority of cases, and almost 100 per cent immunity after the third dose. The global rate of vaccination against neonatal tetanus for pregnant women has risen sharply since 1980, when it stood at just 9 per cent, to 81 per cent in 2007. Nonetheless, this still leaves almost 1 in every 5 newborns without protection. In part, this is due to missed opportunities for vaccinating pregnant women who visit facilities to receive antenatal services, to women arriving too late for immunization, or to the failure to provide post-partum immunization to protect future pregnancies.

Those at risk of tetanus live in communities that have little access to health and immunization services. To reach them, an innovative solution – dubbed the 'high-risk approach' – was initiated. This approach aims to immunize all women of childbearing age living in areas deemed to be high risk with at least two doses of tetanus toxoid (TT) vaccine. The risk factors for tetanus, which include unhygienic delivery practices and lack of immunization, are explained to the communities. Improvements in delivery practices are promoted, and surveillance for neonatal tetanus is strengthened. Booster shots are provided to women with no recorded history of receiving tetanus toxoid vaccine when they were children.

The high-risk approach has been widely adopted, enabling 64 million women to receive at least two doses of tetanus toxoid between 1999 and 2005. The results have been impressive at the country level:

- In *Nepal*, before immunization started in the early 1980s, surveys showed high rates of neonatal tetanus among newborns. After the introduction of immunization of adult women and the implementation of the high-risk approach, the rate had fallen by 2005 to less than 1 death from neonatal tetanus per 1,000 live births in every district.

- A survey conducted in *Egypt* in 1986 indicated that for every 1,000 children born, 7 would die of neonatal tetanus, with rates of 10 per 1,000 live births in rural areas. Following implementation of the high-risk approach, by 2007, the rate was brought down to less than 1 death per 1,000 live births in all districts.

- In the mid-1980s, *Bangladesh* had a high rate of neonatal tetanus, which stood at 20–40 cases for every 1,000 live births in some parts of the country. At that time, only 5 per cent of women of childbearing age were immunized with tetanus toxoid and only 5 per cent of pregnant women were able to have a clean delivery. Adoption of the high-risk approach helped Bangladesh reduce its mortality from neonatal tetanus to less than 1 death per 1,000 live births by 2008.

Some places have used the high-risk approach to deliver other interventions alongside tetanus toxoid vaccine, including measles vaccine (e.g., Kenya, Southern Sudan) and vitamin A (e.g., Democratic Republic of the Congo). Others, such as Ethiopia, Uganda and Zambia, have incorporated the approach in mechanisms for delivering packages of essential interventions. A key benefit of the high-risk approach is that, in addition to reducing neonatal tetanus, it diminishes inequities in access to maternal and neonatal health care within countries and shows that it is possible to deliver health interventions to populations that have often been forgotten or omitted.

See References, page 109.

Antenatal care provides an opportunity to reach pregnant women with multiple interventions, such as immunization, micronutrient supplementation and improved hygiene practices.

vital to their well-being and that of their babies. Nutritional supplements for protein, folic acid and iron provided by skilled health workers or community health workers can have beneficial effects, reducing the likelihood of undernutrition and anaemia in the mother and low birthweight in the newborn.

The minimum number of antenatal care visits during pregnancy recommended by UNICEF and WHO is four. These visits help provide key services to pregnant women, including measures to detect and treat malaria and anaemia; tetanus immunization; management of sexually transmitted infections and antiretroviral therapy for HIV-positive pregnant women; and provision of vital information to pregnant women on risks in pregnancy and delivery. Owing to data limitations, and the fact that many countries are delivering far below the UN interagency minimum recommendation, most of the data relate to women who have received at least one antenatal visit.[9]

In the developing world as a whole, three quarters of pregnant women receive antenatal care from a skilled health provider at least once, though the household surveys that record this data give no indication of the quality of the care or the information conveyed.

In three regions – Latin America and the Caribbean, Central and Eastern Europe and the Commonwealth of Independent States, and East Asia and the Pacific – around 9 out of every 10 pregnant women receive antenatal visits one or more times. These percentages are far lower in the Middle East and North Africa, sub-Saharan Africa (both 72 per cent) and South Asia (68 per cent).

Even at the relatively low coverage rates in these regions, however, antenatal care represents a significant opportunity to reach a large proportion of pregnant women with essential interventions.[10]

Packaging essential interventions, including those for which there is already a strong interest — such as insecticide-treated mosquito nets — has the potential to strengthen demand for, and use of, antenatal services. It may also encourage women to attend clinics and outreach events for antenatal care earlier in their pregnancies.

Ensuring skilled attendance at delivery

Childbirth can be a time of risk not only for the baby but also for the

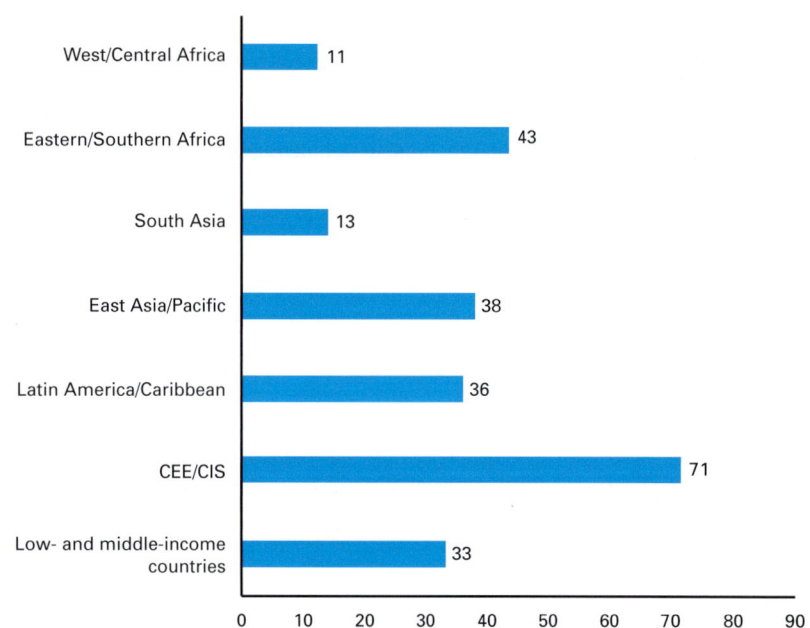

Figure 3.2

Antiretroviral prophylaxis for HIV-positive mothers to prevent mother-to-child transmission of HIV

Region	%
West/Central Africa	11
Eastern/Southern Africa	43
South Asia	13
East Asia/Pacific	38
Latin America/Caribbean	36
CEE/CIS	71
Low- and middle-income countries	33

Estimated percentage of HIV-positive pregnant women who received antiretrovirals for prevention of mother-to-child transmission of HIV, 2007

Source: UNICEF, UNAIDS and WHO, *Towards Universal Access: Scaling up HIV services for women and children in the health sector – Progress Report 2008*, UNICEF, New York, 2008, p.43.

In the least developed countries, 1 in 3 women do not receive any antenatal care during pregnancy, and 3 in 5 women deliver their babies without the assistance of a skilled health worker.

Figure 3.3

Antenatal care coverage

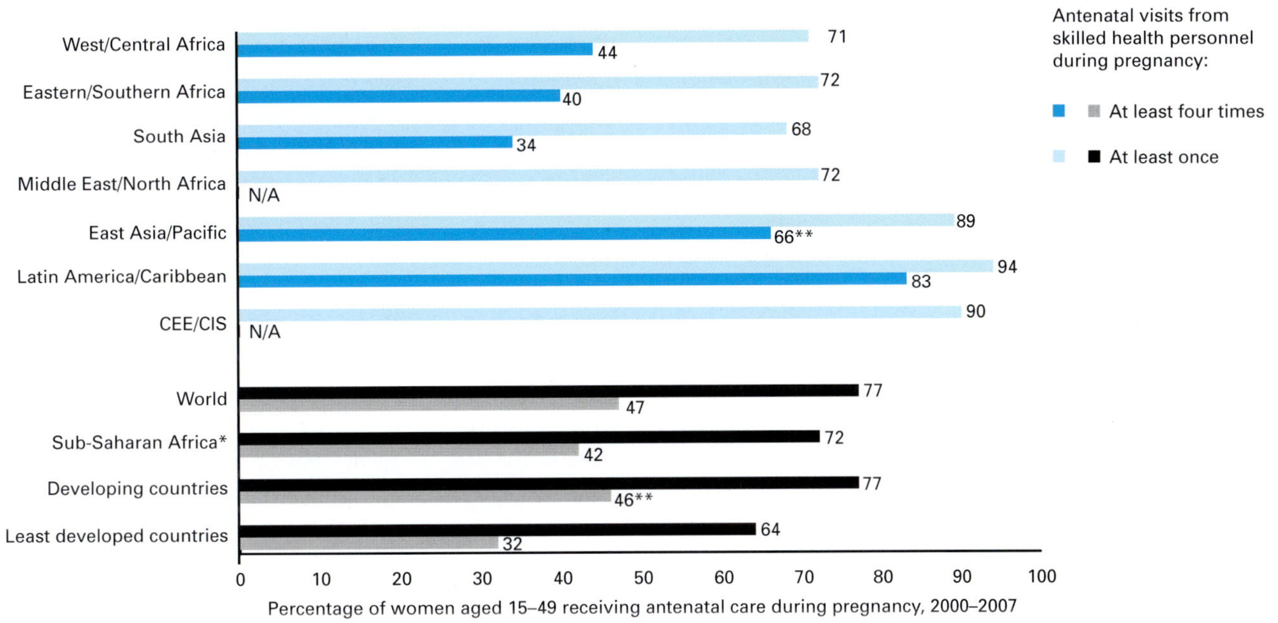

Antenatal visits from skilled health personnel during pregnancy:
- At least four times
- At least once

Region	At least four times	At least once
West/Central Africa	44	71
Eastern/Southern Africa	40	72
South Asia	34	68
Middle East/North Africa	N/A	72
East Asia/Pacific	66**	89
Latin America/Caribbean	83	94
CEE/CIS	N/A	90
World	47	77
Sub-Saharan Africa*	42	72
Developing countries	46**	77
Least developed countries	32	64

Percentage of women aged 15–49 receiving antenatal care during pregnancy, 2000–2007

* Sub-Saharan Africa comprises the regions of Eastern/Southern Africa and West/Central Africa. ** Excludes China.

Source: Demographic and Health Surveys, Multiple Indicator Cluster Surveys and other national household surveys.

mother. Three quarters of all maternal deaths occur from complications either during delivery or in the immediate post-partum period. These complications include: haemorrhage (25 per cent of maternal deaths); infections (15 per cent); complications of abortion (13 per cent); eclampsia or related hypertensive disorders (12 per cent); and obstructed labour (8 per cent).[11]

Reducing maternal deaths from birth complications is possible through increasing the number of births attended by a skilled health worker – a doctor, nurse or trained midwife. Trained health personnel should not only be able to assist with a normal delivery or a delivery with moderate complications, they should also recognize when serious complications arise that require more specialized emergency care. Even skilled health workers, however, require access to essential drugs, supplies and equipment to provide adequate care – particularly when complications such as haemorrhage, sepsis and obstructed labour occur. They also require the skills and judgement to recognize serious complications and to manage an effective referral.

There has been a marked increase in the number of deliveries attended by skilled personnel across the developing world over the last decade, with the notable exception of sub-Saharan Africa. In the 2000–2007 period, skilled health workers attended 61 per cent of the total number of births in the developing world. The improvement has been particularly striking in the Middle East and North Africa, which increased its coverage from 55 per cent in 1995 to 81 per cent in 2000–2007. The two regions with the lowest levels of skilled birth attendance – sub-Saharan Africa (45 per cent) and South Asia (41 per cent) – are also the regions with the highest incidence of maternal mortality.[12]

A quarter of the world's unattended deliveries take place in India, which is also one of the 10 countries that together account for two thirds of births not attended by skilled health workers. India is currently seeking to address the problem by encourging facility-based care with financial incentives[13] (*see Panel on Integrating maternal and newborn health care in India, page 84*).

Worldwide, births in urban areas are twice as likely to be attended by skilled health personnel as those in rural areas. In West and Central Africa, where the disparity is greatest, they are two and a half times as likely. Disparities along economic lines are also notable; for the developing world as a whole, deliveries of women from the poorest households are around half as likely to be attended by skilled health workers as those from the richest households.[14] (*For a fuller discussion of disparities in access to maternity services, see Panel on page 38, Towards greater equity in health for mothers and newborns.*)

WHO has made several recommendations for reducing post-partum bleeding or haemorrhage, a leading cause of maternal death. The most common causes of post-partum bleeding are failure of the uterus to contract sufficiently, tears of the genital tract and retention of the placental tissue. The most widely accepted method of intervention is active management of the third stage of labour, which follows the completed delivery of the newborn child and lasts until the completed delivery of the placenta. Active management involves administering a uterotonic to facilitate contractions for delivery of the placenta and delayed clamping, cutting and traction of the umbilical cord.

WHO recommends active management by skilled attendants for all mothers but does not recommend the package for unskilled attendants. The agency has called for further research on optimal times for cord clamping and what drugs, if any, non-skilled attendants should administer.

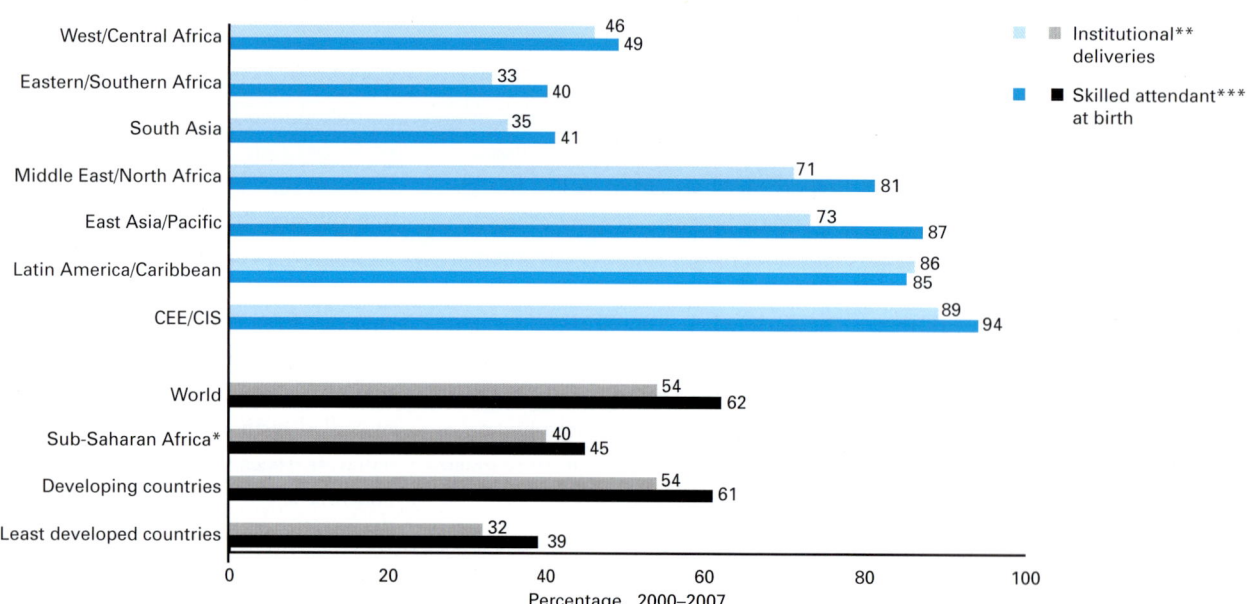

Figure 3.4

Delivery care coverage

Region	Institutional** deliveries	Skilled attendant*** at birth
West/Central Africa	46	49
Eastern/Southern Africa	33	40
South Asia	35	41
Middle East/North Africa	71	81
East Asia/Pacific	73	87
Latin America/Caribbean	86	85
CEE/CIS	89	94
World	54	62
Sub-Saharan Africa*	40	45
Developing countries	54	61
Least developed countries	32	39

Percentage, 2000–2007

* Sub-Saharan Africa comprises the regions of Eastern/Southern Africa and West/Central Africa.
** *Institutional deliveries* refers to the proportion of women aged 15–49 years who gave birth in the two years preceding the survey and delivered in a health facility.
*** *Skilled attendant at birth* refers to the percentage of births attended by skilled health personnel (doctors, nurses and midwives).
Source: Demographic and Health Surveys, Multiple Indicator Cluster Surveys, World Health Organization and UNICEF.

Addressing disparities will be critical to improving maternal health. Women from the poorest quintile of households are only half as likely to be attended by skilled health workers as those from the richest households.

Hypertensive disorders: Common yet complex

Hypertensive disorders are the most common medical problems in pregnancy and account for a significant proportion – between 12 and 20 per cent – of maternal deaths worldwide. They affect women in every region, causing nearly 10 per cent of maternal deaths in Africa and Asia, over 16 per cent in industrialized countries, and more than one quarter in Latin America and the Caribbean. Hypertension in pregnancy can result in a range of conditions, from elevated blood pressure, the least severe, to cerebral haemorrhage, which is fatal. It can result in fetal death, preterm delivery and low birthweight in newborns.

The causes of hypertension are still not fully understood, but research suggests that obesity, high salt intake and genetic predisposition are factors. Some forms of hypertension in pregnancy may arise from the biology of pregnancy itself. Pre-eclampsia, which develops after the first 20 weeks of pregnancy, is defined as pregnancy-induced hypertension accompanied by excess protein in the urine, and brings the greatest risk to maternal and fetal health, particularly when it accompanies chronic hypertension. It is a leading cause of premature births.

Several risk factors predispose mothers to these disorders, including first pregnancy, multiple pregnancy, history of chronic hypertension, maternal age over 35, gestational diabetes, obesity and fetal malformation. One study showed that intervals of 59 months or longer between pregnancies were also associated with higher rates of pre-eclampsia and eclampsia. Researchers have also proposed that hormonal imbalances, calcium deficiency and insulin resistance are possible causes.

Calcium supplementation has been shown to be an effective intervention in developing countries where pregnant women may be calcium deficient, reducing the incidence of pre-eclampsia by 48 per cent. If this intervention has a similar effect on maternal deaths from hypertensive disorders, calcium supplementation could prevent some 21,500 maternal deaths. The Magpie Trial, the largest trial for hypertensive disorders of pregnancy, conducted in 1998–2002 in both industrialized and developing countries, and follow-up studies have produced strong evidence that magnesium sulfate given to women in the pre-eclampsia stage can reduce their risk of progression to eclampsia. Subsequent studies have strengthened the evidence base for this critical and cost-effective intervention.

Ideally, care should begin before conception, so that a reproductive woman's medical history can be tracked and her options for managing chronic hypertension known. Hypertensive women also need information about their risks in pregnancy and changes in their lifestyle that illness may require. Bed rest is a common recommendation for hypertensive pregnant women. Regular examinations by skilled health personnel are required to monitor the onset and development of pre-eclampsia and other hypertensive conditions.

Hypertension in pregnancy has long been understood as an obstetric condition, with interventions focusing mostly on outcomes for the pregnancy and less on long- and short-term effects on the mother. New research has shown, however, that hypertension in pregnancy can also affect the post-natal health of a mother, increasing her risks of developing chronic hypertension and cardiovascular disease. With high maternal mortality and morbidity resulting from these disorders, further research is warranted. Treatment or management of these conditions will have great significance for the continuum of care model of maternal and newborn health care.

See References, page 109.

Providing emergency obstetric and newborn care, and making post-natal care available, are key challenges and opportunities for enhancing maternal and newborn health.

Other risks from childbirth can also be addressed with skilled care. The World Health Organization recommends that a woman with eclampsia or pre-eclampsia be hospitalized in the days leading up to delivery to receive treatment with magnesium sulphate. Most infections are treatable with antibiotics. Some infections, such as tetanus, can easily be avoided through immunization programmes and sterile umbilical cord practices[15] (*see Panel on page 49, Eliminating maternal and neonatal tetanus*).

Providing emergency obstetric and newborn care

Timely care in a medical facility is often necessary to save the life of a woman experiencing birth complications. The quality of care delivered by the facility is critical: To provide adequate assistance it must have adequate medicines, supplies, equipment and personnel. In addition, it should be able to perform potentially life-saving functions such as Caesarean sections, blood transfusions and newborn resuscitation.

Data on emergency obstetric care in developing countries are often scarce. Studies have shown that around 15 per cent of live births are likely to need emergency obstetric care, and Caesarean sections may be required in 5–15 per cent of births. It is evident that there are many important gaps in coverage, especially in rural areas of sub-Saharan Africa, where rates of Caesarean section are around 2 per cent.[16]

Factors hindering the provision of emergency obstetric care include distance, direct user charges, transportation and accomodation costs, knowledge and cultural barriers, among others. Furthermore, the quality of care offered may also prove a deterrent, as shown in a study in northern United Republic of Tanzania, which indicated that the poor quality of care in facilities was the main barrier to access.[17]

Making post-natal care available

There is a clear need for far greater emphasis on post-natal care – an intervention that has long been neglected in many developing countries, and one that represents a gap in the continuum of care. An urgent need is for care in the immediate post-partum period, as evidence indicates that the risks of maternal mortality and morbidity are high in the 48 hours immediately following birth. Post-natal care is often critical for newborns, particularly immediately after birth. Around three quarters of neonatal deaths take place in the first week, with up to half of these occurring within 24 hours of birth.

In many developing countries, mothers are likely to be discharged from a health facility within 24 hours of giving birth or may lack access to skilled professional care. Evidence shows that even once the high-risk period is over, the risks of maternal mortality and morbidity continue for at least 42 days after birth, and can even extend

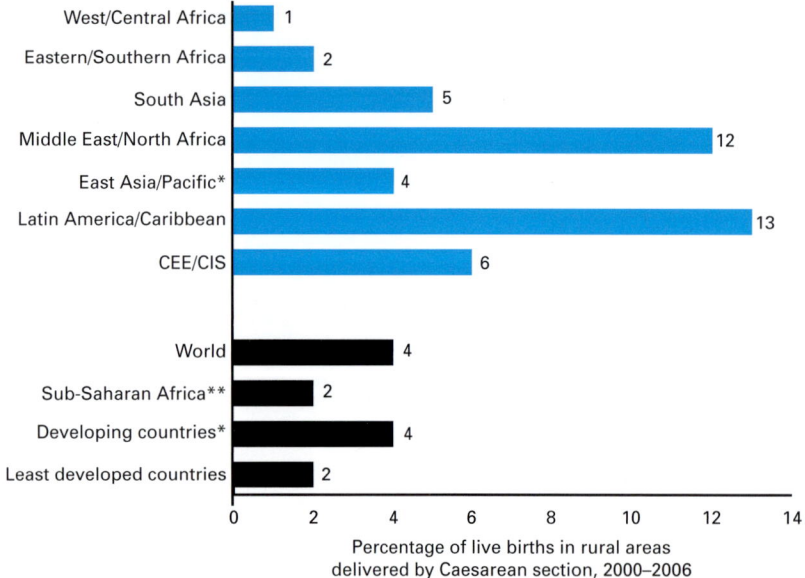

Figure 3.5

Emergency obstetric care: Rural Caesarean section

Percentage of live births in rural areas delivered by Caesarean section, 2000–2006

* Excludes China. ** Sub-Saharan Africa comprises the regions of Eastern/Southern Africa and West/Central Africa.
Source: Demographic and Health Surveys, other national household surveys and UNICEF.

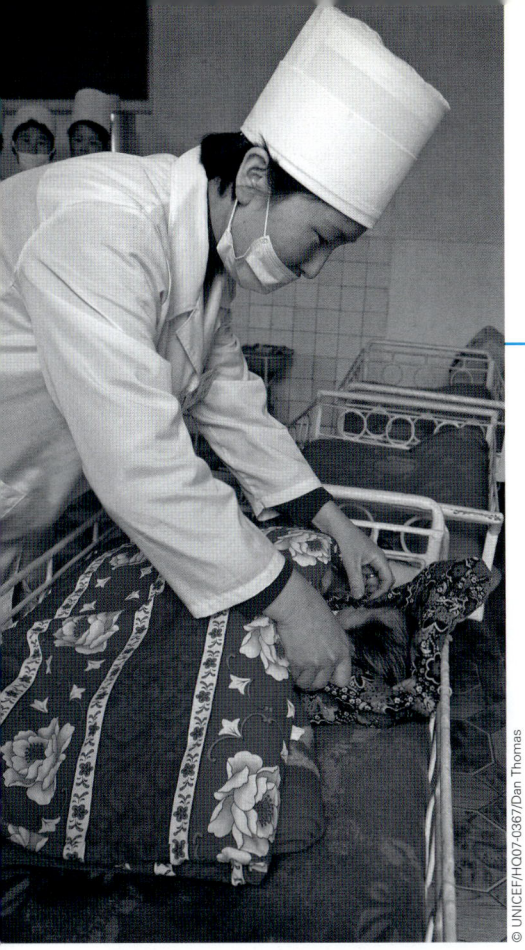

Establishing a continuum of quality maternal and neonatal health care will require the recruitment and training of skilled health personnel and community health workers. *A nurse tends to a newborn baby at a paediatric hospital, Democratic People's Republic of Korea.*

to six months to a year. The main causes of post-partum mortality are severe bleeding, infections and hypertensive disorders. Treating these conditions will require the skilled care and attendance at birth outlined in earlier sections of this chapter.[18]

Routine post-natal visits are necessary in the high-risk post-partum period, when any complications need to be promptly detected and referred to more expert services if required. Even in the absence of complications, these visits can provide essential information and guidance on maternal and newborn health – especially on the care and feeding of babies, the danger signs of illness, referral processes and improved hygiene practices. Studies show that fewer neonatal deaths occur when mother and baby are visited within 48 hours of birth. Mothers who are HIV-positive and babies born prematurely need particular attention.[19] Low birthweight infants require special attention, particularly for temperature management.

(*See Panel on page 62, Kangaroo mother care in Ghana*).

Even mothers who benefit from immediate post-partum care are often neglected in the days and weeks that follow. Their next contact with health workers may be at the six-week period, when the baby is due to receive the first round of immunizations. Evidence shows that mothers seek post-natal care less often than antenatal care or a supervised delivery, even if they are suffering from post-partum bleeding or conditions such as fistula and uterine prolapse.[20]

Effective post-natal care requires care and attention during the immediate post-partum period and also several follow-up visits. Enabling mothers to return to health facilities, or following up with outreach visits in the days and weeks following childbirth, can be challenging – there may be costs or difficulties in arranging transport and visitation, or cultural reasons that make a return to the clinic or hospital unlikely. This is why outreach visits can have a vital part in maintaining maternal and neonatal health, irrespective of where the birth took place. (*See Panel on page 57, The first 28 days of life, and Panel on pages 80–81, Saving mothers and newborn lives – the crucial first days after birth*).

Little is known about the effects and extent of depression during pregnancy and the post-partum period in developing countries. Research has identified partner and social support, life events, the experience of motherhood and infant temperament as critical factors in the onset of depression during the post-natal year.

While it is estimated that around 10–15 per cent of women in industrialized countries may experience depression during the weeks and months after delivery, information on this condition in the developing world is scarce. Small-scale studies from Pakistan and Viet Nam indicate that women who suffer from depression tend to have underweight infants, and research from India suggests that children of depressed mothers may face a higher risk of stunting.[21]

Healthy practices for newborn care

Prevention of newborn deaths requires skilled care more than technology, and demands flexible and responsive systems of intervention. The state of the health system, social context and local practices matter just as much as epidemiological risks. Neonatal health can be improved, for example, by practices that do not have high costs attached, such as clean delivery conditions and the promotion of early and exclusive breastfeeding, and by ensuring that the mother is healthy when she gives birth.

Recent progress has been achieved in providing simple, cost-effective interventions that have a positive impact on neonatal health, including tetanus immunization, the use of insecticide-treated nets to combat

Promoting healthy behaviours for mothers and newborns, particularly in nutrition and hygiene, is vital to reducing health risks and morbidity.

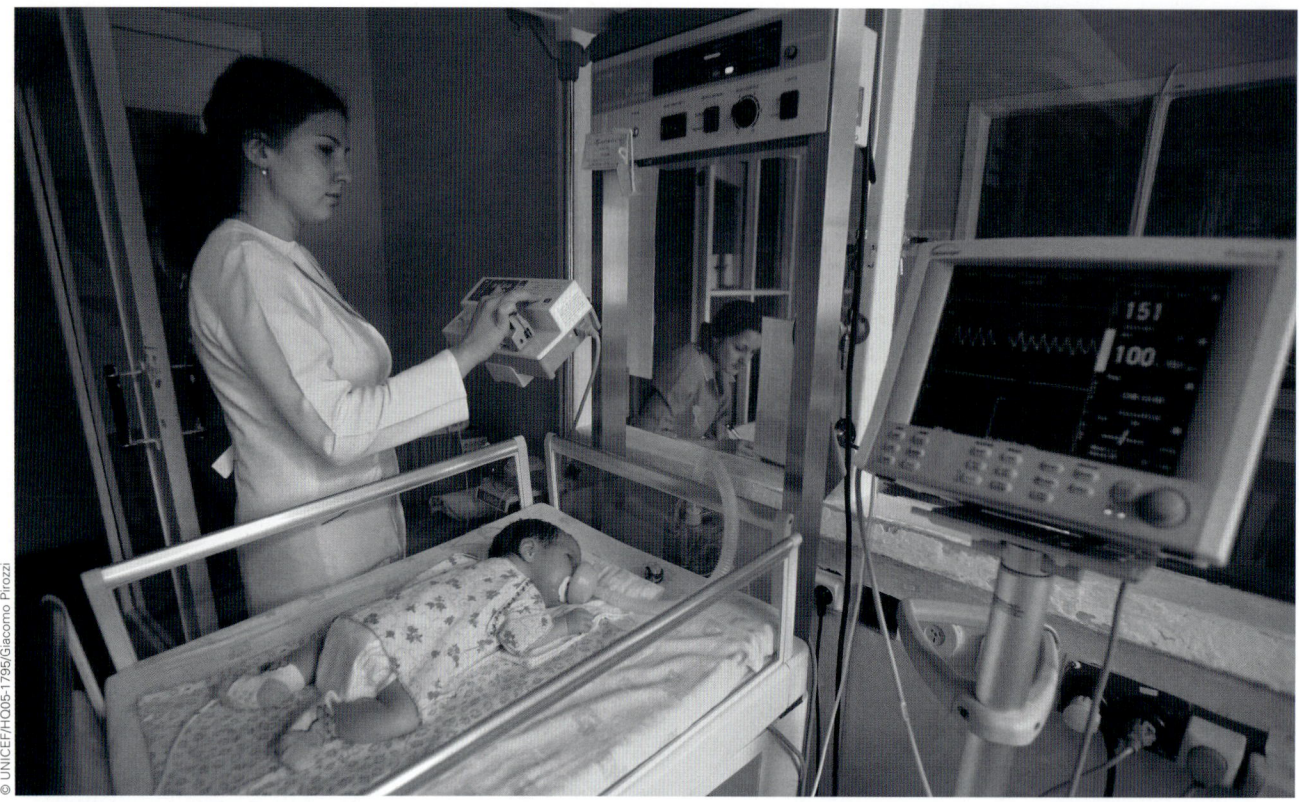

Skilled health personnel, with access to proper equipment and support, can provide critical life-saving interventions when emergencies arise during labour and childbirth. *A newborn is monitored by a medical worker in a children's hospital, Ukraine.*

malaria and micronutrient supplementation. A study tracking coverage of interventions for maternal, newborn and child survival found greater improvement in the delivery of these types of preventive intervention than of curative care. Progress on actions focusing on behavioural changes, such as breastfeeding, was mixed.[22]

Since the early 1990s, the emphasis in coping with these manifold threats to the lives of children has been on a broad, cross-cutting approach that recognizes there is normally more than one contributory cause to any ailment. This approach, introduced by UNICEF and the World Health Organization, became known as the Integrated Management of Childhood Illness (IMCI), and it has met with increasingly positive results. More recently, this integrated model has been incorporated into the maternal, newborn and child health continuum of care.

The continuum of care: Linking lives to places

It is now recognized that linking interventions in packages can also increase their efficiency and cost-effectiveness. In addition, when services are integrated there is both more incentive for people to use them and greater opportunity to extend and enhance coverage. The goal is to develop a comprehensive primary-health-care system that provides women and children with essential interventions and strengthens the links between households and health facilities that have so often been missing in the past.

Household practices and behaviours

When children fall ill, the first point of intervention inevitably lies in the hands of their families, especially their parents, close relatives and guardians. The initial diagnosis of

The first 28 days of life

by Zulfiqar A. Bhutta, Professor and Chairman, Department of Paediatrics & Child Health, Aga Khan University, Karachi, Pakistan

It is widely recognized that a large proportion of child deaths occur in the newborn period, the first 28 days of life. Of an estimated 9.2 million deaths of children under five around the world in 2007, around 40 per cent occurred in the newborn period. In many developing countries, deaths of newborns account for over half of all deaths in infancy, with the vast majority occurring in the first few days of life. The major causes of such deaths are serious infections (36 per cent), prematurity (27 per cent), birth asphyxia (23 per cent) and congenital malformations (7 per cent). These figures do not include an estimated 3 million stillbirths annually. Some 30–40 per cent of these stillbirths may be related to events during labor and delivery, which in turn may result from intrauterine problems and asphyxiation.

The relative lack of progress in reducing newborn deaths is due to several factors. Most important is that, unlike health in the post-natal period (29 days to 59 months), newborn health is closely tied to maternal health. Improving it requires interventions that address complex issues such as maternal empowerment, sociocultural taboos and health-system responsiveness.

Specific factors leading to neonatal deaths include:

- A lack of attention to maternal health, with limited access to skilled care providers.
- The poor state of maternal health care, especially during home births, which are associated with at least half of all newborn deaths.
- Inadequate recognition of newborn illnesses and insufficient care-seeking among families and communities.
- A limited repertoire of interventions for early neonatal disorders such as birth asphyxia and problems due to premature birth.
- A lack of consensus on interventions and delivery strategies to prevent and treat serious neonatal infections – other than neonatal tetanus – in community settings.

Recent years have brought significant improvement in our understanding of neonatal illnesses and mortality. Inequities in distribution of maternal and newborn deaths indicate that most deaths occur in poor, rural populations and in often-ignored urban squatter settlements. Many countries also recognize that reaching the Millennium Development Goal for reducing child mortality will not be possible without improving care for mothers and newborns, focusing efforts on reducing deaths during the first 28 days of life.

The evidence supporting strategies and interventions that use community partnerships has also improved. A number of programmes, largely based in South Asia, have attempted to reduce newborn morbidity and mortality in community settings using innovative approaches. In a landmark study undertaken in rural Maharashtra, India, Dr. Abhay Bang and his colleagues trained community health workers, working with traditional birth attendants, to recognize serious neonatal illnesses such as birth asphyxia or suspected bacterial infections and treat them with home-based resuscitation or oral and injectable antibiotics, respectively. The programme showed a significant reduction in neonatal mortality through these home-based newborn care strategies. More recently, researchers from Johns Hopkins University have demonstrated the efficacy of using trained community health workers to deliver an integrated package of preventive and curative newborn care in Sylhet, rural Bangladesh. While home-based care provision was important in these studies, it is possible that major benefits also accrued from improved family practices and newborn care. In a study in Makwanpur, in rural Nepal, women's support groups, assisted by trained facilitators, effected a significant reduction in neonatal mortality. Further studies have shown that a concerted strategy of community-based education in newborn care can lead to significant change in practices and reductions in neonatal mortality.

All of these recent studies provide evidence that community-based education in improved maternal and newborn care and home-based treatment for newborn infections can significantly enhance newborn survival. To affect public-health systems in the foreseeable future, these strategies need to be replicated at scale using feasible motivation and training of available health-care workers. Such an expansion has taken place in rural Pakistan, where community-based Lady Health Workers work with village health committees and women's groups. A recent evaluation of the Pakistan initiative has shown a significant reduction in perinatal and neonatal mortality and improved care-seeking for skilled maternal care.

This emerging evidence provides support for strategies to improve maternal and newborn health in the very communities and families with the highest burden of mortality and least access to quality health care. The challenge is to integrate effective strategies and interventions across the continuum of maternal and newborn care in both community settings and health facilities. Recent estimates indicate that providing basic preventive and curative interventions for mothers and newborns in primary-health-care settings at pragmatic levels of coverage has the potential to reduce maternal and newborn deaths by 20–40 per cent.

While these measures show promise, particularly when several complementary interventions are packaged together and delivered through a range of health-care providers, important bottlenecks to improved service delivery remain in many developing countries, including poorly functioning health-system facilities and limited numbers of skilled health-care providers. These bottlenecks can and must be addressed through strategies targeted to reach those families, communities and districts most at risk of missing out on basic health care and maternity services. Despite these difficulties, and the still important gaps in our knowledge of how best to tackle difficult newborn problems such as birth asphyxia, the fragility of preterm infants and serious bacterial infections in community settings, one point is clear: We know enough about what works to make a difference. The critical need is to implement what we know and create the policy framework for appropriate maternal and newborn care where it matters: among the rural and urban poor.

See References, page 109.

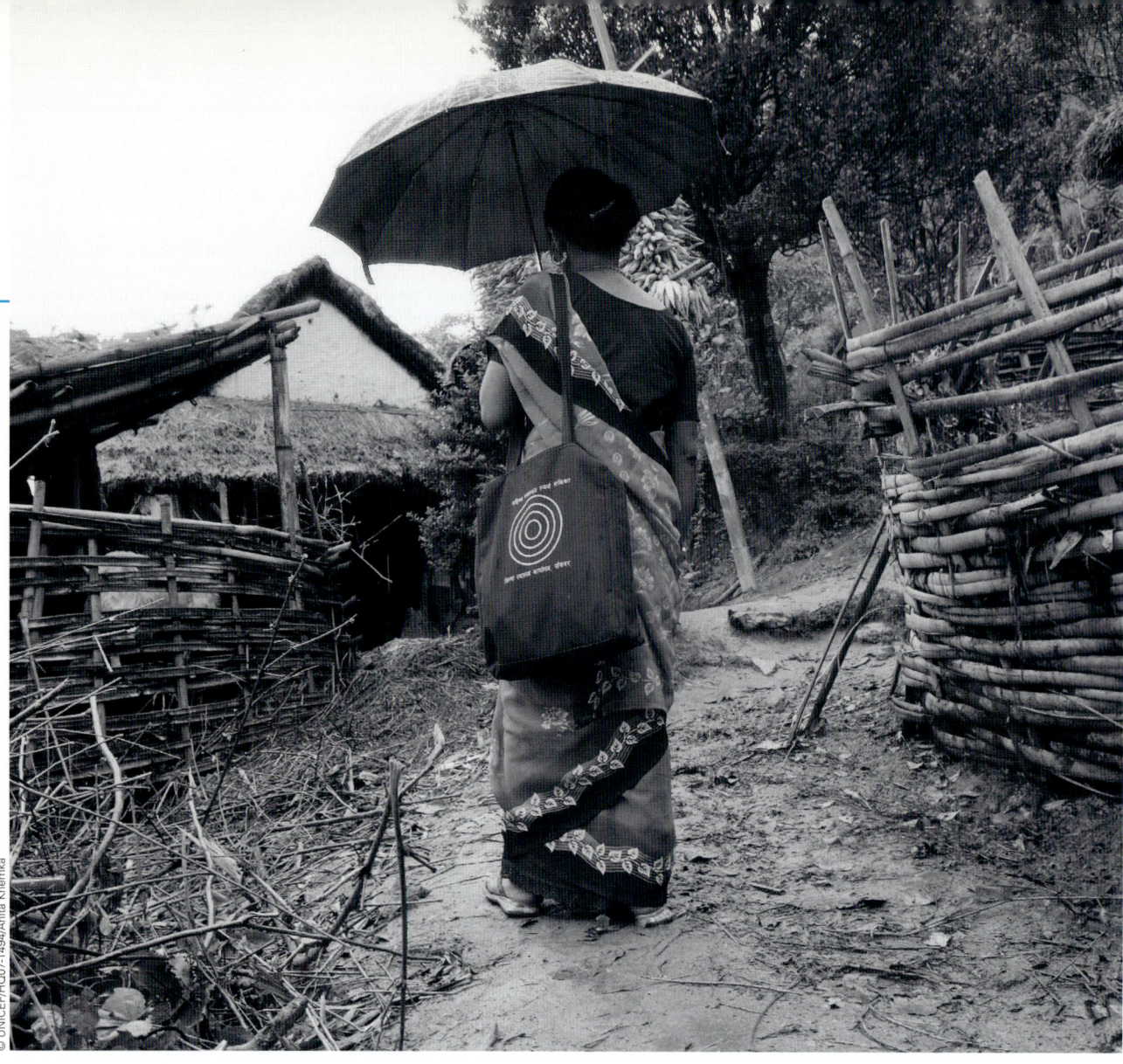

Community partnerships in health care can help expand coverage of essential services and improve practices in health and nutrition. A community health volunteer who is also a trained birth assistant visits a pregnant woman in a village, Nepal.

any childhood illness is most often made not by a doctor or nurse, but by a mother, who assesses the symptoms, decides on their severity and either settles on a form of care and treatment within the home or decides that a trained health worker must be consulted. Irrespective of whether a health worker is sought, it also falls to family members to nurse sick children and to administer any necessary medicines or other remedies.

A similar process often applies to women who are pregnant or have recently given birth, although to a lesser extent. The woman herself will have her own view of the severity of any problem that arises before, during and after birth, but families inevitably play a key role, especially in deciding whether it is necessary to seek external, and often expensive, medical assistance. In addition, sociocultural factors may mean that women need to receive the permission of their husbands or other family members to seek care during pregnancy, childbirth or the post-partum period.

The competence of family members to make judgements on medical matters varies enormously, of course, but no health system can afford to ignore the vital part played by families or household members in identifying and coping with childhood or maternal illness. In addition, although in the developing world as a whole a small majority (54 per cent) of births take place in clinics or hospitals, in both sub-Saharan Africa and South Asia – the regions with the greatest burden of maternal and neonatal mortality – more than 60 per cent of women give birth at home.[23] Even those women who give birth in a health facility are often discharged from hospitals within 24 hours of delivery, and the main burden of post-partum and neonatal care and supervision falls on family members of the mother and newborn.

Community partnerships in health can promote early and exclusive breastfeeding, which provides vital protection for newborns against ill health and disease.

At a more basic level, nutrition and hygiene practices in the household are prime determinants of the health risks faced by mothers and newborns. Inadequate maternal nutrition, unhygienic practices at delivery, and in caring for the umbilical stump or cord, inattention to basic hygiene practices such as hand washing with soap or ashes after using latrines and before preparing and eating meals, and indoor air pollution can accentuate the spread of infections and diseases such as tetanus, diarrhoea and acute respiratory infections. Raising awareness of improved individual household practices and behaviours, such as exclusively breastfeeding newborns and infants up to six months, has considerable potential to improve the health and well-being of families.

Simple messages regarding basic hygienic practices in food preparation – such as keeping food in covered containers to exclude insects and drying cloths used to clean dishes or pans in the sun – can have beneficial results. Improving household knowledge of elementary health, nutrition and environmental health interventions, along with increased empowerment of women to make decisions about their own or their children's health, could have a strong positive impact on health outcomes both for children and new or expectant mothers.

Community partnerships in primary health care

Communities have a vital role in health care and nutrition of mothers, newborns and children. The notion of the community as a cornerstone of primary health care was asserted in the Alma-Ata Declaration of 1978, and it is clear that the goal of health care for all cannot be achieved without community participation, especially in poorer and more remote areas. It is beneficial that communities take an active part in improving health care, hygiene practices, nutrition and water and sanitation services. This is, however, not merely a necessary tool in the absence of more expensive alterna-

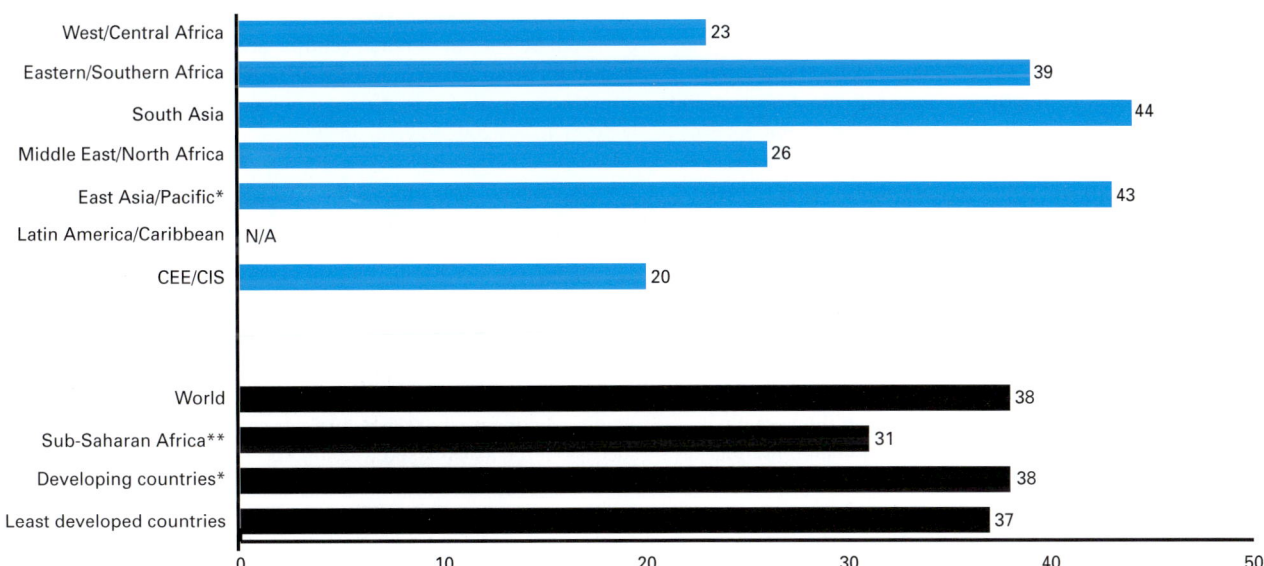

Figure 3.6
Early and exclusive breastfeeding

Region	%
West/Central Africa	23
Eastern/Southern Africa	39
South Asia	44
Middle East/North Africa	26
East Asia/Pacific*	43
Latin America/Caribbean	N/A
CEE/CIS	20
World	38
Sub-Saharan Africa**	31
Developing countries*	38
Least developed countries	37

Percentage of infants less than six months old that are exclusively breastfed, 2000–2007

* Excludes China. ** Sub-Saharan Africa comprises the regions of Eastern/Southern Africa and West/Central Africa.
Source: Demographic and Health Surveys, other national household surveys and UNICEF.

Focus On: Midwifery in Afghanistan

Decades of conflict and instability have disrupted Afghanistan's basic health infrastructure. Women in particular have suffered from a lack of access to health services. As a consequence, maternal mortality among Afghan women is extremely high, standing at 1,800 deaths per 100,000 live births in 2005, according to the latest inter-agency estimates.

Women in Afghanistan face a lifetime risk of death from causes related to pregnancy or childbirth of 1 in 8, the second highest rate in the world. More women die in Afghanistan from these causes than from any other, with haemorrhage and obstructed labour the most common. The proportion of maternal deaths ranges from 16 per cent of all deaths of women of childbearing age in Kabul (the largest urban center in Afghanistan) to 64 per cent in the Ragh district of Badakhshan.

The high rates of maternal death reflect several factors, including limited access to quality maternal health care, particularly in rural parts of Afghanistan; a lack of knowledge of maternal health and safe delivery; and the scarcity of qualified female health providers, since there is a strong cultural preference for women to be cared for by other women. It is estimated that 9 out of 10 rural women deliver their babies at home, without skilled birth attendants or access to emergency obstetric care. Sociocultural factors that inhibit women's mobility without the permission or escort of male relatives can also limit their access to essential services. Other factors contributing to maternal mortality are the low social status of women and girls, poverty, poor nutrition and lack of security.

Improving the survival rates of mothers in Afghanistan is an issue of immense importance. Midwives can provide crucial care. The World Health Organization recommends one midwife or other skilled birth attendant for every 175 women during pregnancy, childbirth and the post-natal period. Using this estimate with the estimated number of births, Afghanistan should have 4,546 midwives to cover 90 per cent of pregnancies. The country actually had only 467 trained midwives in 2002. Fewer than half of health facilities had any female staff. In rural Nooristan, the ratio of male to female health personnel was as high as 43 to 1.

Although much remains to be done to improve maternal and newborn health in Afghanistan, many successful efforts to date have focused on expanding and strengthening midwifery.

Afghanistan's Government is collaborating with local and international partners, including UNICEF, to develop a comprehensive approach that includes strengthening and expanding midwifery education, creating policies to ensure the pivotal role of midwives in providing essential obstetric and newborn care, supporting the establishment of a professional association for midwives, and developing initiatives to increase access to skilled care during childbirth.

The Community Midwifery Education (CME) programme, an 18-month, skills-based training programme that has less stringent entry requirements than previous midwifery programmes, is considered an appropriate approach to scaling up training and deployment of skilled birth attendants. In 2008, there were 19 CME programmes, each with 20–25 trainees. This represents a marked increase in training capacity over 2002, when there were only six nurse midwifery training programmes run by the Institute of Health Science at regional centres, and one community midwifery programme in Nangahar province. The number of midwives available in the country has increased rapidly, from 467 in 2002 to 2,167 in 2008.

The CME encourages applications from women in districts with shortages, with the understanding that they will work in those districts once they are trained. This policy has resulted in a sharp increase in facilities having skilled female health personnel (doctors, nurses or midwives), from 39 per cent in 2004 to 76 per cent in 2006. It is also having a tangible impact on maternal care; the number of deliveries attended by skilled workers has risen from roughly 6 per cent in 2003 to 19.9 per cent in 2006. The success of the skills-based training approach has resulted in the existing midwifery programmes adopting the CME curriculum and certification process.

See References, page 109.

Outreach and outpatient services can act as a bridge between the household and health facilities, providing reproductive, antenatal, intrapartum and post-natal services.

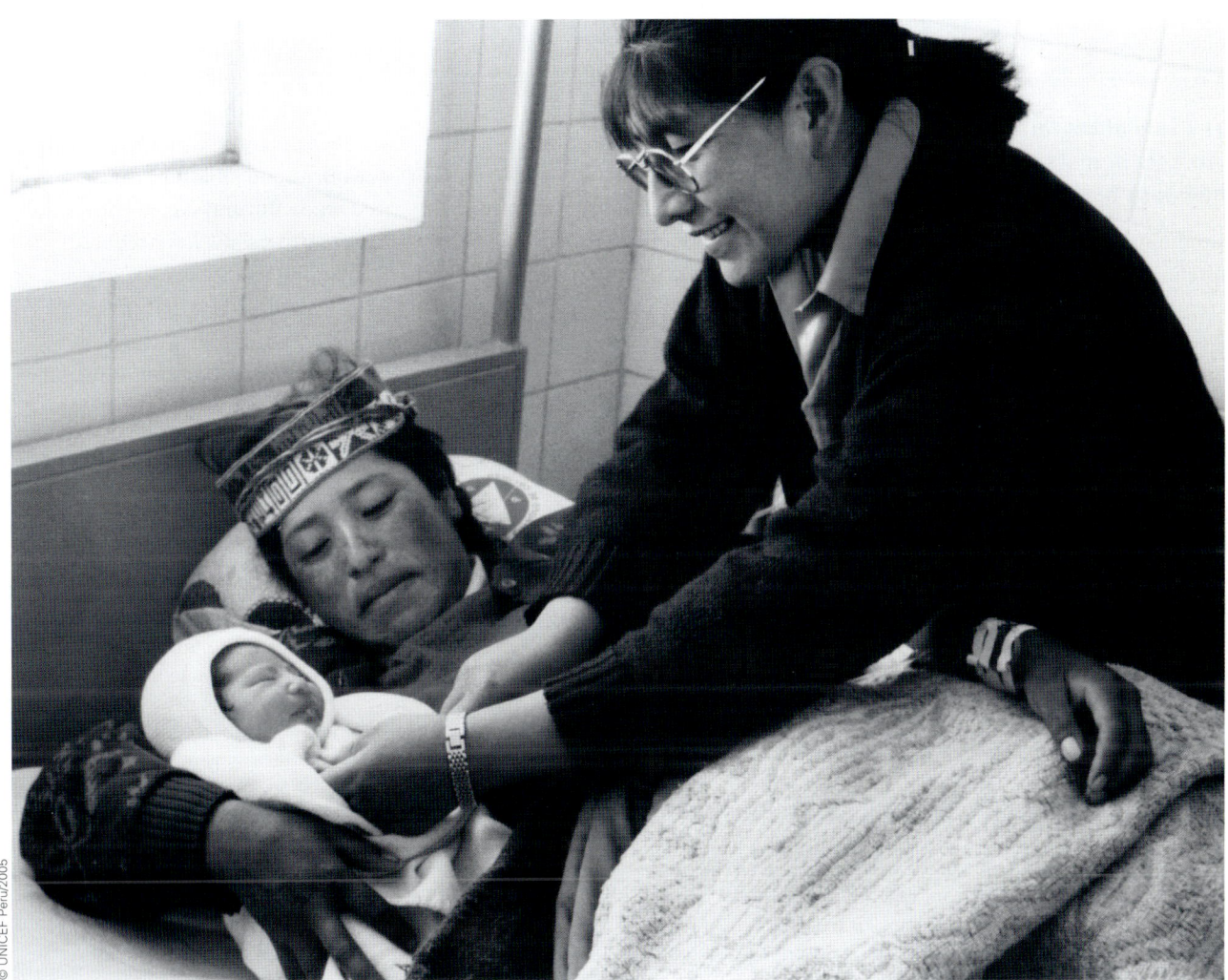

Addressing cultural, social and geographic barriers to health care helps increase access to health services in rural communities. *A mother and her newborn are attended by a health worker in a health centre, Peru.*

tives but rather a desirable route for empowerment and participation.[24]

Community partnerships are especially valuable in improving maternal, newborn and child health. There are almost as many different kinds of community partnerships as there are communities. Some are small and local, while others form part of a national network. Some are entirely voluntary, while others involve payment of some sort. Some operate independently of the national health-care system, while others are fully integrated within it. Programmes seeking to use community partnerships as an approach have to be careful to adapt to the particular local context.

At their best, community partnerships in health and nutrition not only improve people's access to services and facilitate closer contact between health workers and individuals or households, but also encourage behavioural change and social mobilization. At their most challenged, community partnerships are short-staffed, poorly coordinated, underfunded and ill-supplied. Examples of successful community partnerships in health across the developing world demonstrate that the balance sheet as a whole is positive.[25]

The role of community health workers in maternal and newborn health

Community partnerships in health often involve training people as community health workers. These workers undertake basic health care and nutrition activities – whether through home visits or at an established location. Community health workers also lead campaigns for better caring or hygiene practices. Exclusive breastfeeding, hand washing with soap or ashes and the use of insecticide-treated mosquito nets for malaria prevention are three of the most common interventions advocated by community health workers. In addition, many community partnerships in health include workers who advise on prevention of mother-to-child transmission of HIV and contribute to the management of childhood illnesses such as malaria, pneumonia and neonatal sepsis.

Nepal provides one such example. Trained community health workers collaborate with skilled health personnel to provide care to mothers, newborns and children. A randomized study in rural Nepal shows that these partnerships have reduced neonatal mortality by 30 per cent. These findings are complemented by a study in rural India, which shows a 62 per cent reduction in neonatal mortality when community health workers provided home-based care for the newborn, including resuscita-

Kangaroo mother care in Ghana

Kangaroo mother care for low-birthweight babies was introduced in Colombia in 1979 by Drs. Hector Martinez and Edgar Rey as a response to, inter alia, high infection and mortality rates due to overcrowding in hospitals. It has since been adopted across the developing world and has become an essential element in the continuum of neonatal care across the world.

The four components of kangaroo mother care are all essential for ensuring the best care options, especially for low birthweight babies. They include skin-to-skin positioning of a baby on the mother's chest; adequate nutrition through breastfeeding; ambulatory care as a result of earlier discharge from hospital; and support for the mother and her family in caring for the baby.

The most important method of spreading kangaroo mother care has been by means of training programmes. Often, the training remains confined to hospital settings. A new approach was adopted in Ghana under a kangaroo mother care (KMC Ghana) project undertaken in four regions, with the support of UNICEF and the South African Medical Research Council's Unit for Maternal and Infant Health Care Strategies. Instead of merely providing training, a longitudinal, 'open door' approach based on continuous support from health-care facilities was adopted.

Under the programme, kangaroo mother care is singled out for special attention for two to three years. This requires participants to focus on one aspect of newborn care, implement it well and in the process integrate it into the normal spectrum of newborn care practices.

The implementation model identifies specific roles for districts and regions, depending on the way authority is devolved in a country. In Ghana, the region is the nodal point for implementation, with districts being responsible for the actual implementation actions. Although half of all births still occur at home, one of the cornerstones of the KMC Ghana project is the establishment of centres of excellence at regional hospitals and 24-hour, continuous kangaroo mother care in each district hospital.

Implementation is overseen by a KMC Steering Committee in each region, consisting of one member from each of the districts. These representatives, in turn, establish steering committees at the district level. Although the focus is on introducing KMC in district hospitals, other health care facilities and community organizations are also sought as partners.

While a comprehensive evaluation of the KMC Ghana programme has yet to take place, preliminary evidence suggests that it is effective in improving the survival of low birthweight babies and strengthening the bond between mothers and newborns.

See References, page 109.

HIV/malaria co-infection in pregnancy

Co-infection with HIV and malaria presents specific complications for pregnant women and fetal development. HIV lessens pregnancy-specific malaria immunity normally acquired during the first and second pregnancies. Placental malaria is associated with increased risk of maternal anaemia and HIV infection, especially among younger women and those experiencing their first pregnancy. The role of co-infection in mother-to child transmission of HIV is unclear, with some studies reporting an increase and others reporting no change. The potential risks of adverse drug interactions have critical implications for effective management of co-infection, and call for increased research.

Although malaria affects Asia, Latin America and the Caribbean, and sub-Saharan Africa, the largest burden of co-infection lies in Africa, the continent with the greatest burden of malaria, and where more than three quarters of all HIV-infected women live. Variations exist across the African continent. Most affected by HIV/malaria co-infection are the Central African Republic, Malawi, Mozambique, Zambia and Zimbabwe, where some 90 per cent of adults are exposed to malaria and average adult HIV-prevalence surpasses 10 per cent. In parts of southernmost Africa, where the HIV epidemic is most severe, there is a lower incidence of malaria, although outbreaks do occur in particular areas, such as Kwazulu-Natal, South Africa.

Data for other regions are not as clear, but the overlap of infections may be present in the general populations of Belize, El Salvador, Guatemala, Guyana and Honduras – and, to a lesser extent, Brazil. Research indicates that certain populations, such as migrant goldmine workers in Brazil and Guyana, may have greater risk of co-infection. The HIV epidemic is generalized in Asian countries such as Myanmar and Thailand, but malaria transmission is unstable and heterogeneous across this region, as in Latin America and the Caribbean. The most common species of malaria in each region also differs – *P. falciparum* in Africa, *P. vivax* in Asia and Latin America and the Caribbean – and the effects of the disease may vary by the degree of immunity a women has achieved by the time she becomes pregnant. Women in Asia are less exposed to intense malaria transmission and therefore have less opportunity to develop acquired immunity. This is also true of areas of unstable malaria transmission in parts of southern Africa. Most studies of malaria in pregnancy are from Africa, and more are needed from other regions and *non-falciparum* species.

Malaria sufferers with severe anaemia who require blood transfusions, particularly children, also are at higher risk of acquiring HIV. Every year, between 5,300 and 8,500 children in areas of endemic malaria in Africa become infected with HIV from blood transfusions administered for severe malaria.

Regional differences notwithstanding, co-infection affects all pregnant women in similar ways. HIV in pregnancy combined with malaria increases the risk of severe anaemia and reduces any acquired immunity that women living in areas of stable malaria transmission may have developed – effectively meaning that HIV-positive women in their second, third and fourth pregnancies have the same low immunity to malaria as women in their first pregnancy. Pregnant women infected with HIV become twice as susceptible to clinical malaria, regardless of gravidity. In these women, malaria can restrict fetal growth, cause preterm delivery and low birthweight in newborns and reduce the transfer to children of maternal immunities and cellular responses to infectious diseases such as streptococcus pneumonia, tetanus and measles. Recent evidence suggests that HIV-positive mothers with malaria are more likely to have low-birthweight infants; in turn, low-birthweight infants were shown to have significantly higher risks of mother-to-child transmission of HIV compared with infants of normal birthweight.

The effects of malaria on HIV are less clear, though episodes of acute malaria can increase viral load and hasten disease progression. Malaria infection during pregnancy may increase the risk of mother-to-child transmission of HIV in utero and during birth, and higher viral load can result in greater risk of transmission during breastfeeding. Some research shows that viral loads can return to pre-episode levels following malaria treatment, which suggests that management of malaria may be critical to slowing the spread of HIV and its progression to AIDS.

One of the most pressing questions about co-infection concerns drug therapies. The World Health Organization recommends that all pregnant women in areas of high HIV prevalence (>10 per cent) receive at least three doses of sulfadoxine-pyrimethamine as intermittent preventive treatment (IPT), even in asymptomatic cases, unless they are receiving cotrimoxazole for the treatment of opportunistic infections of HIV.

Many African governments use artemisinin-based combination therapy for malaria case management in pregnancy; with research still limited, WHO continues to recommend this treatment be used for uncomplicated malaria in pregnancy during the first trimester, if it is the only effective treatment available. In cases of severe anaemia, treatment with either artemisinin-based therapy or quinine, should be administered, although the former is preferred in the second or third trimester. There is little published information on the risks of co-administration of antiretrovirals and antimalarials, including artemisinin derivatives, but artemisinins have not yet been observed to have important toxicities when co-administered with antiretrovirals or when given in early pregnancy.

See References, page 109.

The challenges faced by adolescent girls in Liberia

by the Honourable Vabah Gayflor, Minister of Gender and Development, Liberia

Ensuring that adolescent girls have a supportive environment for their growth and development and are protected from abuse, exploitation, violence and premature entry into adult roles such as marriage and labour is particularly challenging in my country, Liberia.

An adolescent girl living in Liberia:

– *has probably not been to primary school;* the net primary school enrolment for girls stands at only 39 per cent, according to the latest national estimates.

– *is unlikely to go on to secondary school;* just 14 per cent of girls of secondary school age are enrolled in secondary education.

– *is at high risk of being illiterate*, like 24 per cent of adolescent girls and young women aged 15–24 in the country.

– *has a high risk of suffering rape* – the most frequently reported crime, with girls aged 10–14 the most frequent victims of rape.

– *probably has limited knowledge of HIV and AIDS;* only 21 per cent of young women aged 15–24 have comprehensive knowledge of HIV and AIDS.

– *has a high probability of either being married or in union;* 40 per cent of women aged 20–24 in Liberia were married before the age of 18.

– *faces the strong likelihood of being pregnant;* the adolescent birth rate for girls aged 15–19 stands at 221 per 1,000 – the second highest rate in the world.

– *is unlikely to give birth in a hospital or health facility*, as only 37 per cent of births take place in institutional settings.

– *will possibly have to give birth without the assistance of a skilled health worker*, which only attend 51 per cent of births.

– *runs a high risk of death from pregnancy and childbirth;* the maternal mortality rate stands at 1,200 per 100,000 live births.

– *has an even higher risk of death from maternal causes if under 15;* girls aged 10–14 are five times more likely to die from causes related to pregnancy and childbirth than those of ages 20–24.

– *may be left with a delivery-related injury if she survives her pregnancy*, such as fistula or uterine prolapse.

– *faces a high lifetime risk of death from her first and subsequent pregnancies;* the lifetime risk of maternal deaths stands at 1 in 12.

– *may see her child die within the first year of life*, with almost 1 in every 10 infants dying before their first birthday.

– *will probably not have support from a partner, even if she is married.*

– *has little or no recourse to protection from further abuse, exploitation and disempowerment.*

Creating a supportive environment for adolescent girls in Liberia begins with protecting them from violence and abuse, and ensuring that they obtain a quality education.

It will also necessitate ensuring that families do not allow their girls to marry before age 18 or allow them to be engaged in exploitative labour.

It requires that knowledge of HIV and AIDS be promoted among young people, and that victims of sexual violence have recourse to justice.

It necessitates investment in reproductive, maternity and basic health care for millions of adolescent girls.

Most of all, it demands that communities and society respect the rights of women and girls, and have the courage to address customs and practices that harm and discriminate against them.

Under the leadership of President Ellen Johnson-Sirleaf, the Government of Liberia is striving to provide the protection adolescent girls need and to help them acquire the skills that will enable them to protect themselves. We welcome the support of the international development community in assisting us to act quickly and effectively.

See References, page 109.

Facility-based care is essential for referrals and providing a range of routine and emergency services for mothers and newborns.

tion for birth asphyxia and treatment of sepsis with antibiotics.[26]

Community partnerships in health care can help expand coverage of essential services and improved practices in health and nutrition. Perhaps even more importantly, such partnerships can also enable health systems to reach out to their communities, however poor or marginalized they may be.

Outreach and outpatient services

Outreach and outpatient services, such as antenatal care and immunization, are delivered on a routine basis through one of two modes: stationary clinics visited by pregnant women and their children, or mobile services whereby health workers undertake essential interventions to mothers and children in their communities. In almost all cases, recipients are not assessed as clinical cases but receive a standardized service. Many of these interventions do not need to be delivered by skilled medical staff to prove beneficial, but can be dispensed by semi-skilled health workers and by community health workers with some training. This, in turn, makes it easier and more cost-effective to increase coverage of outreach-based services to large sectors of the population.[27]

Outreach and outpatient services can act as a bridge between home and community care and facility-based care. They are vital mechanisms for delivering antenatal and post-natal care, as well as promoting sexual and reproductive health. For example, antenatal care can of course be offered at clinics or hospitals, but it is entirely appropriate as an outreach service.

Antenatal outreach services should screen for and treat disorders such as anaemia, hypertension, diabetes, syphilis, tuberculosis and malaria, as well as check the baby's position. They should also provide tetanus immunization, distribute insecticide-treated mosquito nets and offer intermittent preventive treatment of malaria in malaria-endemic areas, in addition to counselling on such matters as diet, hygiene, the danger signals in pregnancy and breastfeeding. It is also important, however, not to overburden outpatient or outreach services to the point at which they become overstretched.[28]

Outreach services can also be adapted to provide post-natal care, as mentioned earlier in this chapter. Key services include recognizing and checking for danger signs for mothers and newborns, guidance on feeding – particularly early and exclusive breastfeeding – and caring for the newborn, referral for treatment of mother or baby if appropriate, and support and counselling on healthy practices.[29]

Reproductive health is another area appropriate to outreach and outpatient services. Outreach services can raise awareness of options for reproductive health services and practices, including birth spacing. They can also detect sexually transmitted infections and treat them promptly. Many outpatient or outreach services in reproductive health currently offer only poor-quality interventions, however, which deter people from using them.[30]

Facility-based care

Health facilities generally provide the broadest range of preventive and curative treatments for maternal and child health, and potentially the most skilled pool of health-care workers. These facilities generally fall into two main categories: clinics and hospitals. The facility closest to the community is likely to be a clinic providing immediate, generalized care, possibly overseen by a nurse. Clinic staff can often cope with uncomplicated births and offer support and advice on the care of the newborn. They should also be able to deal with some of the key complications – able, for example, to remove the placenta manually, or to offer resuscitation to a newborn. Given the potential risks associated with labour and childbirth, however, staff in clinics, as well as those engaged in outreach attendance at birth, need the skilled knowledge to recognize swiftly when a complication in the delivery, or the degree of sickness in the newborn, is beyond their competence and to refer it to a higher level.

That next level is likely to be a district hospital where doctors can offer medical diagnosis, treatment, care, counselling and rehabilitation services. In some health systems there may be a referral hospital providing complex clinical care, but in many communities across the developing world, the facility-based health needs of mothers and infants are met by clinics or the district hospital, if at all.[31]

Access to emergency obstetric care can pose a major challenge for pregnant women living in rural areas, owing to the distance to be covered to reach a suitable facility and the lack of transport or adequate roads by which it can be reached. Even if transportation vehicles and infrastructure are available, travel and accommodation costs, together with indirect costs such as the income foregone by accompanying family members, may prove prohibitive. Families living in geographically isolated communities therefore face elevated risk of maternal and neonatal mortality when birth complications arise. A recent study of maternal deaths in Afghanistan, for example, showed that physical remoteness added to the epidemiological risks that women faced.[32]

Geographical distance is not the only impediment to accessing health-care facilities, however; there are cases where women living in the vicinity of a health facility will only visit for antenatal care but not the delivery itself. Cultural reservations about a woman's delivery being attended by strangers, and economic costs of skilled attendance at delivery, are examples of deterrents that impede usage of health-care facilities. Lack of health-care personnel and inadequate medical equipment and drugs can also deter families from seeking an institutional delivery. One particular challenge is to lower the incidence of facility-acquired diseases – a serious risk in sub-Saharan Africa – that can increase the risk of infection from blood transfusions and the reuse of needles.[33] Despite these impediments, it is clear that upgrading maternity clinics, health centres and hospitals to provide at least basic emergency obstetric care would be a major step towards reducing maternal and neonatal mortality.

The continuum of care: Practical steps towards primary health care for mothers and newborns

Health-care services function best when they link care in the home through the community to outreach services and beyond to clinics and hospitals. This is by no means a new insight: The evidence and knowledge have been available for decades. Their application has the potential to reduce markedly the toll of preventable maternal and neonatal deaths. The challenge now is to put in place the levels of investment in health services that will guarantee a continuum of care. Chapter 4 outlines a framework for devising strategies and apportioning resources to deliver the improvements in maternal and neonatal health that the developing world urgently requires.

THE STATE OF THE WORLD'S CHILDREN 2009

4 Strengthening health systems to improve maternal and newborn health

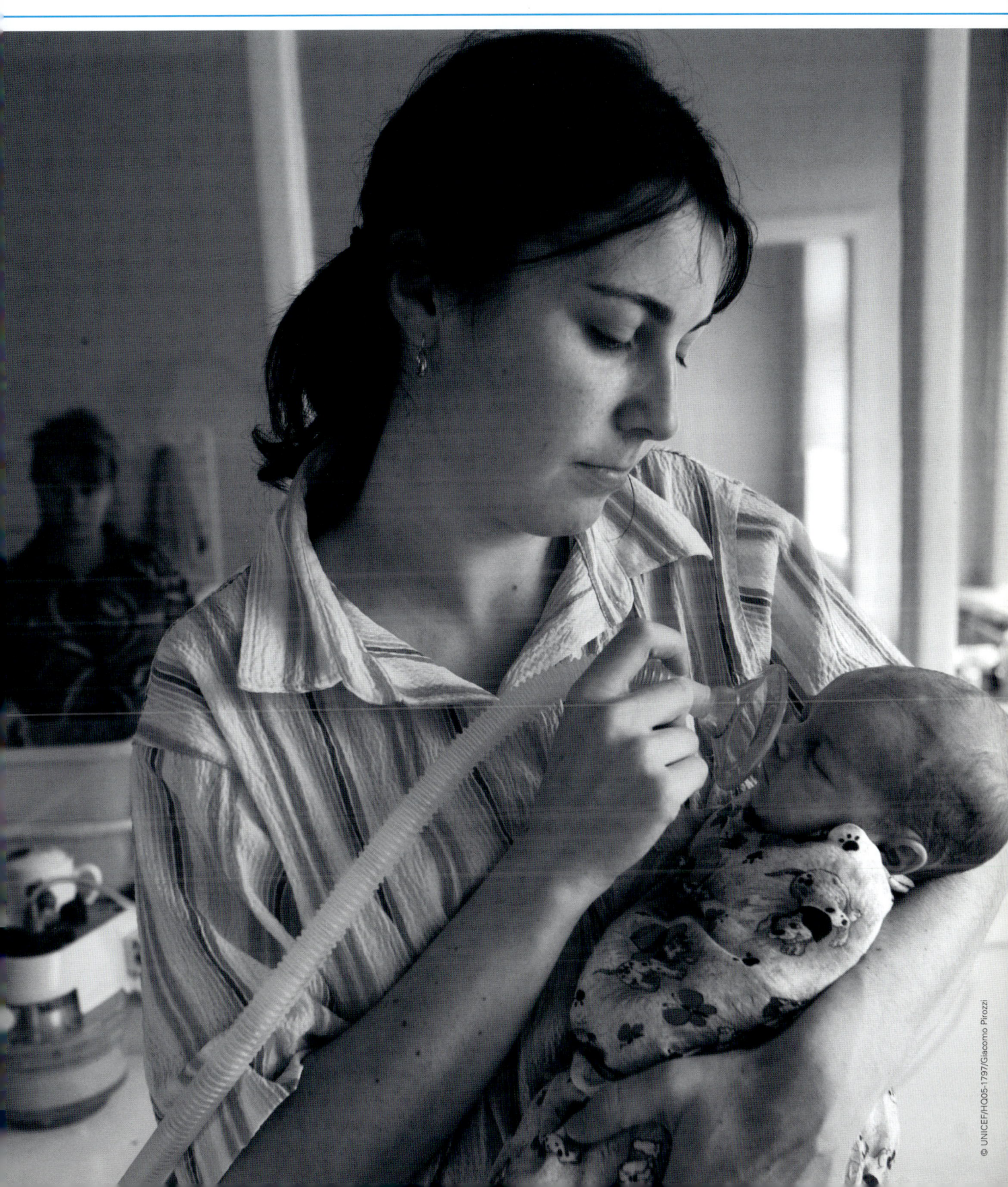

Establishing effective continua of care will involve taking practical steps to strengthen health systems. The key elements for health systems development – deepening the evidence base, expanding and enhancing the health workforce, upgrading and broadening infrastructure and logistics, providing equitable financing solutions and stimulating demand for care through social mobilization, ensuring the quality of care and fostering political commitment and leadership through collaboration – are increasingly accepted by national governments and local and international agencies. Chapter 4 of The State of the World's Children 2009 examines each of the first six steps, illustrating their practical application through country examples. The seventh step – political leadership and commitment – is addressed in the final chapter of the report.

Meeting Millennium Development Goal 5 will be challenging. As a whole, the world is far behind on improving maternal health, with little progress achieved in sub-Saharan Africa in particular since 1990. Even within those developing countries and regions that have seen more progress, pockets of poverty and marginalization continue to exclude many from essential maternity and basic health-care services. (*See Chapter 1 for a full description of trends in maternal mortality.*)

Faster progress and major improvements in maternal and newborn survival and health are possible through packaging and scaling up proven, affordable interventions, delivered through a continuum of care and underpinned by a supportive environment for the rights of women and children.

Policy recommendations on the frameworks required to accelerate progress are being continually enriched through data collection, research and analysis, monitoring and evaluation, and collaborative actions. Chapter 4 contributes to these efforts by summarizing a series of practical steps towards strengthening health systems to support the continuum of care outlined in Chapter 3. These involve the following actions:

- Enhancing data collection and analysis of trends, levels, risks, causes of and interventions for maternal and newborn mortality and morbidity.
- Expanding the primary health-care workforce in developing countries and enriching skills levels.
- Mobilizing societies to demand better maternal and newborn health care and a supportive environment for the rights of women and children.
- Establishing practical, equitable and sustainable financing mechanisms for basic health care and maternity services.
- Investing in infrastructure, logistics, information and communications technology, facilities and management capacity to ensure quality care and effective referral.
- Improving the quality of care across the health system.
- Fostering political commitment and leadership through stronger collaboration between partners.

This chapter examines the first six of these steps, illustrating their practical application through country examples. The seventh step will be addressed in Chapter 5.

Step 1: Enhancing data collection and analysis

Since no single indicator can adequately describe the varied dimensions of either maternal or newborn health, a wide array of indicators is useful to guide and monitor programmes. Vital information for policies and programmes includes demographics, nutritional status, socioeconomic status, health-care provision, care-seeking practices and the application of improved health and nutrition practices.

Good data on maternal and newborn health and survival form the foundation for sound policies, effective programmes and collaborative partnerships.

These measures strengthen understanding of the burden, trends, risks and causes of maternal and newborn mortality and morbidity. But much more needs to be done. Gaps in knowledge of many aspects of maternal and newborn health – from the estimation of mortality figures to risks to pregnancy posed by HIV and AIDS, to name but two elements – remain significant. Health information systems remain incomplete in many developing countries, complicating efforts to determine the status of maternal and newborn health and apply the most appropriate strategies and interventions.[1]

Strengthening the knowledge base that forms the foundation for policies, programmes and partnerships is therefore an essential component for developing health systems. Work has begun on the process of enriching data collection. The World Health Organization has developed guidelines to assist governments and other agencies in expanding data collection and improving data quality on maternal health. WHO recommends that health information systems should strive to capture data in five key areas relevant to maternal and child health:

- Maternal and newborn mortality rates.
- Factors or determinants contributing to morbidity and mortality.
- Community perceptions of these health problems and appropriate actions, including types of services and attitudes towards care seeking.

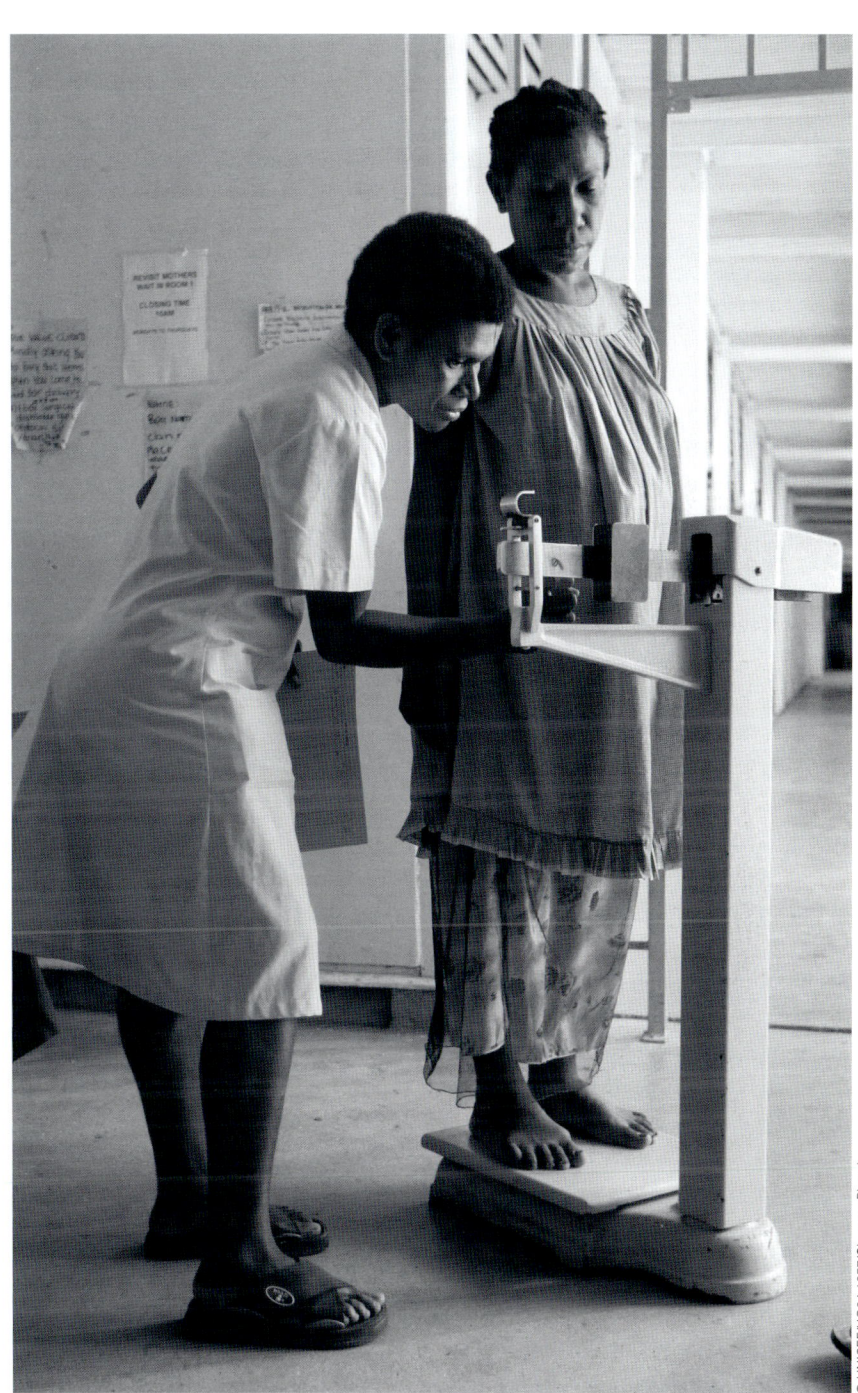

Providing essential care such as immunization and micronutrient supplementation to pregnant women protects them against disease and undernutrition. *A health worker provides consultations that include weight and blood-pressure measurements, tetanus vaccination and iron supplementation, Papua New Guinea.*

STRENGTHENING HEALTH SYSTEMS TO IMPROVE MATERNAL AND NEWBORN HEALTH

A wide array of methods is being employed to enhance data collection on maternal and newborn survival, including censuses, household surveys, and facility-based data gathering.

Figure 4.1

Emergency obstetric care: United Nations process indicators and recommended levels

UN process indicator	Definition	Recommended level
1. Amount of EmOC services available	Number of facilities that provide EmOC	Minimum: 1 comprehensive EmOC facility and 4 basic facilities for every 500,000 people
2. Geographical distribution of EmOC facilities	Facilities providing EmOC well-distributed at subnational level	Minimum: 100% of subnational areas have the minimum acceptable numbers of basic and comprehensive EmOC facilities
3. Proportion of all births in EmOC facilities	Proportion of all births in the population that take place in EmOC facilities	Minimum: 15%
4. Met need for EmOC services	Proportion of women with obstetric complications treated in EmOC facilities	Minimum: 100% (estimated as 15% of expected births)
5. Caesarean sections as a percentage of all births	Caesarean deliveries as a proportion of all births in the population	Minimum: 5% Maximum: 15%
6. Case fatality rate	Proportion of women with obstetric complications admitted to a facility who die	Maximum: 1%

Source: United Nations.

- Availability of and access to quality health-care services.
- Quality of care.[2]

A number of tools exist to facilitate the collection of this information, including censuses, verbal autopsy, death registration, surveys or studies, data obtained from health facilities and health surveillance. Since each method has strengths and weaknesses, more than one mechanism should be employed to assess maternal and newborn health.

Censuses, questionnaires and household surveys

National censuses are a key source of data and information on maternal health. Often they provide the only household-level survey large enough to allow for the measurement of geographic and socio-economic variations in maternal mortality. A census may include follow-up questions aimed at assessing the timing of deaths of women of child-bearing age in each household within the past 12 months. It should be noted, however, that some countries are not using their censuses to collect this information, missing out on an opportunity to collect valuable information on maternal health.

Verbal autopsy is another method of gathering information on mortality and morbidity. The World Health Organization has developed three verbal-autopsy questionnaires – one to ascertain deaths within the first four weeks of life, another for children aged four weeks to 14 years, and a third for persons aged 15 and over – with the goal of helping standardize measurement criteria and methods. This level of scrutiny takes into account the critical issue of timing that has in the past not been adequately emphasized.[3]

Obtaining information on cause of death can be challenging. According to the World Health Organization, only 31 of its 193 member states report high-quality cause-of-death statistics. Several countries are now using surveillance tools such as Demographic Surveillance Systems in

Household surveys such as DHS and MICS are providing vital data on a wide range of outcome and coverage indicators.

smaller geographic areas to ascertain cause of death. Methods used include follow-up investigations of deaths using verbal autopsy to ask family members, health-care providers and community members to explain circumstances of death. These systems are called sample vital registration with verbal autopsy systems. A no-blame policy, in which the respondents are not held liable for answers to survey questions, is pivotal to enlisting and retaining community support for these endeavours.[4]

A number of factors influence maternal and newborn health outcomes, including biological factors such as nutritional status; socioeconomic determinants such as income and education; health-seeking behaviours and healthy practices; barriers to accessing health services; and behavioural risk factors such as domestic violence and smoking. Household surveys and studies are the primary methods used to assess the frequency of these types of determinants, which can then be analyzed to better understand the population for which health programmes are intended.

Important periodic cross-sectional household surveys include the Demographic and Health Surveys (United States Agency for International Development), Multiple Indicator Cluster Surveys (UNICEF) and Reproductive Health Surveys (Centers for Disease Control). These international surveys provide comprehensive quantitative data on a wide range of health topics. Since 1995, nearly 200 MICS have been conducted in 100 countries.

Facility- and community-based data collection

Data derived from health facilities across the wide range of public and private health-care providers are also useful in assessing the state of maternal and newborn health. The number of deaths in facilities can be readily monitored and provide opportunities to learn about improvements needed to avert further deaths, particularly those in institutional settings, in a process known as 'maternal death review or audit'. This type of data can also provide insights into the 'near-misses' – life-threatening complications that heightened the risk of mortality but which ultimately did not result in death – that are important for improving service quality.[5]

Governments, research institutions and other agencies also conduct health surveillance, defined by the Centers for Disease Control as "the ongoing, systematic collection, analysis, interpretation, and dissemination of data regarding a health-related event that is for use in public health action to reduce morbidity and mortality and improve health."[6] This method of data gathering can be combined with others to assess the

Figure 4.2

Distribution of key data sources used to derive the 2005 maternal mortality estimates

Total number of countries: 171

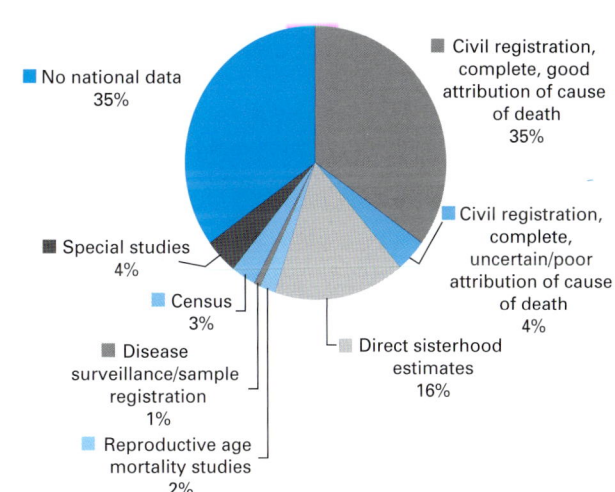

Source: World Health Organization, United Nations Children's Fund, United Nations Population Fund and the World Bank, *Maternal Mortality in 2005: Estimates developed by WHO, UNICEF, UNFPA and the World Bank*, WHO, Geneva, 2007, p. 9.

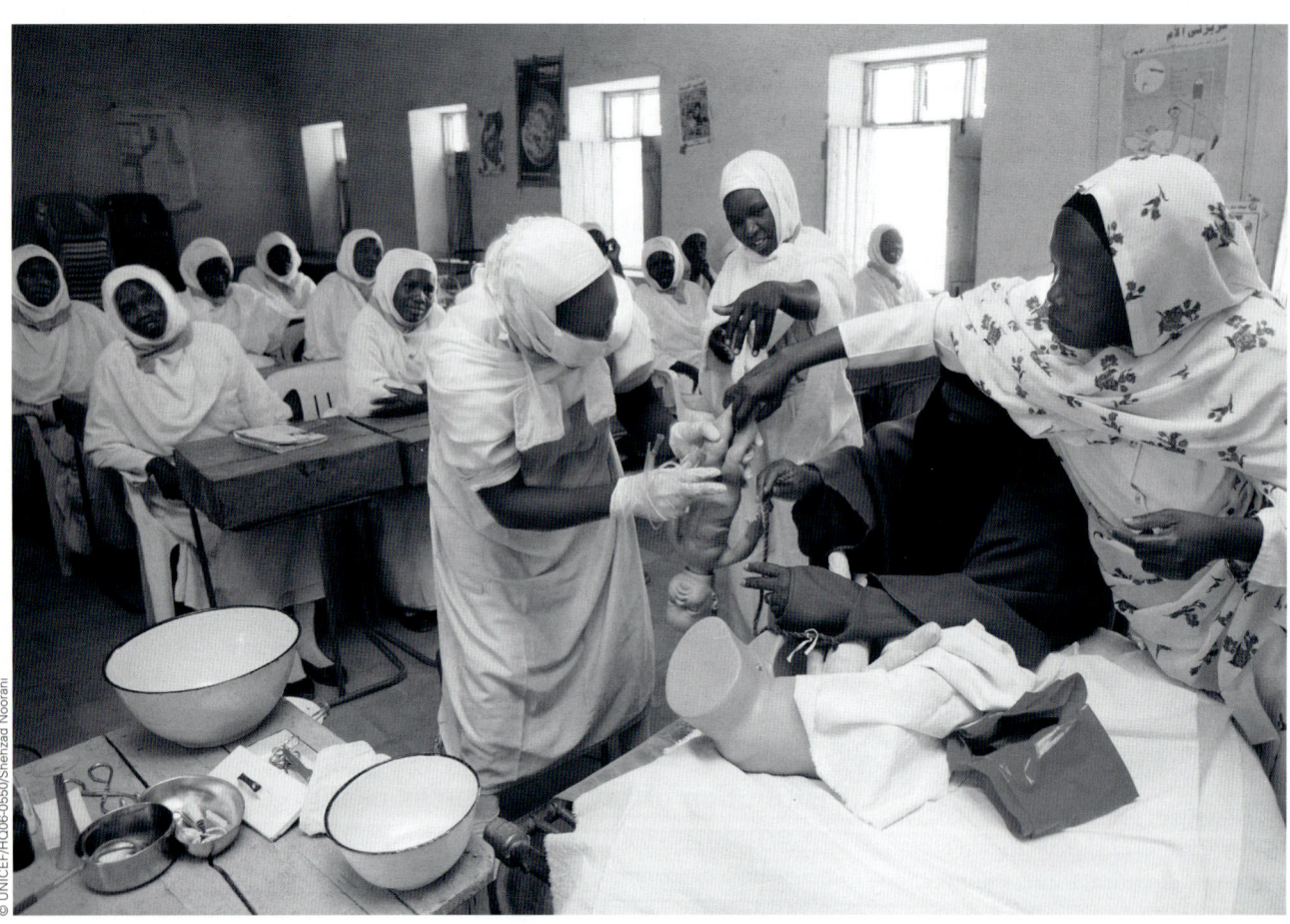

Increasing the number of births attended by skilled health workers can reduce maternal deaths arising from complications during childbirth. *Two teachers demonstrate proper procedures for holding a baby after delivery during a training session for women at a midwives training centre, Sudan.*

health of a population over time and by geographical area.

Other aspects of maternal health care are also being measured, with strong support from international agencies. Facility-based data are being collected by UNICEF and its partners to provide indicators for emergency obstetric care. Needs assessment for emergency obstetric care has also been undertaken by UNICEF, the United Nations Population Fund and Columbia University in the Averting Maternal Death and Disability Project.[7]

The Health Metrics Network, an international partnership dedicated to helping countries strengthen their health management information systems, has developed a tool to assess the completeness and quality of such systems (*see Panel on Enhancing health information systems: The Health Metrics Network, page 104*). The World Health Organization has led the development of a guide entitled *Beyond the Numbers*, which describes methods that can be used to relate the story of a woman's death as part of efforts to reduce maternal mortality. These methods included community-based verbal autopsies, facility-based maternal death or near-miss reviews, clinical audits, and larger regional or national confidential enquiries.[8] In Mozambique, a review of maternal deaths in health facilities has provided valuable insights into the preventable factors behind these deaths and guided policy and system responses.[9]

Using critical link methodology in health-care systems to prevent maternal deaths

by Rosa Maria Nuñez-Urquiza, National Institute of Public Health, Mexico

Critical link methodology (CLM) examines each maternal death as a sentinel event. It reviews all the health-care interactions between a woman and health personnel prior to her death, providing a timeline of health-seeking actions and corresponding care provision across the health system.

CLM assesses health care through three dimensions:

- clinical performance (delays, omissions and compliance with quality standards compared to established guidelines).

- internal hospital organization.

- continuity of care between health-care facilities.

Through this process of review, CLM focuses on those crucial interventions that, if provided in an expeditious manner, can avert future maternal deaths. It enables safe motherhood committees to shift their focus from a medical cause of death to a managerial perspective of missed opportunities. This change in perspective is highlighted through the following lines of enquiry:

- *During which interactions between the woman and the health system could the condition leading to her death have been better addressed?*

- *Based on this analysis, what specific steps must be done differently in the future to prevent the deaths of women in similar circumstances?*

- *To sustain these specific changes, what processes in each care unit require modification to ensure quality of care, and what factors of the health system should be redesigned to ensure the continuity of care during obstetric emergencies?*

Furthermore, the comparison of near-miss cases (complications that lead to severe morbidity but which ultimately do not prove fatal) with cases of maternal mortality highlights the imperative of timely provision of care. This has resulted in a new category of analysis: therapeutic time interval, which calls for clinical research to establish the time interval during which interventions are effective. The therapeutic time interval helps demonstrate that even when appropriate treatment is provided, it may fail to save women's lives unless applied in a timely manner.

From single-case red alerts to further research

Open and regular communication between CLM field supervisors and federal authorities ensured that alerts detected by individual case studies spurred further analysis of routine data systems (hospital registries of 1,029,000 obstetric patients yearly from 617 public hospitals) to explore the magnitude and distribution of these gaps in maternal care across the health system.

One such example is provided by a CLM study of women with post-partum haemorrhage who died as they were transferred from community hospitals to referral hospitals. The assessment identified the lack of stabilization of women prior to transportation as a fatal omission. In the seven states where the percentage of maternal deaths due to post-partum haemorrhage was above the national average, up to 60 per cent of maternal deaths occurred while transporting patients to larger hospitals. When ambulances and trained personnel were provided in one of those health districts, the maternal mortality rate from post-partum haemorrhage fell by 30 per cent the following year.

CLM is helping to redesign the way facilities are networked in each district health system. In addition, applying CLM necessitates involving a broader group of stakeholders than those traditionally engaged in safe motherhood committees, i.e., heads of clinical laboratories and blood banks, as well as health district administrators.

One outcome of CLM is that the reproductive health divisions at both the Ministry of Health and the Instituto Mexicano de Seguridad Social (IMSS, the Mexican social security system) now report the Causes of maternal deaths not only as medical causes, like "pre-eclampsia, sepsis, etc.," but also by detected failures in the process of care. For example, the report of maternal mortality of a given district or state health system will now state, "15 per cent of maternal deaths due to lack of IV solutions in health centres leading to failure to stabilize the women before transfer" or "10 per cent of maternal deaths due to delays in bringing in the surgeon on call to district hospitals during weekends." Seeing beyond the medical causes helps to diagnose health-system failures which, if immediately addressed, will avert maternal deaths.

See References, page 111.

New technologies are also showing potential to assist in data collection on maternal and newborn health.

Methods have also been devised to assess the quality of care delivered by health providers. Two such frameworks include the Performance Quality Improvement method developed by the United States Agency for International Development, and the client-oriented, provider-efficient services (COPE) method developed by EngenderHealth.[10]

In addition to new measurement tools, new technologies are also being applied to assist in intelligence gathering. For example, surveys using digital technologies show hope for improving data collection in the remotest areas.

In one study conducted by the Initiative for Maternal Mortality Programmed Assessment (IMMPACT) in eastern Burkina Faso, 127 interviewers using personal digital assistants captured data from 86,376 households in just over three months. Each unit cost approximately US$ 350, amounting to US$ 60,000 for the equipment; although no cost-effectiveness analysis was completed, a paper approach would have required over 1 million printed pages, 100 global positioning satellite receivers and 20 desktop computers and cost more. The PDA experiment had the advantage of immediacy of data entry, often cited as a problem in paper-based surveys. It also trained and employed local schoolchildren with the requisite linguistic competence and familiarity with mobile phones.[11]

It is apparent that there are numerous means of data collection that can provide useful information to guide programmes and policies. Dissemination and analysis of this data is essential, at local, national and international levels, to inform resources allocation and policy responses, and achieve the greatest impact in reducing maternal deaths.

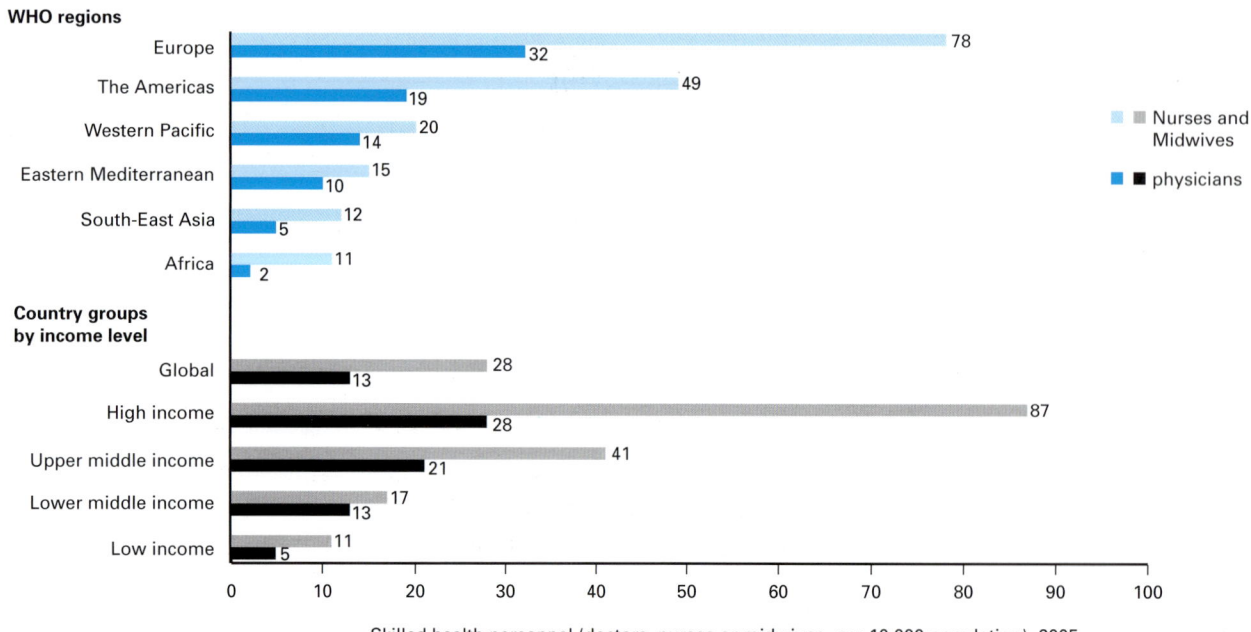

Figure 4.3

Skilled health workers are in short supply in Africa and South-East Asia in particular

Skilled health personnel (doctors, nurses or midwives, per 10,000 population), 2005

Source: World Health Organization, *World Health Statistics 2008*, WHO, Geneva, 2008, pp. 82–83.

New directions in maternal health

by Mario Merialdi, World Health Organization, and Jennifer Harris Requejo, Partnership for Maternal, Newborn and Child Health

Twenty-one years ago, the global health community came together under the auspices of the Safe Motherhood Initiative to focus on maternal mortality, whose upper and lower bounds represent the starkest disparity in international public health. Yet by 1990, the baseline year for the Millennium Development Goals, more than half a million women, 99 per cent of them in developing countries, were still dying every year due to complications related to pregnancy and childbirth. Maternal mortality estimates for 2005 indicate that around 536,000 women continue to die each year in pregnancy and childbirth, equivalent to roughly one woman dying every minute from largely preventable causes. These deaths, which are heavily concentrated in the most disadvantaged population groups within low-resource countries, are reflective of a persistent, unjust, social inequality that is long overdue for greater attention. These deaths are disproportionately occurring in sub-Saharan Africa, which accounts for half of annual maternal deaths, and South Asia (35 per cent), leaving the world a long way from its target of reducing the maternal mortality ratio by three quarters between 1990 and 2015 (Millennium Development Goal 5, Target A).

Despite the disappointing lack of progress in reducing maternal mortality since the launch of the Safe Motherhood Initiative, important advances in maternal health have been achieved on several fronts. An unprecedented amount of resources apportioned to health at the international level, combined with renewed political commitment to primary health care and with new complementary initiatives focusing specifically on maternal, newborn and child health, suggests that momentum is building to address the historically neglected issue of maternal mortality. Other developments in this direction include the adoption of the continuum of care as a core framework for public health programs; the establishment of the Partnership for Maternal, Newborn and Child Health in 2005 to guide and promote the continuum; ratification of the Maputo Plan of Action to implement the continental framework for sexual and reproductive health and rights in Africa; the addition of a new MDG 5 target (5.B) that seeks universal access to reproductive health by 2015; and the inclusion of maternal survival in the Countdown to 2015 assessments. These developments are testament to the revitalized focus in the global health community on maternal and newborn survival and well-being.

Improvements in procedures for estimating maternal mortality, new estimates of the incidence of abortion and increased efforts to map the global burden of maternal ill-health are important epidemiological advancements that will enable better decision-making by governments and their partners. The growing recognition of the causal role of undernutrition in maternal mortality has resulted in renewed interest in micronutrient supplementation during pregnancy and a stronger emphasis on the need to address underlying and basic factors, such as poverty and gender discrimination and disempowerment – including limited access to education for many girls and young women and their high exposure to infections. A broad consensus has also emerged about the core health-sector strategies required to reduce maternal mortality. Comprehensive reproductive health care is now considered to include family planning, skilled care for all pregnant women during pregnancy and delivery, and emergency care for all women and infants with life-threatening complications. Coverage indicators for proven interventions and approaches linked to each of these three pillars – including antenatal care, availability of emergency obstetric care, Caesarean section rates, contraceptive prevalence, skilled attendance at delivery, post-natal care and unmet need for family planning – are now being tracked in the Countdown to 2015 initiative, by national governments, UN agencies, international health partnerships and non-governmental organizations.

Improvements in documenting the global distribution of maternal mortality and morbidity, and identifying and tracking effective interventions, have been complemented by important research findings on ways of countering maternal health risks. Several interventions, shown to improve maternal survival in epidemiological studies and appropriate for universal application, are now ready for wide-scale implementation. These include magnesium sulphate and calcium supplementation for the prevention of hypertensive disorders of pregnancy, effective dissemination strategies for guidelines on the prevention and treatment of post-partum haemorrhage, and the recommended provision of at least four antenatal visits to pregnant women and one post-partum visit to new mothers. Increasing awareness of the inextricable link between maternal and newborn health has also resulted in the introduction of effective programmes for the prevention and treatment of malaria and HIV, through measures to expand provision of insecticide-treated mosquito nets and intermittent preventive treatment of malaria in pregnancy, interventions to prevent mother-to-child transmission of HIV, preventive measures to avoid HIV infection – particularly among young people – and antiretroviral treatment for HIV-positive women and children.

Key areas of promising research include activities focused on developing strategies for ensuring the delivery of comprehensive packages of maternal and newborn health services along the continuum of care. An essential component of these strategies is the establishment of mechanisms for integrating services traditionally delivered through vertical approaches – such as immunization and micronutrient supplementation – with antenatal and post-natal care as part of health-system strengthening. Recent years have also witnessed an encouraging trend towards the establishment of collaborative partnerships between international organizations, governmental agencies, research institutions, non-governmental organizations and the private sector to promote multi-country research projects on major complications in pregnancy and childbirth – including preterm delivery, stillbirths, impaired fetal growth, hypertensive disorders, post-partum haemorrhage and obstructed labour and obstetric fistula.

The growing political and financial support for programmatic and research initiatives aimed at improving maternal and newborn health, and the shift from single issue, sectoral approaches to health care to collaborative forms of delivering primary health care in a continuum of care, raises hopes and expectations that the long-awaited gains in maternal, newborn and child health that are so critical for the well-being and development of populations will become increasingly apparent in the near future.

See References, page 111.

Strengthening the health system in the Lao People's Democratic Republic

The Lao People's Democratic Republic is a mountainous, largely rural, country in South-East Asia with an average gross national income per capita of less than US$ 600 in 2007. Nearly 40 per cent of the population in this ethnically diverse nation – which comprises nearly 50 different ethnic groups – lives below the poverty line. Although the country is on track to meet Millennium Development Goal 4, having managed to reduce its under-five mortality rate by 57 per cent between 1990 and 2007, significant health challenges remain for mothers and newborns.

Chief among them are undernutrition, improving feeding and hygiene practices, immunization, environmental health and ensuring adequate skilled health personnel to deliver quality health services. More than 1 in 7 newborns suffer from low birthweight, a condition that is often associated with poor maternal nutrition. Exclusive breastfeeding, at 23 per cent according to the latest estimates, is far below the regional average of 43 per cent for East Asia and the Pacific. Only 60 per cent of the population have access to improved drinking-water supplies, and just 48 per cent have access to adequate sanitation facilities. Access to both of these critical services is far lower still in rural areas. In 2007, only 40 per cent of infants under age one were immunized against measles and just 47 per cent of pregnant women were immunized against neonatal tetanus. With maternal mortality standing at 660 deaths per 100,000 live births in 2005, the Lao People's Democratic Republic has the highest rate of maternal deaths in the region. The lifetime risk of maternal death stood at 1 in 33 in 2005.

Notwithstanding these challenges, advances are steadily being made to expand health services to the country's large rural population. One such programme involves Save the Children Australia, which has worked with the Provincial Health Office and other partners in Sayaboury to expand and enhance primary-health-care infrastructure in four three-year phases. Their goals are:

- **Phase I:** Strengthen the provincial management team responsible for training district teams and village health volunteers and traditional birth attendants, develop fixed and mobile maternal and child health clinics and provide essential equipment.
- **Phase II:** Integrate primary health care at all levels – provincial, district and village.
- **Phase III:** Expand programmes into four remote districts.
- **Phase IV:** Strengthen the skills of health workers through adoption of the Integrated Management of Childhood Illness framework.

The programme also prioritizes education for women in improved nutrition practices, including breastfeeding and complementary foods, since studies have shown strong linkages between inappropriate feeding practices and child undernutrition in the Lao People's Democratic Republic. The dissemination of other health information, including clinical care and immunization, is also an important component of the programme.

The Sayaboury programme has shown significant success, at a highly affordable cost of around US$4 million over a 12-year period, representing a per capita expenditure of just US$ 1 per year. The district's maternal mortality ratio fell from 218 per 100,000 live births to 110 per 100,000 live births between 1998 and 2003. The median age at which infants received complementary foods increased from 2.8 months in 1999 to 3.7 months in 2001, while the rate of exclusive breastfeeding for the first four months rose from 28 per cent in 1999 to 66.2 per cent in 2004. Vaccination coverage remained inadequate, however, with only 50 per cent of children under age one receiving three or more doses of diphtheria, pertussis and tetanus vaccine – the benchmark indicator for routine immunization coverage – in 2007.

Complementing efforts to improve maternal and newborn health, the Caring Dads communication campaign encourages fathers to support pregnant women and mothers in caring for themselves and their babies. The Ministry of Health, in collaboration with UNICEF and the Lao Trade Union, has collaborated on comprehensive methods to advocate for greater involvement by men in family care. These campaigns are aimed primarily at wage-earning fathers, who have been identified as the group most likely to engage in commercial sex, the source of the growing HIV prevalence within the country. While the Lao People's Democratic Republic has a lower adult HIV prevalence rate than some of its neighbouring countries, poverty and cross-border migration are contributing to the spread of the virus. Posters and booklets on themes such as the Caring Dad in Pregnancy have been reprinted because of unexpectedly high demand.

Such programmes aimed at community initiatives in health, together with expanded immunization and supplementation campaigns supported by UNICEF in 2007 and health infrastructure-building, are steadily beginning to help reduce the still high burden of maternal and newborn deaths in the Lao People's Democratic Republic.

See References, page 111.

Addressing the health worker crises is critical to improving maternal and newborn health. The greatest shortages are in Africa and Asia.

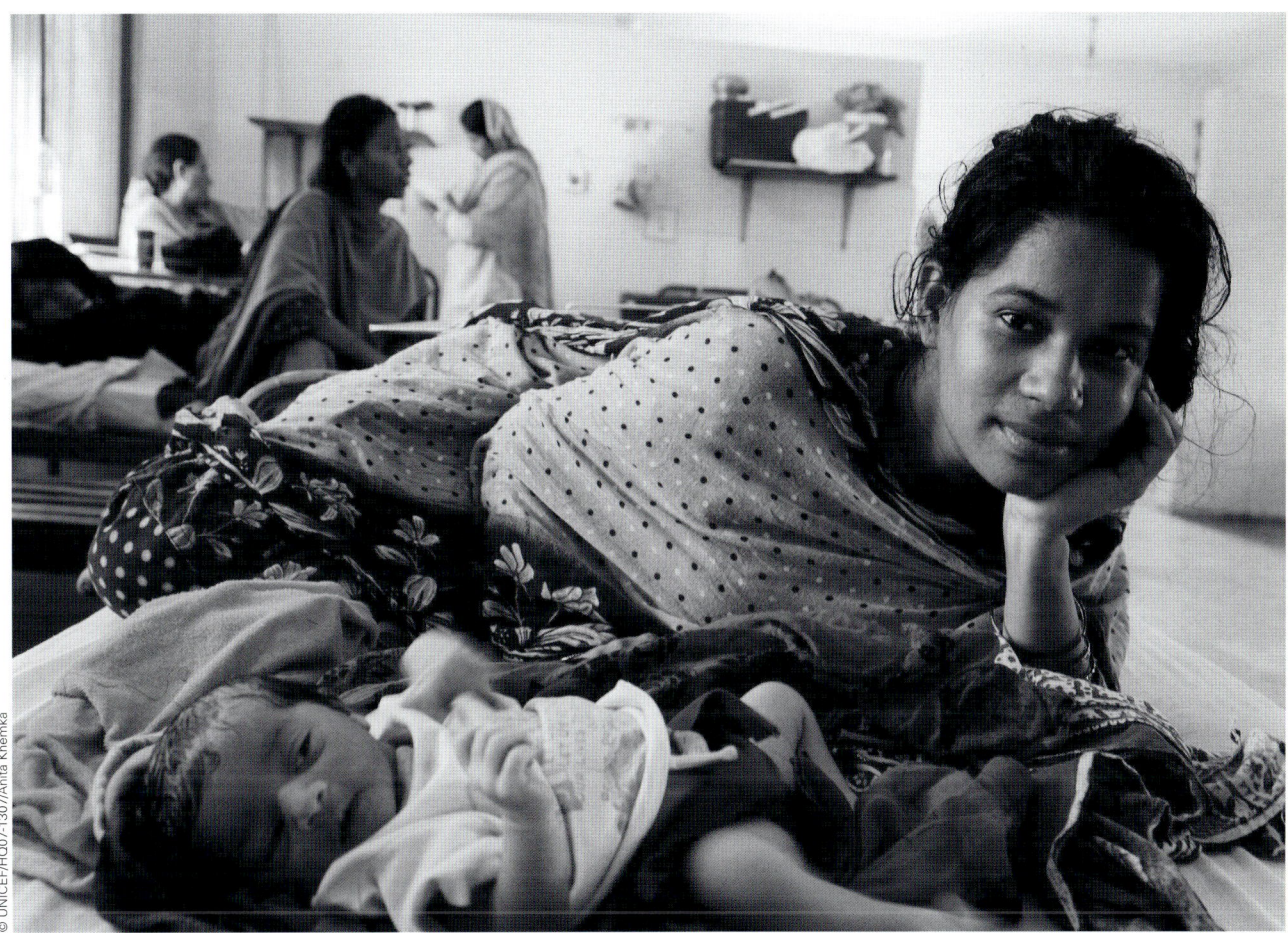

Averting maternal death helps safeguard the survival and health of newborns. *A mother lies in bed with her newborn daughter in a maternity ward after a successful delivery, Pakistan.*

Step 2: Enhancing human resources, training and supervision

Many developing countries are facing an acute shortage of skilled health workers. Mass migration, AIDS and armed conflict are among the key factors debilitating national health workforces, which in turn is constraining progress in reducing maternal and newborn mortality and morbidity. Furthermore, the distribution of health workers is uneven, with greater concentration in developed countries compared to developing countries, and in urban areas relative to their rural counterparts within countries.

In 2006, research by the World Health Organization recommended that countries should have an average of 2.28 health-care professionals per 1,000 population to achieve adequate coverage of skilled health personnel at delivery. Of the 57 countries that fall below this threshold, 36 are in sub-Saharan Africa. The greatest shortage of health workers in absolute terms is in Asia, especially India, Indonesia and Bangladesh, but the largest relative need is in sub-Saharan Africa, where the number of health workers must increase by 140 per cent to reach the requisite density.[12] In the *World Health Report 2005*, the World Health Organization estimates that increasing coverage of maternal health care for women by

57 countries – 36 in sub-Saharan Africa – have less than the WHO minimum threshold of 2.28 health workers per 1,000 population that would provide adequate skilled assistance at delivery.

2030 would require coverage levels to rise threefold, with 334,000 skilled health attendants needed to reach 73 per cent coverage of births worldwide by 2015 – along with thousands more doctors, surgeons, anaesthetists, technicians and maternity units within facilities.[13]

No substitute exists for the presence of skilled health workers at delivery, which has been a common factor across a set of countries with diverse profiles that have succeeded in lowering maternal mortality rates. A skilled birth attendant is defined by the World Health Organization as "an accredited health professional – such as a midwife, doctor or nurse – who has been educated or trained in management of uncomplicated deliveries and post-natal care and in the identification, management and referral of complications in women and newborns."[14] Yet the skills of health workers who fall into this category vary widely by country, and not all health workers described as 'birth attendants' have the skills required.

Midwives or other mid-level providers who have been trained for shorter periods and require lower entry education qualifications should form one cadre within a spectrum of health workers who can undertake different roles, distribute workloads, and build a referral system for pregnant women and newborns. It is also critical to ensure that trained birth attendants are supported by an

Figure 4.4

Uptake of key maternal, newborn and child health policies by the 68 Countdown to 2015 priority countries

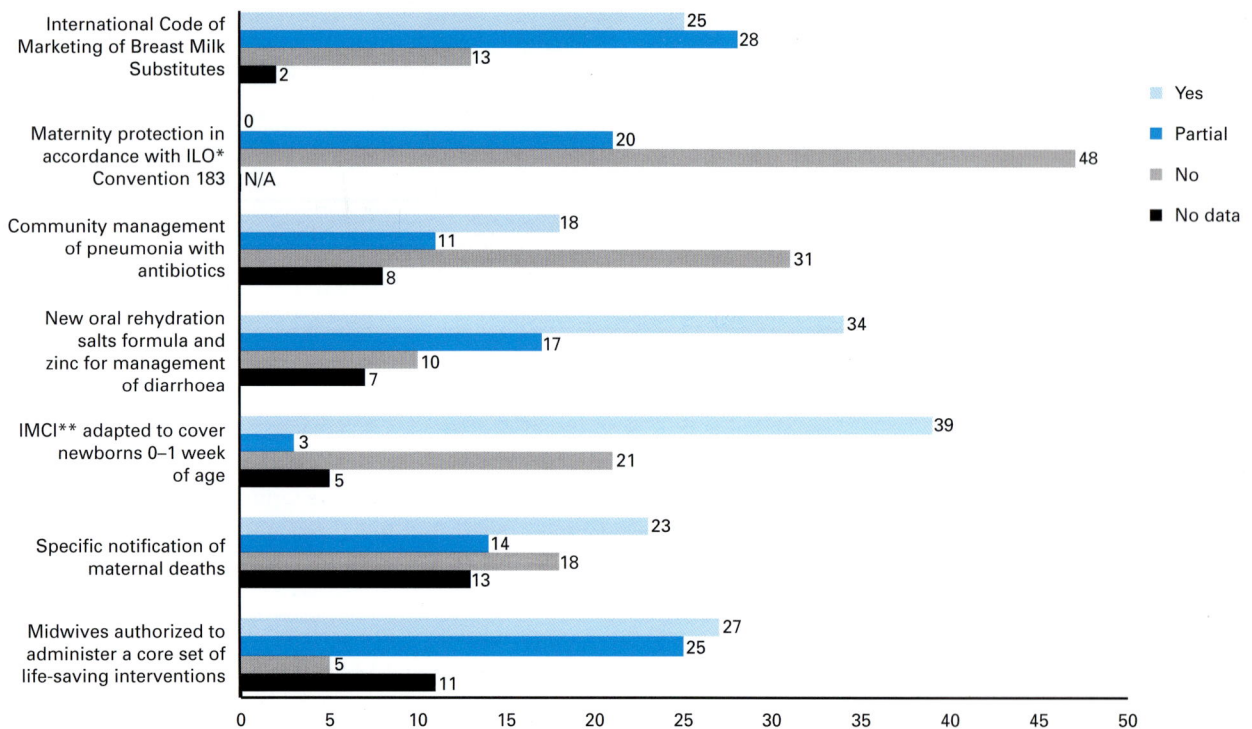

* *ILO*: International Labour Organization
** *IMCI*: Integrated Management of Childhood Illness
Source: Countdown to 2015, *Tracking Progress in Maternal, Newborn and Child Survival: The 2008 report*, UNICEF, New York, 2008, pp. 200–201.

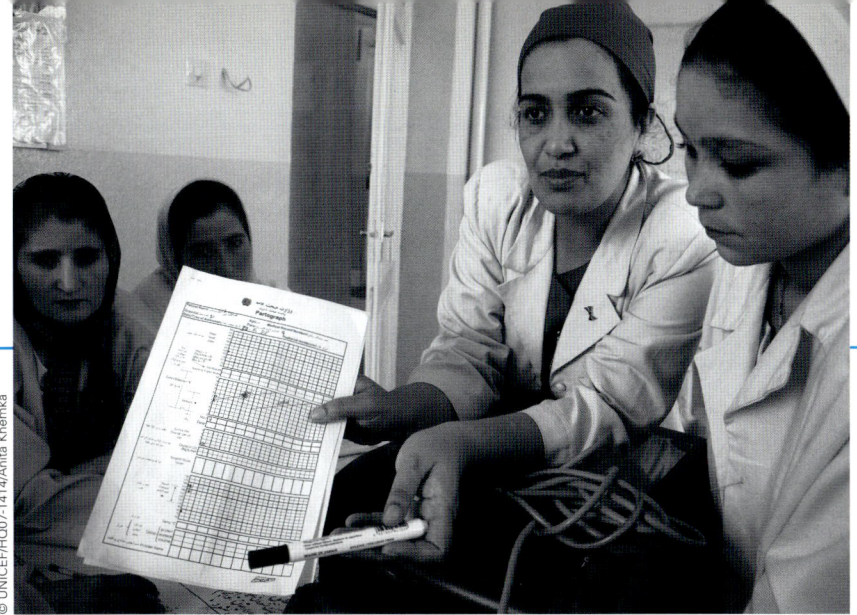

Strengthening the health workforce through recruitment, training and retention of skilled health personnel and community health workers is a key challenge for countries across the developing world. *A doctor conducts a midwifery training course at a hospital, Afghanistan.*

environment that enables their skills to be used. This requires effective teams, supplies, supervision and referral systems. In Mozambique, for example, midwives and nurse midwives have helped obstetricians provide cost-effective quality emergency obstetric care functions in under-serviced areas.[15] In Peru, community health workers pay monthly visits to 'high risk' households – defined as homes including children under one, pregnant women and women of childbearing age – and assist babies with breathing difficulties.[16] The distribution of responsibilities can give pregnant women and children more care while alleviating overdependence on an overworked, small staff.

Countries also face the challenge of developing worker-retention strategies that adequately remunerate health workers and respond to their needs. In Mali, for example, the Ministry of Health offers newly graduated doctors training, accommodation, equipment, and transportation in exchange for service in rural areas.[17] In Pakistan, the Punjab Safe Motherhood Initiative rotates postgraduate doctors from

Figure 4.5

Asia has among the lowest levels of government spending on health care as a share of overall public expenditure

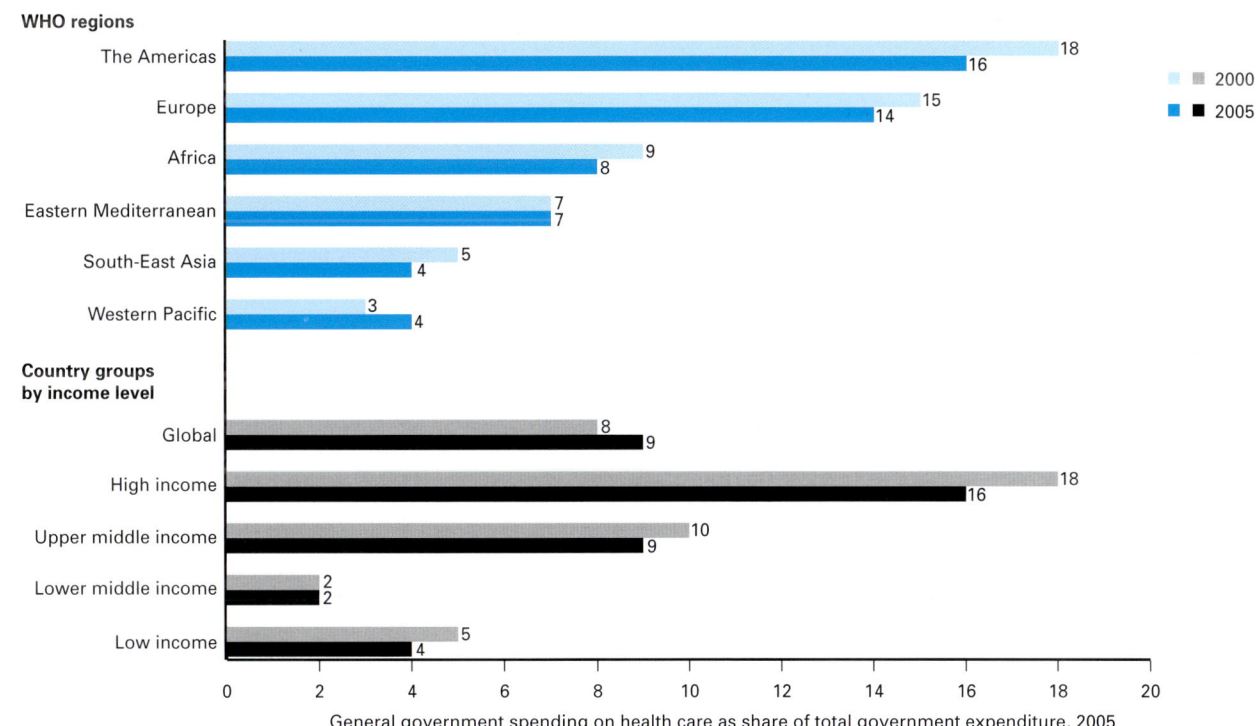

Source: World Health Organization, *World Health Statistics 2008,* WHO, Geneva, 2008, pp. 90–91.

Saving mothers and newborn lives – the crucial first days after birth

by Joy Lawn, Senior Research and Policy Advisor, Saving Newborn Lives/Save the Children-US, South Africa

Investing in post-natal care can generate high returns in maternal and newborn survival

Across the human lifespan, an individual faces the greatest risk of mortality during birth and the first 28 days of life – the neonatal period. Each year, nearly 4 million newborns die during this period – equivalent to around 10,000 per day. Three quarters of these deaths take place within one week of birth, and 1–2 million die during the first day following birth. Most of these deaths occur at home, are unrecorded, and remain invisible to all but their families. Millions more suffer severe illness each year, and an unknown number are affected with lifelong disabilities. Moreover, the risks of maternal mortality and morbidity also are highest at birth and in the immediate post-natal period.

For babies and mothers facing such complications as neonatal sepsis or post-partum haemorrhage, delay of even a few hours before appropriate care is delivered can be fatal or result in long-term injuries or disability. Important new data from Bangladesh show that a home visit on the first or second day after birth can reduce neonatal deaths by two thirds, but later visits are less effective at reducing mortality. The early post-natal period – the first seven days of life – is also the critical period for initiating high impact life-saving behaviours, including exclusive breastfeeding. Optimal breastfeeding does not start at the six-week visit for infant immunization – evidence shows that effective support and counselling in the first days of a child's life directly increase rates of exclusive breastfeeding. Other key behaviours during the neonatal period, such as hygienic cord care and keeping the baby warm, can make the difference between life and death – particularly for babies who are born prematurely. The post-natal period is also a critical time for preventing mother-to-child transmission of HIV and for providing women with access to family planning options.

Coverage gap for early postnatal care

Providing effective care for mothers and newborns during the early post-natal period has the potential to generate the greatest gains in survival and health of any period in the continuum of care. Despite this promise, however, the first days following birth are the time when coverage of appropriate services and behaviours is currently lowest. Among the 68 priority countries identified by the Countdown to 2015 initiative, a median of just 21 per cent of women received post-natal care.

Changing paradigms in post-natal care

Growing recognition of the critical importance of providing care to mothers and newborns, and the substantial gaps in coverage that currently exist, along with evidence generated mostly from trials in South Asia, have prompted paradigm shifts. Three tenets have emerged:

- **Who for?** Integration of post-natal care for mothers and newborns provides more effective and efficient care than separate approaches to post-partum and newborn care.
- **Where?** Routine post-natal visits should be provided at home or close to home, both to promote healthy behaviours and to link with curative care – instead of just hoping that the mother or baby will be brought to a health facility if problems arise.
- **When?** Early contact with mothers and babies is critical, ideally within 24 or at most 48 hours of birth for the first visit – instead of the more common visit six weeks after birth. The indicator measuring post-natal care published by the Countdown to 2015 in its 2008 report focuses on care within two days of birth. Large-scale surveys are changing to measure this indicator in more countries and communities.

Closing the gap between policy and action

Changing policies and indicators to reflect the importance of post-natal care is necessary, but not sufficient, to save lives. Services must also be scaled up to ensure high coverage and quality care during this period. While the content of a post-natal care package is fairly clear, the most effective delivery mechanism will vary, especially to provide services in remote rural areas and to reach newborns and mothers immediately after birth. Figure 4.5 maps delivery options with conditions of access to health facilities and human-resource availability in facilities and at community level. Many of the tasks involved in post-natal care can be delegated to an extension worker who is adequately supervised and effectively linked with the health system.

Case management of neonatal infections is an urgent priority

While early post-natal care visits for preventive care are immensely important, these are most effective at reducing mortality rates when integrated with curative care. Almost one third of newborn deaths result from infections; in poor, high-mortality settings, this proportion is far higher. Many of these babies are born preterm.

With an effective post-natal care package, infections in newborns will be identified early. In most countries, however, newborn illness can only be treated through referral to a health facility; even then, only a low percentage of those referred will actually seek the care. One option is to have first level, routine IMCI health-care workers begin antibiotic treatment. In countries where community health workers already provide case management for pneumonia or malaria, case management of neonatal infections may also be considered to bring care closer to home. Several Asian studies have shown how such strategies can result in large reductions in neonatal mortality, and community case management of neonatal sepsis is now being scaled up in Nepal, linked to case management of childhood pneumonia. Of the 68 Countdown priority countries, 39 have changed policy to include case management of neonatal sepsis within the Integrated Management of Childhood Illness framework. The key challenge now is to identify the appropriate providers of such care in each country.

Closing the knowledge gap

Almost all (98 per cent) of newborn deaths occur in low- and middle-income countries. Yet most research and funding have focused on incremental advances in highly technical care for the 2 per cent of newborn deaths occurring in high-income countries. An increasing number of studies are providing new guidance on the 'how, who, when and where?' questions for provision of life-saving interventions where the majority of newborn deaths occur and particularly where access to health facilities is low. A network of studies is under way in eight African countries examining nationally adapted packages and potentially scalable cadres of workers. Analysis of lives saved and costs will help guide policies and programmes to improve maternal and newborn care in the earliest days of life.

See References, page 111.

Figure 4.6

Post-natal care strategies: Feasibility and implementation challenges

	Possible strategies for post-natal care contact	Mother-friendly	Provider-friendly	Implementation challenges
1	Mother and baby go to facility	*	***	Requires mother to go to the facility within a very short time after birth. More likely following a facility birth, but still challenging in first days after birth.
2	Skilled provider visits the home to provide post-natal care for mother and baby	***	*	Conditional on sufficient human resources, which is challenging. Providing post-natal care may not be highest priority for skilled health personnel in settings where their attendance at birth is still low. Many post-natal care tasks can be delegated to another cadre. A skilled provider may be able to provide home visits during the post-natal period if rural health facilities are quiet during afternoons.
3	Community health worker visits home to see mother and baby	***	*	Requires sufficient numbers of community health workers with adequate training, supervision and incentives.
4	Combination: Facility birth and first post-natal care visit in facility, then home visit within two to three days, with subsequent post-natal care visits at a health facility	**	**	Requires team approach between facility-based and community health workers, sufficient human resources, management and supervision, effective referral systems and an efficient information tracking system so that the progress of the mother and baby is easy to track.

Note: * Low degree. ** Moderate degree. *** High degree

Source: Lawn Joy, and Kate Kerber, editors, *Opportunities for Africa's Newborns: Practical data, policy and programmatic support for newborn care in Africa*, Partnership for Maternal, Newborn and Child Health, Cape Town, 2006.

Initiatives to include community partnerships in supporting maternity services are showing promise in several developing countries.

sub-district hospitals to the district hospital in Sheikhupura, providing quality obstetric and emergency care 24 hours a day.[18] Other non-financial incentive schemes, such as short-term rotation of midwives, training opportunities and psychosocial support groups, have been used in southern and eastern Africa, with varying degrees of success, but larger-scale implementation and further research are required to fully evaluate their impact.[19]

Step 3: Fostering social mobilization

Supply-side measures cannot be successful without strengthening demand for quality health care at the level of households and communities. Social inclusion must be prioritized and individual families – particularly women – and communities must be included and treated as partners in health-care provision. Numerous cases show that negative experiences from contacts with formal health-care facilities can dissuade families and even entire communities from seeking care.

One of the most important interventions to improve maternal and neonatal health is the recognition of preventable risks. Entrenched cultural attitudes and beliefs often surround pregnancy and childbirth, and women themselves may be blamed for their own ill health and disease, and the mortality and morbidity of newborns. Where stillbirths and newborn deaths are common, they may not be seen as preventable. While communities cannot be forced to accept alternative practices, they can become partners in the promotion of their own health and well-being and that of their mothers and children.

Although health education is central to fostering healthy practices and behaviours and appropriate knowledge for care seeking, partnerships that involve key community stakeholders directly in health

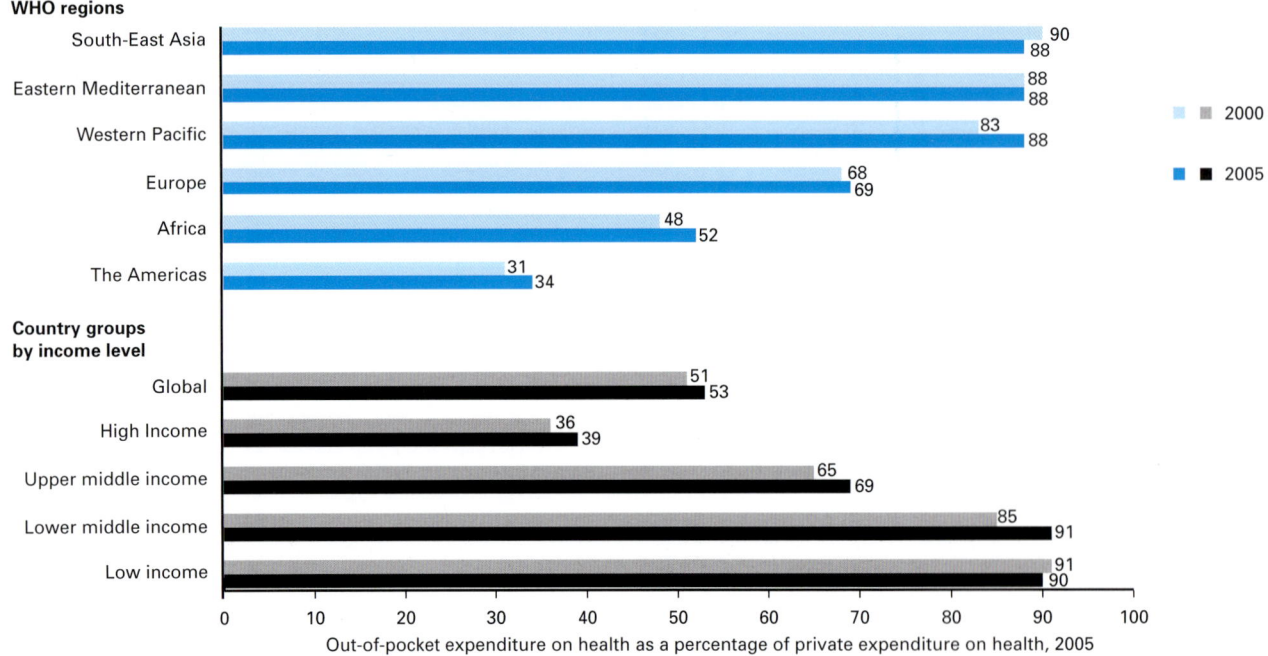

Figure 4.7

Lower-income countries pay most of their private health-care spending out of pocket

Out-of-pocket expenditure on health as a percentage of private expenditure on health, 2005

Source: World Health Organization, *World Health Statistics 2008*, WHO, Geneva, 2008, pp. 90–91.

Mobilizing families, including men and other relatives, to recognize and respond to health risks is essential to strengthen the supportive environment for maternal and newborn health.

Burundi: Government commitment to maternal and child health care

Burundi is one of the world's least developed countries. Protracted civil war and halting political restructuring have stymied economic and social progress. Poverty rates are soaring, with nearly 88 per cent of Burundians living on just US$ 2 a day. Undernutrition affects 66 per cent of the population, and more than half of children under age five suffer from moderate or severe stunting. In 2005, women faced a lifetime maternal death risk of 1 in 16. The adjusted maternal mortality ratio stood at 1,100 deaths per 100,000 live births in 2005, and the neonatal mortality rate was 41 per 1,000 live births in 2004.

Burundi has learned through experience the importance of providing affordable, quality health care for the poor in general, and for mothers and children in particular. In February 2002, the Government implemented a cost-recovery programme that required patients to pay for medical consultations, tests and drugs. The initiative aimed to generate resources for a nascent health-care system and was implemented in 12 of 17 rural provinces, covering 5 million of the country's 8.5 million inhabitants. The programme's introduction increased the numbers of patients who were unable to pay for the medical services they received in public hospitals, and many of them were subject to detention in the facility. Women who had delivered by Caesarean section comprised an estimated 35 per cent of indigent hospital patients included in a 2006 Human Rights Watch report on patient detentions; 10 per cent of the indigent patients in the study were children. In addition to the burdensome expenses, health-care services for women and children were often of poor quality.

The current Government, led by President Nkurunziza, has begun to take steps towards tackling this health-care crisis. In 2005, when Burundi joined the International Monetary Fund-World Bank 'Heavily Indebted Poor Countries Initiative' with interim debt relief in 2005, the health budget was tripled. In 2006, the Government took the critical step of announcing free health care for pregnant women and children. A new policy, 'Road Map for the Reduction of Neonatal and Maternal Mortality', was drawn up and launched in that same year with the assistance of the United Nations Population Fund, World Health Organization, World Food Programme and UNICEF. Another important step was taken in 2007, when Burundi was one of eight countries to join the International Health Partnership, a country-led and outcome-driven collaboration between governments, international organizations and non-governmental organizations. A major objective of this partnership is to identify a set of key goals, which include raising the number of institutional deliveries and increasing services to prevent mother-to-child transmission of HIV.

Burundi's National Reproductive Health Policy now includes newborn care as a critical strategy in reducing child mortality. A central feature of this policy will include scaling up services to prevent mother-to-child transmission of HIV. The median HIV-infection prevalence rate for young pregnant women aged 15–24 in Bujumbura stood at 16 per cent in 2005. One area for future programming may be securing greater male support for prevention of mother-to-child transmission strategies.

The country has also embarked on providing badly needed basic health care that will positively affect women and children. Immunization programmes have provided tetanus toxoid vaccine to nearly three quarters of women in high-risk districts. Such efforts have galvanized stakeholders at the national and local levels. But sustained governmental prioritization of health care for the poor will be necessary for the continued support of international and grass-roots actors in building Burundi's health infrastructure.

See References, page 112.

Financing quality health care is a global challenge. Almost one third of the 68 priority Countdown to 2015 countries spend less than the initiative's minimum threshold of US$ 45 per person each year.

provision are also important. One such example is under way in Burundi, where traditional birth attendants have been included in institutional deliveries as assistants to formal health-care workers and new mothers, who share food and other gifts rather than paying the attendants money.[20]

Health systems can also enlist communities through inclusion rather than coercion. Policymakers in Ecuador took such an approach by legally integrating intercultural approaches in reproductive and sexual health, with the aim of encouraging greater participation of indigenous women in sustainable health development. This strategy may help address the belief of some indigenous women that their cultural practices, such as vertical positioning during delivery, were excluding them from modern health services.[21]

Engaging men and other family members

The goal of greater unity requires not just inclusion of more women but of men as well. Studies suggest that men perceive a myriad of complications that result in maternal mortality, yet they do not always recognize their own roles in preventing these deaths. More extensive research on men's roles in maternal and child survival and health is needed because most currently available studies focus on economic provision and less on disease prevention, care, nutrition, and other health determinants.[22]

Just as male and female parents can be mobilized, so, too, can other family members. In many societies where extended kin live in close proximity, in-laws and other older relatives have influence in health-care decision-making. In Mali, for example, the involvement of grandmothers in community education led to increased awareness of good nutrition for mothers and babies and the detrimental effects of heavy work for mothers as well as greater involvement by fathers in the care of their partners and newborns. The programme also improved relations between women and their

Figure 4.8

Low-income countries have only 10 hospital beds per 10,000 people

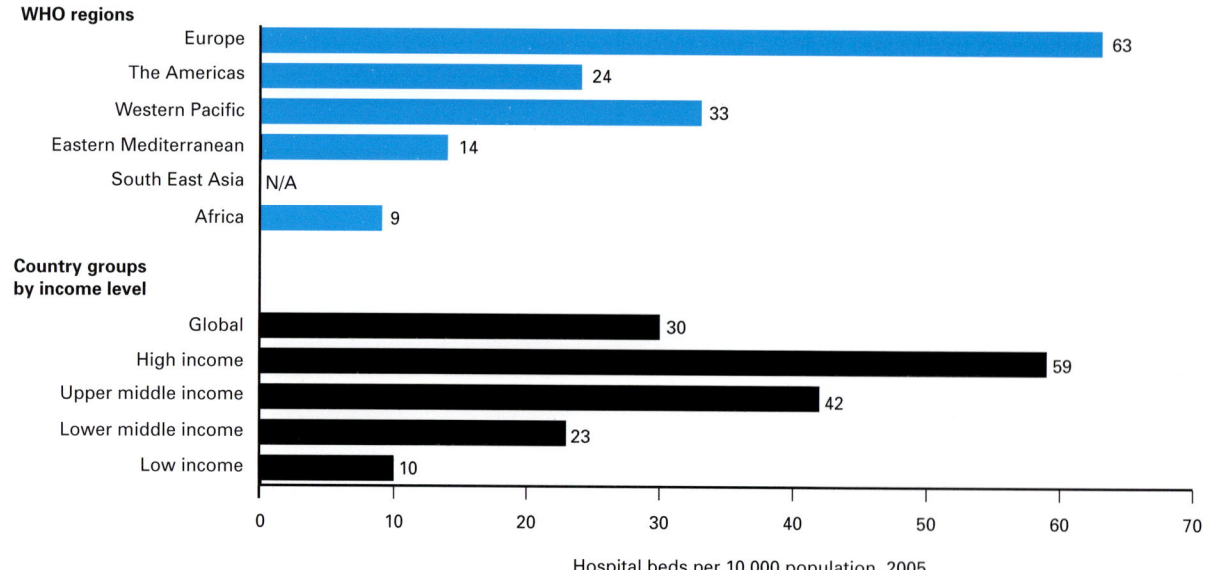

Source: World Health Organization, *World Health Statistics 2008,* WHO, Geneva, 2008, pp. 82–83.

84   THE STATE OF THE WORLD'S CHILDREN 2009

Integrating maternal and newborn health care in India

India's progress is critical to improving maternal and newborn health on a regional and global scale. According to the latest international estimates, India's maternal mortality ratio stood at 450 per 100,000 live births in 2005, while the neonatal mortality rate was 39 per 1,000 live births in 2004. Both figures represent reductions of rates in previous years. Yet even as its economy grows rapidly – with real gross domestic product expanding at an average annual rate in excess of 9 per cent in 2007–2008 – widening disparities are prevalent in health outcomes between income groups and between social and caste groups. Growing inequities, combined with shortages in the provision of primary health care and the rising cost of care, are complicating the country's efforts to meet the health-related Millennium Development Goals.

With a total population of roughly 1.1 billion, broad environmental and sociocultural diversity and an intricate political system comprising 28 states and 7 union territories, India's efforts to manage its citizens' health care have been largely decentralized. The Government of India has emphasized expanding primary health care, which is, by constitution, under the purview of the states. Beginning in 2000, it began a greater push to provide care to women and children in rural areas and in poor-performing states such as Bihar, Orissa and Rajasthan. It has also encouraged private health care, which few can yet afford, while spending on public health care has fallen to just 2 per cent of gross domestic product.

To address the widening disparities, the Government of India has issued a commitment to 'inclusive growth'. One such initiative is Janani Suraksha Yojana, a government-sponsored project under the National Rural Health Mission that provides cash incentives for antenatal care during pregnancy, assisted institutional delivery, and post-partum care by field-level workers. The benefits extend to all pregnant women aged 19 and older living below the poverty line in 10 states, for up to two pregnancies. Women who are not enrolled in the programme but who experience complications such as obstructed labour, eclampsia and sepsis are also eligible for benefits. The programme also includes a mechanism for accrediting and compensating participating private practitioners.

According to one follow-up study undertaken in select districts in Rajasthan in 2007–2008, Janani Suraksha Yojana has increased access to antenatal and post-natal care. The review also revealed that 76 out of 200 participants in the study, or nearly 40 per cent, were girls under 18, the legal age of marriage in India. The programme is successfully expanding access to care while allowing the Government to monitor more closely the situation of girls and women.

Some states have also taken the initiative to inaugurate health partnerships with the private sector. In Gujarat state, one of India's most developed provinces, the shortage of skilled health-care providers has prompted the state government to join with private hospitals to provide free obstetric care for pregnant women living below the poverty line, especially those of scheduled castes and scheduled tribes. Chiranjeevi Yojana – meaning 'a programme for long life' – was launched in 2005 and operates through a memorandum of understanding between the Government of Gujarat and private obstetricians. For every delivery, the Government pays Rs 1,795 (US$ 40), which also includes Rs 200 towards transportation costs for each patient and Rs 50 for the person accompanying the beneficiary, to compensate for the loss of earnings.

In 2006, a United Nations Population Fund study of Chiranjeevi Yojana reported that the programme had successfully raised the number of births delivered in health facilities, and that private practitioners were mostly enthusiastic about their participation in the initiative. It also noted the reluctance of patients to utilize facilities for births, and that their spouses and in-laws had great influence on decision-making, which limited their ability to actively seek healthcare. The study made several recommendations, including the establishment of an independent body to ensure quality control and equitable implementation.

The Gujarat Government's initiative is a departure from previous practice in that it took sole responsibility for the reimbursement of private health-care providers, rather than relying on intermediary parties such as insurers. The state government is working with professional agencies such as associations of obstetricians and academic organizations to plan and implement the new arrangements.

Showing remarkable successes, the programme has been expanded from five to all 25 districts of Gujarat. Between January 2006 and March 2008, 180 doctors were enlisted. Nearly 100,000 deliveries were performed, with each doctor performing an average of 540. While a promising experience, ongoing monitoring and evaluation are required to ensure improvements are made and the desired impact is achieved.

See References, page 112.

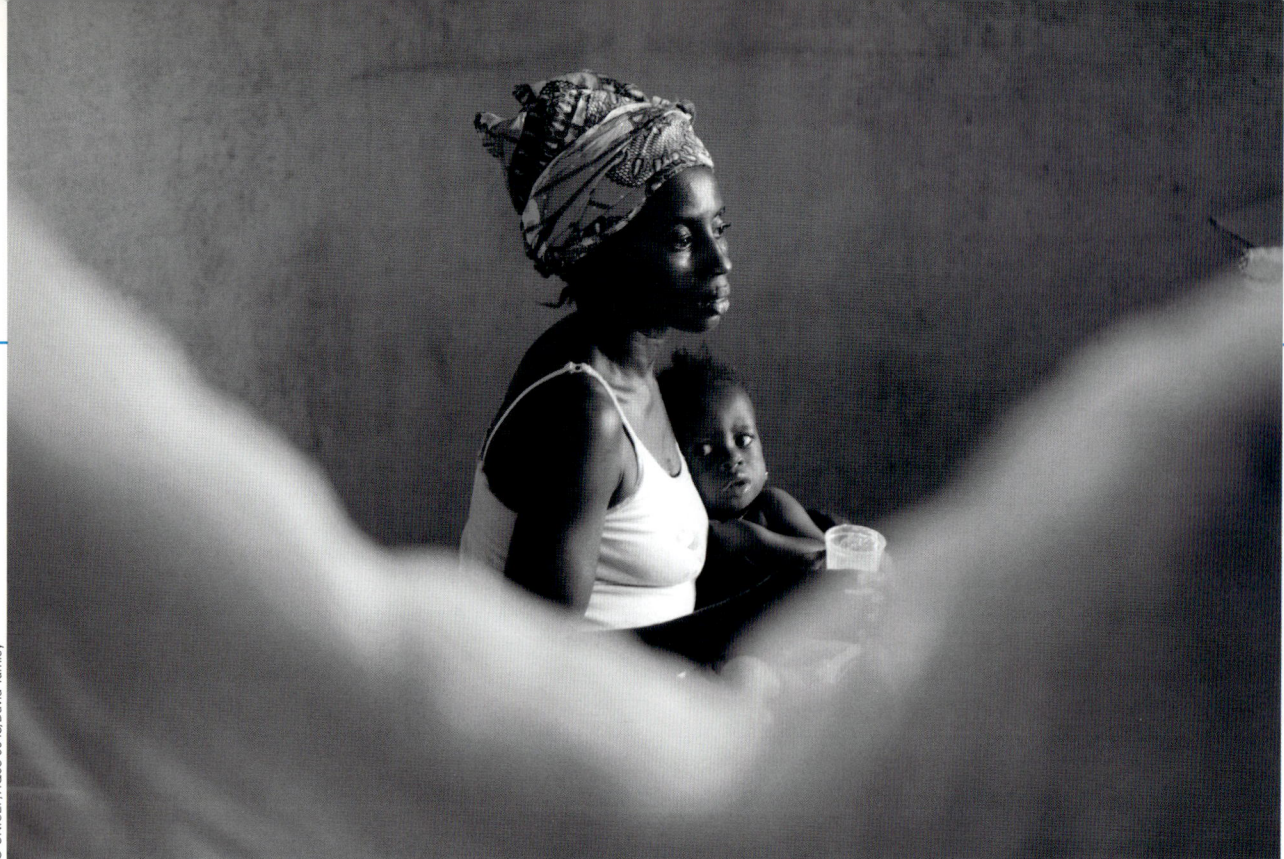

Strengthening and integrating maternal and neonatal care requires national and international commitment and global health partnerships among agencies and institutions. *A woman holds her toddler and a cup of complementary food, Sierra Leone.*

mothers-in-law, reducing shame and mistrust that had created distances between them.[23]

Step 4: Ensuring equitable and sustainable financing

Financing quality health care is a global challenge for industrialized and developing countries alike. Although there are no internationally agreed thresholds on minimum per capita total spending, the Countdown to 2015 initiative has estimated that per capita spending of less than US$45 is insufficient to provide quality basic health care services. Among the 68 priority countries for maternal, newborn and child health identified by the Countdown to 2015 initiative, 21 have spending of less than US$45 per capita.[24]

Public expenditure on health can be a key determinant of health system capacity. Countries with low rates of spending per capita may be associated with poor health outcomes, gaps in staffing, and weak investment in health-care infrastructure and logistics.[25] Data from the Pan-American Health Organization have shown that in 2004, the average expenditure on public health was just 2.6 per cent of gross domestic product for low- and middle-income countries as a whole, in sharp contrast to the near 7 per cent of GDP spent by high-income countries. South Asia had among the lowest rate of spending, at just 1.1 per cent of gross domestic product. While sub-Saharan Africa spends slightly more of its GDP on health care (2.4 per cent in 2004), only a few countries in this region are meeting the commitment made in the 2001 Abuja Declaration of apportioning 15 per cent of their national budgets to health care spending.[26]

Countries and donors are increasingly recognizing the pivotal importance of maternal and newborn health care in equitable social and economic development. Many governments, even in low-resource areas, are exploring different strategies for helping families manage the costs of routine and emergency obstetric and newborn care. Various options are possible, including reducing or eliminating direct user charges; implementing social protection initiatives such as cash transfers and vouchers on either a conditional or unconditional basis; and introducing national or community health insurance or subsidizing private provision of health care for poor households.[27]

Direct user charges

A key area of debate in health financing is direct user charges, which are an important barrier to accessing health services, particularly for poor people. Removing user fees has the potential to improve access to health services, especially for the poor. Several countries across the developing world have already abolished, or are in the process of eliminating,

Options for improving equity in maternal and newborn health care include increasing health budgets, eliminating direct user charges, implementing insurance initiatives and cash transfer programmes.

some or all direct charges – often with encouraging increases in access to health-care services. These countries range from Burundi in Eastern Africa (*see Panel on page 83*) and Ghana in West Africa to selected districts of Nepal.[28]

No systematic evaluation of user fee removal across developing countries has taken place so far. Preliminary evidence suggests that in countries where user fee removal was not supported by other policy measures, such as increased national budgets for health care or careful planning and deliberate implementation strategies, health system problems tended to increase and performance weakened. In countries where fee removal was carefully planned and managed, however, there are signs of increased utilization of services and indications that the poor may have benefited most, although the incidence of catastrophic expenditures among the poor did not fall.[29]

The experiences of Uganda and South Africa suggest that for fee removal to be effective, it needs to be part of a broader package of reforms that includes increasing budgets to offset lost revenue, maintain quality and respond to increased demand. It also requires clear communication and wide stakeholder buy-in, careful monitoring to ensure that official fees are not replaced by informal fees, and appropriate management of the alternative financing mechanisms that are replacing user fees.[30]

It should be emphasized that user fees are not the only barrier that the poor face. Other cost barriers include informal fees; the cost of medicines, laboratory and radiology tests not supplied in public health facilities; travel, food and accommodation; and charges in private health-care facilities. These costs generally make up a significant proportion of the total costs that households face and disproportionately affect the poor.[31]

In addition, a number of quality, information and cultural barriers must also be overcome before the poor can access adequate health services. The evidence indicates that the poor are disproportionately affected by these non-cost barriers.

Although user fees are only one of many barriers facing the poor, they are among the most amenable areas for policy action. As the recent experience from Uganda has shown, the policy process of fee elimination can have a catalytic effect in allowing governments to confront other issues, such as drug supply and procurement, budget allocation or financial management, which pose further barriers to progress.[32]

Clearly, removing user fees is not a simple exercise. Countries that seek to move in this direction require support in planning and implementing this policy change, and need to link the removal of direct user charges to broader measures for strengthening health systems.

It should be noted that the context for user fee removal is critical, and no blanket policy is likely to address the needs of each country. Careful analysis of the country-specific situation, the equity implications of alternative financing and delivery strategies and the multiple financial and non-financial barriers to access is required to support decisions on the most appropriate course of action.

Insurance and transfers

National health insurance schemes such as Bolivia's social insurance for maternal and child health-care services can increase access for the poorest women to antenatal and delivery care.[33] Yet this form of financing is hard to expand in countries with limited formal sector employment, low incomes, dispersed households and minimal infrastructure.

Community health insurance schemes, which operate more informally and on a smaller scale than social insurance schemes, have increased institutional-delivery rates by 45 per cent in Rwanda and by 12 per cent in the Gambia.[34] A cost-sharing scheme in an urban district of Burkina Faso increased the number of emergency referrals from 84 to 683 in a year.[35] It may be difficult to expand such schemes for wider coverage, however, and they require government or donor support because they may not be self-financing and are dependent on effective community mobilization.

Conditional cash transfers and voucher schemes are being piloted

Financing and development strategies should take account of the national and local context, and also focus on indirect barriers to access, such as transport costs and infrastructure.

to generate demand for specific services among the poor. Cash transfers have increased antenatal care during the first trimester among poorer women in Mexico by 8 per cent and in Honduras by 15–20 per cent.[36] India has provided financial incentives for deliveries in facilities for women from marginalized groups in priority districts. While these initiatives have increased access to health-care services, effective improvements in maternal health outcomes may not be realized without concomitant improvements in quality of services. Continued monitoring and evaluation of these financing innovations are required to inform appropriate scale-up by policymakers.

Private-sector providers

The private sector has become an important health-care provider, particularly in Asia, but the evidence base to measure its effectiveness is still limited, with most evaluations measuring short-term changes in provider behaviour, not health outcomes or other impacts on beneficiaries. The private sector is heterogeneous in nature and encompasses a variety of providers, including traditional healers and birth attendants, church-based hospitals, spas and corporate global entities that may operate without regulation and oversight. In many low-income countries, private providers work in environments where formal regulatory controls, whether in the form of professional associations, legislative enforcement or government taxation, are weak.[37]

Attention to the emerging public-private mix in health systems is urgently required as inequitable financing profiles and the unregulated nature of the private sector can affect government commitments to health care, public confidence and socio-economic disparities. Findings from studies of private services in India, Indonesia and Mexico show the challenges of assessing quality of care across the public and private sectors and the importance of taking into consideration the national context before drawing definitive conclusions about either sector.[38] Governments face the challenge of improving the regulation of private health-care providers, using international guidelines to develop national policies that mandate minimum standards for such services as antenatal care, case management of HIV and AIDS, maximum acceptable rates for Caesarean-section deliveries and other critical issues in maternal and newborn care.

Step 5: Strengthening infrastructure, transportation, logistics, supplies and the referral process

Strengthening health systems to support maternal and newborn care requires investing in sectors that support essential maternity and basic health-care services. In addition to enhancing information systems, it is also imperative to expand human resources, foster social mobilization and establish equitable financing, and develop infrastructure, supplies, logistics, transportation and the referral process. Greater investment in expanding health-care facilities is urgently needed, particularly in low-income countries. The latest WHO estimates indicate that there are just 10 hospital beds per 10,000 population in low-income countries, compared with almost six times that number for higher-income countries.[39]

Where facilities exist, governments and other supervising agencies must ensure that they are properly functioning and maintained. In Uganda, where declines in maternal mortality have been registered, a review of emergency obstetric care facilities showed that in 54 districts out of 56 throughout the country, over 97 per cent of facilities expected to provide basic emergency services were not able to do so. Lack of running water, electricity, and functioning operating theatres were among the key impediments to service delivery.[40] Further reviews are urgently required to ensure that existing facilities are upgraded and new ones are established in a sustainable manner. Funding for medical supplies, including essential medicines, is a further priority. The UN inter-agency list of essential medicines for reproductive health serves as a useful guide to the minimum number of effective, cost-saving drugs that should be available.[41]

Plans for health infrastructure development should consider the best means of improving transportation systems to aid women and

Enhancing the quality of care is required both to ensure safety and well-being, and to encourage greater use of health-care services.

children in accessing routine and facilities-based emergency care and, in some environments, to enable mobile healthcare teams. Programmes in India (*see Panel on page 84*) and rural Nepal offer examples of how incentives can be offered to finance transportation for pregnant women.[42]

Improving transportation infrastructure will also assist in strengthening the referral process, which remains a neglected and under-researched element of emergency maternal-newborn services and of health systems more broadly. Yet it is often a crucial element for the survival of mothers and newborns.

Reducing the time between referral and getting women to facilities is often critical to their survival. In a study in rural west Maharashtra, India, the distance to general health services was 3 km for women who died from complications and 2.5 km for women who survived similar complications. But the distance to reach appropriate treatment for birth complications was 63.5 km for women who died and 39.3 km for women who survived. A study in Karnataka, India, showed that referrals of women for emergency obstetric care reflected multiple, but haphazard and frequently futile, attempts to get effective care from a range of poorly functioning government services and informal and private providers. Although informal networks connected private providers, there was no feedback or learning mechanism for referral in government services.[43]

To be more responsive and effective, referral systems must at a minimum ensure: communication between facilities to prepare for urgent cases, transportation and clinical stabilization of patients, accompaniment during referral, follow-up of each case and the ability to move care to a patient if it is too risky to transport the patient. More broadly, referral systems must assess population needs and health system capabilities, encourage active collaboration between referral levels and across sectors, formalize communication and transport arrangements, develop protocols for referrer and receiver, ensure accountability for provider performance and supportive supervision, provide protection against the financial costs, and develop indicators to monitor effectiveness.

Step 6: Improving the quality of care

Definitions of quality maternity and neonatal care have expanded from an exclusive focus on biomedical outcomes to a more inclusive approach that also takes into consideration patient rights and satisfaction, standards, equity, and the responsibilities and rights of health institutions and workers. Good quality care provides a minimum level of care to all pregnant and intrapartum women and neonates, while having the capacity to attend to those requiring emergency or more specialized services. Such care should strive to obtain the best possible medical outcome; satisfy providers, patients, and families; maintain sound managerial and financial performance; and develop existing services in order to raise the standards of care provided to all women.[44]

While existing health systems in industrialized and middle-income countries may need reform to provide more accessible and better maternity and neonatal services, emerging health systems may build quality of care mechanisms into new programmes. In Côte d'Ivoire, for example, a national programme was launched in 2000 to integrate prevention of mother-to-children transmission of HIV into existing maternal health services. A recent study has shown that the programme has improved overall quality of care in many areas, including administration of oxytocin in the third stage of labour and checking the uterus post-partum.[45] Such programmes offer staff new training opportunities and greater investment in their own responsibilities as well as critical opportunities to save lives.

Various organizations have underscored the need for emergency obstetric care by engaging in quality of care measures in such diverse countries as Mali, Peru and Viet Nam. Building on the foundation for emergency obstetric care, these measures improved and simplified reporting and monitoring mechanisms, developed protocols and standards in

Improving maternal and newborn health will require collaboration, commitment and creativity. International and national efforts are becoming increasingly cooperative in meeting the challenges of the Millennium Development Goals and other internationally agreed objectives. It is time to apply the same determination, evidence, innovation and resources that enabled swift and sustained gains to be made in many aspects of child survival to maternal and newborn health. The final chapter of The State of the World's Children 2009 *examines the collaborative partnerships and programmes that are striving to create supportive environments, establish continua of care and strengthen health systems to improve maternal and newborn health. It explores ways of strengthening collaboration, enhancing aid effectiveness and applying resources and commitment to achieve concrete results.*

The halfway point for meeting the health-related Millennium Development Goals has come and gone. The report card on progress to date has been mixed. Much has been done in recent years to accelerate advances in maternal, newborn and child health, coordinate actions and scale up essential interventions. Concrete gains have been achieved, particularly in reducing the number of deaths of children between 29 days and five years of age (the post-neonatal period) in many developing countries. International assistance for maternal, newborn and child health has risen, encouraging higher aid inflows, strengthening partnerships and consolidating frameworks for action.

The challenge is to build on these gains over the remaining years to 2015 and beyond. Particular attention must be given to the needs of Africa and Asia, the two continents that have the greatest burden of maternal and neonatal deaths. Within all developing regions, including those broadly on track to meet all or some of the health MDGs, there are countries, communities and socio-economic groups that are falling behind in their efforts to meet the goals and merit stronger efforts in support of maternal and newborn health.

The need for collaborative action is paramount. Meeting the challenge of improving maternal and newborn health will require creative, consistent and concerted efforts at the macro level to create supportive environments for women and girls, establish continua of care and strengthen health systems.

This report has reiterated a widely known truth: There is nothing mysterious about maternal and neonatal mortality. The reasons women and babies die from causes related to pregnancy and childbirth – and why millions of children die during the first 28 days of life – are well understood. Addressing them requires good data and analysis, sound strategies, adequate resources, political commitment and collaborative partnerships. As outlined in previous chapters, the weaknesses of health systems in individual countries require country-specific actions where the mix of corrective action depends on country profiles, policy choices, specific cost functions and the creation of a supportive environment for maternal and newborn health based on respect for the rights of women and children.

To this end, the final chapter of *The State of the World's Children 2009* focuses on recent developments in global health partnerships, briefly exploring three key areas: collaboration; aid effectiveness; resources and commitment for results.

Strengthening collaboration

Recent years have seen an expansion of global health partnerships, spurred in part by the emphasis on collaboration embodied in MDG 8 – which seeks to develop a global partnership for development – and the 2002 Monterrey Consensus on Financing for Development. These initiatives are having a crucial effect in several areas, particularly research, evaluation and prevention and treatment of communicable diseases such as AIDS, tuberculosis, measles and malaria.

One example relates to measles: In 2007, Africa was able to report a 91 per cent drop in measles deaths between 2000 and 2006. This unprecedented success resulted from a concerted drive by national governments and international partners to boost measles immunization.[1]

Prevention of malaria, too, is being addressed through distribution of insecticide-treated mosquito nets, increasingly available free through mass campaigns. The drive to combat HIV and AIDS, meanwhile, is making progress on many fronts. In 2007, 33 per cent of the estimated 1.5 million HIV-positive pregnant women in low- and middle-income countries received antiretroviral therapy to prevent transmission of HIV to their children, up from 15 per cent in 2005. In addition, the number of children receiving antiretroviral therapy has almost tripled, from 75,000 in 2005 to 200,000 in 2007.[2]

These are but three of the examples of how coordinated action between national governments and international partners is delivering concrete improvements in the lives of mothers, newborns and children.

Maternal and newborn health has drawn specific attention from global health partnerships and initiatives in recent years. This has led to the formation of several new collaborations that complement the work of longstanding partnerships in efforts to accelerate progress towards MDG 5.

The increase in global health partnerships for maternal, newborn and child health is not without challenges, however. Depending on the definition used, global health partnerships number over 100, and developing countries have sometimes reported difficulties in interacting with the large number of initiatives.[3] Further, while there is a consensus around the imperative of creating effective continua of care for mothers, newborns and children, the challenge remains to complement vertical flows of aid on disease-specific interventions with a strengthening of integrated approaches, combined with health-systems development.

Integrating the work of global health partnerships in establishing national continua of care is a key challenge for the coming years. Several bilateral donors are already taking steps to harmonize their collaboration and improve the effectiveness of their contributions through partnerships. These include the Global Campaign for the Health Millennium Development Goals, led by the Government of Norway; Providing for Health Initiative, led by Germany and France; the Catalytic Initiative to Save a Million Lives, led by Canada; and GAVI's Health Systems Strengthening Window.

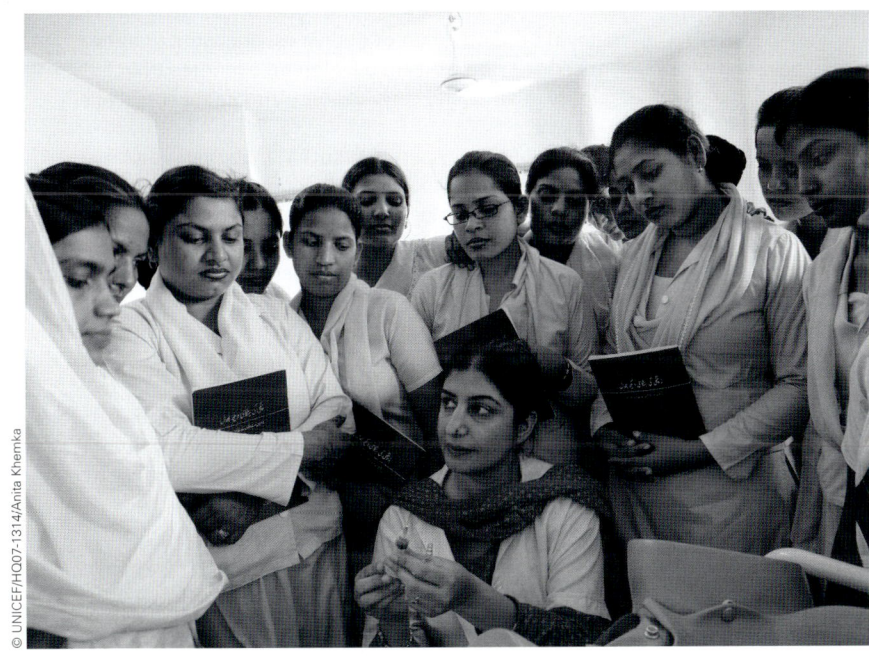

Comprehensive reproductive health care; skilled care during pregnancy; delivery by a trained midwife, nurse or doctor; and emergency obstetric care for life-threatening complications should be available to expecting mothers and newborns. *A doctor leads a training session for nursing students as part of Woman's Right to Life and Health Initiative, Pakistan.*

Focus On

Working together for maternal and newborn health

by Sarah Brown, Patron of the White Ribbon Alliance for Safe Motherhood and wife of Gordon Brown, Prime Minister of the Government of the United Kingdom.

Much of my work over the past few years has focused on preventive programmes to improve the health of infants born prematurely or following difficult pregnancies. Increasingly, by working together, the medical community in the developed world is improving interventions to ensure that a newborn arriving in difficult circumstances receives the necessary care in the first crucial stages of life to survive and enjoy quality of life.

However, the state of infant survival in the developing world sits in stark contrast to the situation in industrialized countries like the United Kingdom. As a representative of the international advisory board of the Royal College of Obstetricians and Gynaecologists, I have observed the training programmes that the RCOG conducts in numerous countries in Africa and Asia at first hand. What this practical experience has brought home to me is the realization that you cannot start saving the most vulnerable infants and children without first ensuring the health of their mothers.

The reason is simple: It is the mothers who do the work of raising their children, feeding them, getting them into school and taking them for their vaccinations. By contrast, children who have lost their mothers are almost five times more likely to die in infancy than those who still have their mothers, and motherless newborns are ten times more likely to die.

The scale of this problem becomes evident when you look at annual numbers of maternal deaths, which are little changed in almost 20 years. Across the world this year, more than half a million mothers will lose their lives in pregnancy and childbirth, and almost all of these deaths will occur in poorer countries. In addition, for every mother who dies, 20 women are left suffering from injuries and disabilities as a result of complications in childbirth.

It is vital that we – governments, non-governmental organizations, faith-based organizations, private-sector companies and committed individuals – all work together to ensure that in every country and community around the globe, women have access to essential primary health care and skilled health workers. This is what will save the lives of mothers – and so bring better life chances to newborns and children otherwise at grave risk.

If we get this right, we will save lives at every stage of the life cycle. Millennium Development Goal 5, which seeks to improve maternal health, lies at the heart of all of the MDGs. Access to skilled health workers supports the continuum of care women and their children need. Mothers give birth safely when they can access antenatal support and skilled care during childbirth and the critical time afterwards. A well staffed, well stocked health centre will also ensure that infants receive essential vaccinations and that the necessary medications are available to keep them from dying from malaria or pneumonia.

We must do more than focus on vertical solutions. All active organizations working to eradicate poverty and disease and to improve health care and education must find the opportunity to integrate delivery. We need to maximize the effectiveness of precious resources and respond to genuine local need. We have seen the difference that effective health services can make. The evidence is clear.

Japan reduced its maternal mortality rate by two thirds in the decade following 1945. It achieved this by introducing community health workers that provided consistent health care from pregnancy right through to when a child starts school. Mothers were educated on their rights and the importance of quality health care through a mother-and-child handbook of which the Japanese are rightly proud. Also important to this achievement was the vital injection of political will and momentum that continue even today. International leadership is critical to focusing attention and channelling resources for maternal health.

Right now, as we count down to the MDG deadline in 2015, we have worldwide momentum. Right now we can achieve worldwide change. Never before has this issue had so much visibility and support from so many different sources around the world. At the G8 Summit in Japan this year, for the first time, maternal health was on the agenda.

However, we must understand that governments cannot dramatically reduce maternal mortality on their own. Non-governmental organizations are increasingly making maternal health a priority and working together. They are joining grass-roots organizations, such as the White Ribbon Alliance for Safe Motherhood, whose members have been campaigning in more than 90 countries for progress. An impressive start has been made by the world's midwives, obstetricians and gynaecologists. Their professional organizations, led by the International Federation of Gynaecology and Obstetrics and the International Confederation of Midwives, are committed to working together to help developing countries train health workers in antenatal care, delivery and infant care skills.

We can all play our part in reducing maternal mortality. Individuals can campaign for change, communities can raise awareness among their men and women, and non-governmental organizations, private-sector organizations and governments can work together to find practical solutions.

Let each of us bring our skills to the table and work together to raise the bar in maternal and child health around the world.

We must work together to ensure that there is access to well-trained health workers in every country and community that needs them, and that each government is ready to put them to work.

We owe it to the millions of mothers who have lost their lives unnecessarily over the last 20 years. We owe it to the thousands of pregnant women around the world giving birth every day in fear of their lives.

We owe it to the next generation of children born in the poorest countries of the world – children who need, and deserve, their mothers.

For their part, the work of the eight major international health agencies – the World Health Organization, UNICEF, the World Bank, GAVI, the United Nations Population Fund, the Joint United Nations Programme on HIV/AIDS (UNAIDS), the Global Fund to Fight AIDS, Tuberculosis and Malaria, and the Bill & Melinda Gates Foundation – is being enriched by increased dialogue through the informal Health-Eight (H8) group. The H8, which held its inaugural session in July 2007, meets twice a year to examine the challenges to expanding key health interventions and accelerating progress towards the health-related MDGs.[4]

The International Health Partnership (IHP), launched in September 2007, is a coordinating partnership that brings together governments, donors and international agencies to harmonize their efforts and support national health development plans. Country and global compacts are the key mechanisms by which the IHP aims to support this process. In August 2008, Ethiopia became the first country in which the Government and partners have signed a country compact with the IHP. Mozambique also endorsed a country compact in September 2008, and other countries in Africa and Asia are set to sign agreements in the coming months.[5]

Improving the effectiveness of international aid

Several high-level forums have set out to tackle the problem of aid effectiveness. Based on the 2005 Paris Declaration on Aid Effectiveness, a set of best practices for global health partnerships has been generated with a focus on harmonization of efforts, alignment of support with national strategies and systems, country ownership, mutual accountability and managing for results. The OECD Development Assistance Committee has also responded to the need for further practical guidance. In September 2008, a third High Level Forum on Aid Effectiveness took place in Accra, Ghana. The Accra Agenda for Action, endorsed by the Forum's participants, deepened and strengthened the commitment. It underlined the need to accelerate aid effectiveness in three key areas: strengthening country ownership, building more effective and inclusive partnerships, and focusing on development results – and openly accounting for them.

Within the area of partnerships, the Accra Agenda for Action recommended that partnerships adopt five key tenets to improve aid effectiveness. These include:

• **Reducing the cost fragmentation of aid** through enhancing the complementarity of donor efforts and promoting a better division

Strong public investment in the overall health system and unified national and international action and commitment will lead to improved maternal and neonatal survival and health. A nurse attends a newborn at a UNICEF-supported health centre for mothers and children, Albania.

Key global health partnerships for maternal and newborn health

In recent years, global health partnerships have emerged to lend attention to, and raise resources for, maternal and newborn health. Some of the key partnerships are highlighted below.

- **The Partnership for Maternal, Newborn and Child Health** is a global health partnership launched in September 2005 that brings together maternal, newborn and child health organizations into an alliance of some 240 member groups. The Partnership, hosted and administered from Geneva by the World Health Organization, advocates for greater investment and commitment to saving the lives of mothers and children. In July 2008, it issued a Global Call asking G8 leaders to fund basic health services for women, newborns and children and urging organizations and individuals to sign on to its demands for political leadership and investment.

- **Deliver Now for Women + Children Campaign** is a new advocacy drive to eliminate maternal and child deaths and improve the health of women and children around the world, co-ordinated by the Partnership for Maternal, Newborn & Child Health. It is a response to concern that the world is lagging far behind in reaching the Millennium Development Goals (MDGs) for reducing maternal and child deaths.

- **The Global Campaign for the Health Millennium Development Goals** was unveiled on 26 September 2007 by Norwegian Prime Minister Jens Stoltenberg at the Clinton Global Initiative in New York. The Global Campaign is supported by several governments, including the UK, Norway, Canada, France and Germany, as well as a number of prominent global health and advocacy organizations. It attaches special importance to the health of women and children, "whose needs remain the most neglected." The Global Campaign brings together a number of related initiatives including:

    - **The International Health Partnership,** launched in London by UK Prime Minister Gordon Brown in September 2007, aims to help build national health systems in some of the poorest countries in the world.

    - **The Catalytic Initiative to Save a Million Lives,** launched by Canadian Prime Minister Stephen Harper in November 2007, aims to strengthen health systems by training frontline health workers and delivering affordable healthcare services directly to local communities.

    - **Innovative Results-Based Financing,** launched by Norway and the World Bank in November 2007, seeks the most cost-effective ways of obtaining better health outcomes.

    - **Providing for Health Initiative,** launched by Germany and France in 2008, aims to strengthen health systems by putting appropriate social health protection mechanisms in place with a view to achieving universal coverage.

- **Women Deliver** was launched in London in October 2007 to mark the 20th anniversary of global efforts to reduce high rates of maternal and newborn death and disability in the developing world – and to apply the knowledge gained from two decades of study and experience. The initiative aims to reframe maternal health as a basic human right and an integral strategy for achieving just development, reducing poverty and ensuring environmental sustainability. The organizing partner is Family Care International.

- **Saving Newborn Lives** is a Save the Children project to improve newborn survival in high-mortality countries. Since its launch in 2000, the initiative has reached more than 20 million mothers and babies with critical health services in 18 countries in Asia, Africa and Latin America.

- **The White Ribbon Alliance for Safe Motherhood** is an international coalition of individuals and organizations formed to promote safe pregnancy and childbirth for all women. Members of the Alliance take action in their own countries to make this issue a priority for their governments and other international organizations.

- **The Initiative for Maternal Mortality Programme Assessment** (IMMPACT) is a global research initiative whose aim is to promote better health for mothers-to-be in developing countries. By carrying out studies of different strategies, and judging their effectiveness and the value for money they represent, IMMPACT aims to improve measurement and the supporting evidence that will help in the assessment of each strategy's potential.

- **Countdown to 2015** was formed in 2005 by a group of scientists, policymakers, activists and institutions to track progress towards Millennium Development Goal 4. Coverage reports were made available at a conference for 60 priority countries for child survival initiatives. The second conference, held in April 2008, expanded the mandate of the Countdown to include maternal and neonatal survival, and the number of countries tracked in reports increased to 68.

- **Averting Maternal Death and Disability** is a global programme run by the Mailman School of Public Health, Columbia University, New York, that contributes to reducing maternal mortality and morbidity through research, advocacy, policy analysis and programme support. In recent years, the programme has operated in around 50 countries across the developing world.

See References, page 112.

Greater political and institutional commitment to maternal and newborn health is being complemented by rising financial flows to these areas.

of labour between partners. Discussions on improving the divisions of labour across countries will begin in June 2009.

- **Increasing aid's value for money** by untying aid, promoting local and regional procurement, and respecting international agreements on corporate social responsibility.

- **Working with all development actors** by recognizing the importance of South-South cooperation, encouraging developing countries to utilize their international cooperation programmes to assist other developing countries, and deepening triangular cooperation. Global funds and programmes are urged to support country ownership, align and harmonize their assistance, ensure mutual accountability and continue their focus on achieving results.

- **Deepening engagement with civil society organizations** through inviting them to examine how they can apply the Paris Declaration principles to their own activities, engage in a multi-stakeholder process to promote their development effectiveness, and provide a supportive environment that enables them to optimize their contributions to development.

- **Adapting aid policies for countries in fragile situations** through monitoring implementation of the Principles for Good International Engagement in Fragile States and Situations, conducting joint capacity and situation analysis, fostering collaboration between donors and national governments to formulate a set of practical objectives that can address the root causes of conflict and fragility, encouraging the participation of women, and working on flexible, rapid and long-term funding modalities.

These actions are particularly relevant for global health partnerships because the health sector has been chosen by donors and partner countries to monitor progress on implementing the Paris Declaration. Steps are already being taken to strengthen and harmonize aid directed towards the health sector. Important advances include: a stronger focus on harmonized approaches, capacity-building and result-based financing; compacts for mutual accountability in several countries; improvements in harmonization and alignment of aid; adoption of core principles of global health partnerships for operations at the country level; and the establishment of H8 and the International Health Partnership to ensure that aid interventions become more cohesive and comprehensive.[6]

Sustained engagement and refinement of the best-practice principles are steadily consolidating a framework for the actions of global health partnerships and a set of indicators of progress and targets that can be measured nationally and monitored internationally.

Figure 5.1

Key global health initiatives aimed at strengthening health systems and scaling up essential interventions

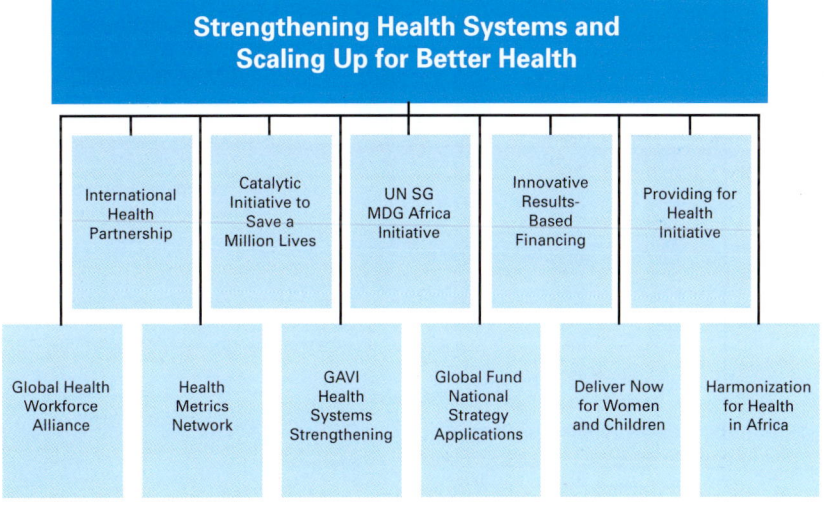

Source: International Health Partnership, <www.internationalhealthpartnership.net/ihp_plus_about_initiatives.html>, accessed 1 September 2008.

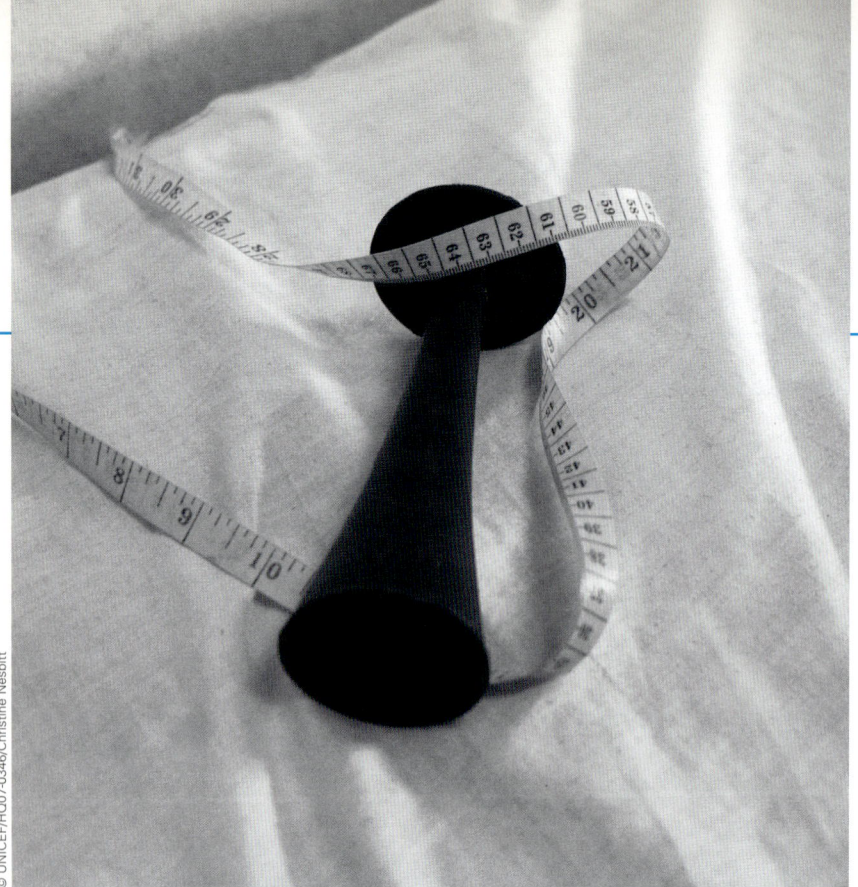

Investing resources at both national and international levels to train and retain skilled staff is vital to improving maternal and neonatal health. *A measuring tape and a traditional fetal stethoscope lie on an examining table in a maternity ward that offers antenatal and neonatal services, as well as services to prevent mother-to-child transmission of the HIV virus, Nigeria.*

Figure 5.2

Official development assistance for maternal and neonatal health has risen rapidly since 2004

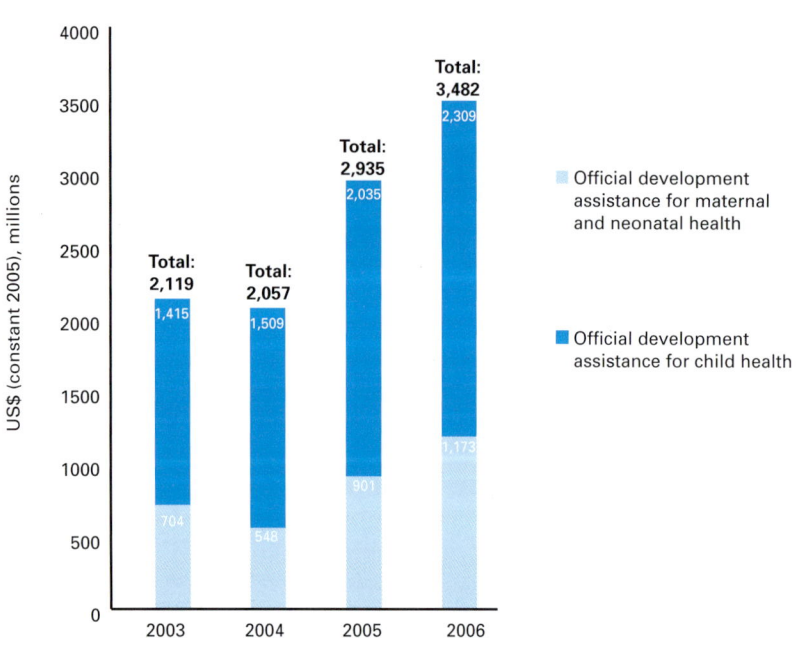

Source: Greco, Giulia, et al., 'Countdown to 2015: Assessment of donor assistance to maternal, newborn, and child health between 2003 and 2006', *The Lancet*, vol. 371, 12 April 2008, p. 1269.

Deepening global political commitments and resources for better health outcomes

Measures to improve the quality of aid are being complemented by growing political commitment and higher financial flows directed at maternal and newborn health. Several years ago, issues of maternal and child health were rarely addressed by world leaders. Today, maternal and child health are on the agenda of world leaders and major conferences, including the G8.

At the 2008 G8 summit meeting, the issue of maternal mortality was discussed, and the Partnership for Maternal, Newborn and Child Health asked leaders to increase spending on maternal and child health care and family planning by US$10.2 billion per year.[8]

In parallel with the 2008 G8 Summit, a G8 Health Experts Group was established. The group set out principles for action, pledging to take comprehensive action to address the health-related Millennium Development Goals, and underlining the importance of both disease-specific initiatives and health-systems strengthening. It also emphasized the need for a longer-term perspective that extends beyond the 2015 MDG deadline, and the imperative of mobilizing a wide range of stakeholders.

Action was pledged in five key areas: health systems strengthening;

Focus On: Partnering for mothers and newborns in the Central African Republic

The Central African Republic is among the world's lowest income countries, with a gross national income per capita of US$360 in 2007. Located in the heart of the African continent, the country has endured a decade of conflict. The worst-affected regions are located in the northeast and northwest, where rebel groups and government forces frequently clash. This ongoing violence has resulted in mass displacement and disruption of public infrastructure such as health care services, especially in the northern region.

Maternal and neonatal survival and health remain at risk from poverty and conflict. The lifetime risk of maternal death is 1 in 25, and UN inter-agency estimates put the country's maternal mortality ratio at 980 maternal deaths per 100,000 live births in 2005. The neonatal mortality rate was 52 per 1,000 live births in 2004, above the West and Central Africa average of 44 per 1,000 – which itself was the highest regional aggregate for this indicator in the developing world. Only 53 per cent of women in the country are attended by a skilled health worker at delivery.

Maternal and infant health is undermined by poor control of communicable diseases, insecurity and the lack of comprehensive maternal health programmes. Among other infectious diseases, tetanus is an important cause of neonatal death. Cases are prevalent in poor, remote and disenfranchised communities where unhygienic obstetric and post-natal practices prevail and access to maternal tetanus toxoid immunization during pregnancy is poor.

Despite the challenges posed by ongoing insecurity, international agencies are collaborating with the Government to tackle maternal and neonatal tetanus as part of a wider effort in support of maternal, newborn and child health. In January 2008, the Ministry of Health, together with the World Health Organization, the United Nations Population Fund and UNICEF, launched the Mother and Child Survival Campaign. The first phase of the campaign prioritized immunization, resulting in the vaccination of 700,000 women of reproductive age against tetanus. A second round of immunization was held in March, and the campaign is set to reach 1.5 million women and children across the country. The tetanus immunization campaign represents an important initial step in the drive to reduce maternal and neonatal deaths.

The Central African Republic and its partners face the challenge of consolidating these gains and strengthening the health system to deliver maternity services and basic health-care interventions that can help improve maternal and newborn health. Enhancing security will also be pivotal to widening access to women and children.

See References, pages 112.

---

maternal, newborn and child health; infectious diseases – including AIDS, tuberculosis, malaria, polio and neglected tropical diseases; promotion of a cross-sectoral approach – including the empowerment of women, reduction of gender inequalities and violence against women, and health; and resources. Developing countries were encouraged to allocate more of their own resources to health care, and the G8 reiterated its commitment to working towards the goal of providing at least US$60 billion for combating major infectious diseases and strengthening health systems.[9]

Disease-specific funds, such as the Global Fund to Fight AIDS, Tuberculosis and Malaria, the GAVI vaccine initiative and the US government's AIDS and malaria programmes provide opportunities to leverage significant resources for maternal and newborn health, through stronger health systems and service provision. These funds contribute to better trained health personnel, more reliable commodity supply systems, improved labs and diagnostics and more home and community based services, even as they focus on fighting specific diseases.

The World Health Organization, UNICEF, the United Nations Population Fund and the World Bank have reinvigorated their commitment to improve maternal and newborn health (*see Panel on page 102*), and major global health partnerships and programmes are mobilizing sizeable resources to support specific programmes and integrated approaches to health-service delivery. The increased political will and commitment evident in low-income, middle-income and donor countries to accelerate progress on maternal and child health is significantly enhancing collaboration and cooperation and creating a global compact.

Financial flows for maternal, newborn and child health

Greater political and institutional commitment to maternal newborn and child health is reflected in sharply rising aid flows to these areas. The latest estimates indicate that global official development assistance to maternal, newborn and child health rose by 64 per cent between 2003 and 2006. Specifically, funds apportioned to child health rose by 63 per cent, while those assigned to maternal and newborn health increased by 66 per cent. Disbursements for maternal, newborn and child health from GAVI and the Global Fund to Fight AIDS, Tuberculosis and Malaria rose by 200 per cent over the same period.

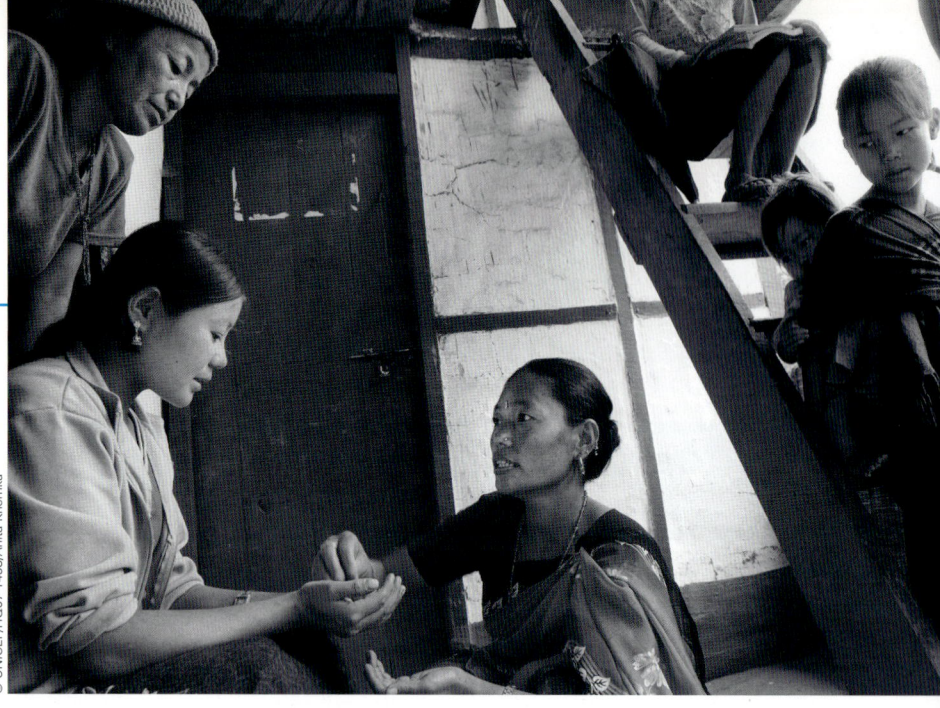

Both community workers and trained medical staff have vital roles in ensuring the continuum of care that runs from the home and the community right through to the clinic and the hospital. *A community health volunteer gives a pregnant woman vitamin A, iron and folic acid supplements, during a home visit, Nepal.*

Figure 5.3

Nutrition, PMTCT and child health have seen substantial rises in financing

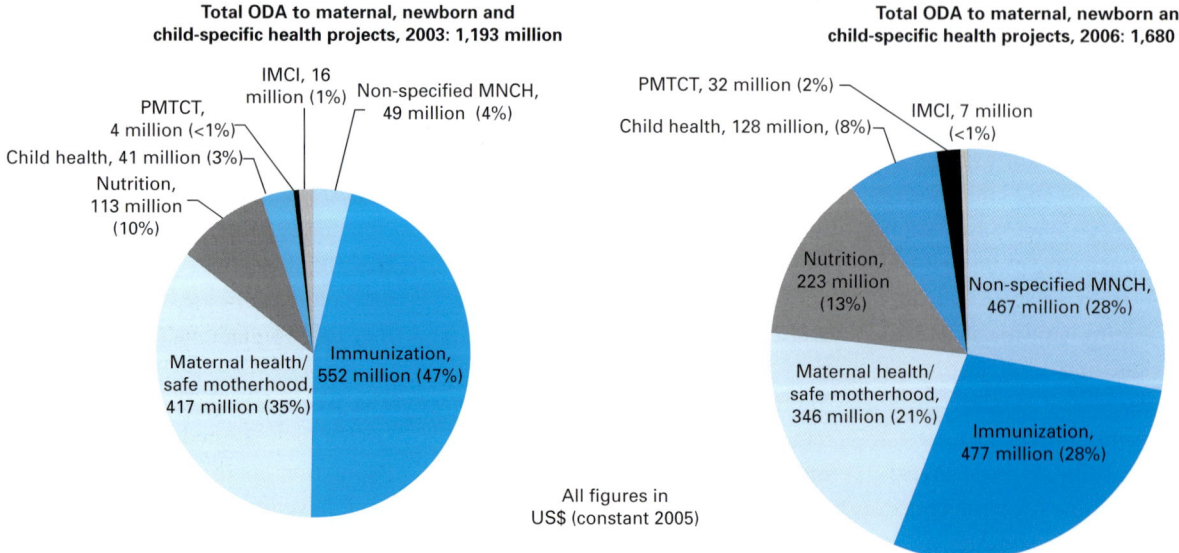

All figures in US$ (constant 2005)

Source: Greco, Giulia, et al., 'Countdown to 2015: Assessment of donor assistance to maternal, newborn, and child health between 2003 and 2006', *The Lancet*, vol. 371, 12 April 2008, p. 1269.

IMCI: Integrated Management of Childhood Illness
MNCH: maternal newborn and child health
PMTCT: prevention of mother-to-child transmission of HIV

The opportunity to save the lives of thousands of women and millions of children lies within reach.

There remains ample scope to further increase resources directed to maternal and newborn health. Recent analysis of official development assistance (ODA) flow to these areas indicates that aid to maternal, newborn and child health-related activities accounted for just 3 per cent of gross ODA disbursements. Moreover, the funds apportioned to maternal and neonatal health activities are lagging behind those devoted to child health. Figures for 2006 indicate that global ODA to maternal and neonatal health reached US$1.2 billion, roughly half the sum apportioned to child health. While this represents a sharp increase since 2003, when global ODA for maternal and newborn health stood at US$704 million, the 2006 figure translates into just US$12 per live birth.

Research also shows that some countries experience sharp fluctuations in aid inflows to maternal, newborn and child health between years, complicating efforts for effective planning for strategic priorities in developing countries – particularly those where aid dependency is greatest. And despite recent enhancements in the frameworks for aid effectiveness and moves towards sector and budget support, the bulk of financing for maternal, newborn and child health is apportioned through project funding.

With the bulk of financing still going to support projects, funding of health system development – such as training, staffing, management and logistics, urgently required to accelerate progress on maternal and newborn health – remains limited in relative terms.[10] Enhancing the predictability and sustainability of aid flows will be critical to ensuring that the progress achieved in maternal, newborn and child health is both maintained and deepened. Reduction of the transaction costs for national governments in their relations with global health partnerships and programmes must also be tackled, with implications

Figure 5.4

Financing for maternal, newborn and child health from global health initiatives has increased sharply in recent years

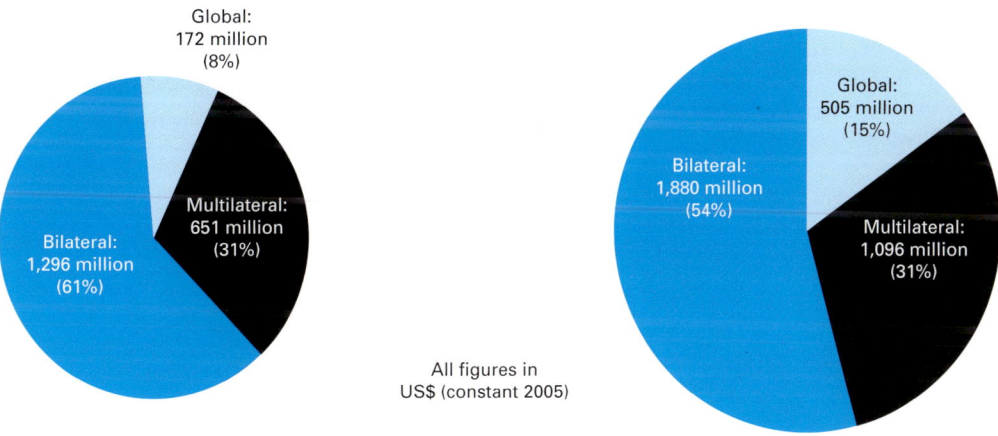

Source: Greco, Giulia, et al., 'Countdown to 2015: Assessment of donor assistance to maternal, newborn, and child health between 2003 and 2006', *The Lancet*, vol. 371, 12 April 2008, p. 1269.

UN agencies strengthen their collaboration in support of maternal and newborn health

At the High Level Event on the Millennium Development Goals held in September 2008 at the UN General Assembly, the four major health agencies – the World Health Organization, UNICEF, United Nations Population Fund and the World Bank – made a joint declaration of their intent to intensify and harmonize their efforts towards Millennium Development Goal 5, the goal that has made the least progress. The main objective of this renewed commitment to collaborative action is to coordinate efforts at the country level and jointly raise the required resources.

The four agencies pledged to strengthen support to countries with the highest levels of maternal mortality – especially the 25 countries with the most elevated maternal mortality ratios or numbers of maternal deaths. Based on their comparative advantage, core specialties and experience, and collective strengths, the agencies plan to jointly contribute to capacity building, health systems development and costing and financing of maternal, newborn and child health plans.

Strengthening national capacity
The agencies will work with governments and civil society to enhance national capacity in the following ways:

- Conduct needs assessment and ensure that health plans are MDG-driven and performance-based;

- Cost national plans and rapidly mobilize required resources;

- Scale up quality health services to ensure universal access to reproductive health, especially for family planning, skilled attendance at delivery and emergency obstetric and newborn care, ensuring linkages with HIV prevention and treatment;

- Address the urgent need for skilled health workers, particularly midwives;

- Address financial barriers to access, especially for the poorest;

- Tackle the root causes of maternal mortality and morbidity, including gender inequality, girls' low access to education – particularly at the secondary level, child marriage and adolescent pregnancy;

- Strengthen monitoring and evaluation systems.

Core agency functions and responsibilities in the continuum of maternal and newborn care
In an earlier document on joint country support for accelerated implementation of maternal and newborn continuum of care published in July 2008, the four agencies also pledged to work with governments to strengthen the continuum of maternal and newborn care. Based on their comparative advantages and expertise, the core functions to be undertaken by each agency were also specified:

World Health Organization: policy, normative, research, monitoring & evaluation.

United Nations Population Fund: reproductive health commodity security, support to implementation, human resources for sexual and reproductive health including maternal and newborn health, and technical assistance on building monitoring and evaluation capacity.

UNICEF: financing, support to implementation, logistics & supplies, and monitoring & evaluation.

World Bank: health financing, inclusion of maternal, newborn and child health in national development frameworks, strategic planning, investment in inputs for health systems, including fiduciary systems and governance, and taking successful programs to scale.

In addition, focal agencies, or shared focal agencies, were identified for each component of the maternal and newborn continuum of care to ensure optimal support, accountability and enhanced coordination. The identification of agency responsibilities, outlined in *Figure 5.5*, does not preclude the involvement of other agencies in each area, but rather implies that the focal agency or agencies will coordinate the UN response to support the national health plan in that area. Furthermore, the work of each agency will continue to be guiding by the prevailing situation in each country, the existing strengths and experience of each agency within the country, and other contextual factors such as sector-wide approaches (SWAps) and other national health plans or compacts. In each case, the government will continue to lead and coordinate the process.

See References, page 112.

Figure 5.5

Focal and partner agencies for each component of the continuum of maternal and newborn care and related functions

Area	Focal agencies	Partners
Continuum of maternal and newborn care		
Family planning	UNFPA, WHO	UNICEF, World Bank
Antenatal care	UNICEF, WHO	UNFPA, World Bank
Skilled attendance at birth	WHO, UNFPA	UNICEF, World Bank
Basic emergency obstetric and newborn care	UNFPA, UNICEF	WHO, World Bank
Comprehensive emergency obstetric and newborn care (C EmONC)	WHO, UNFPA	UNICEF, World Bank
Post-partum care	WHO, UNFPA	UNICEF, World Bank
Newborn care	WHO, UNICEF	UNFPA, World Bank
Maternal and neonatal nutrition	UNICEF, WHO, WB (for maternal nutrition)	UNFPA
Additional areas of maternal and newborn health work		
Girls' education	UNICEF	UNFPA, World Bank
Gender/culture/male involvement	UNFPA, UNICEF	WHO, World Bank
Gender-based violence	UNFPA, UNICEF	WHO
Adolescent sexual reproductive health – young people	UNFPA, UNICEF, WHO	World Bank
Communication for development	UNFPA, UNICEF	WHO, World Bank
Obstetric fistula	UNFPA	WHO
Prevention of unsafe abortion/post abortion care	WHO	UNFPA
Female genital mutilation	UNFPA, UNICEF, WHO	World Bank
Maternal and newborn health in humanitarian situations	UNFPA, UNICEF, WHO	World Bank
Sexually transmitted infections	WHO	UNFPA, UNICEF
HIV/AIDS and integration with family planning	As per UNAIDS *Technical Support Division of Labor*	
Pre-and-in-service training of human resources for MNH	WHO, UNFPA	UNICEF, World Bank
Regulations/legislation for human resources for health	WHO	UNFPA, UNICEF, World Bank
Essential drug list	WHO	UNFPA, UNICEF
Road maps' development and implementation	WHO, UNFPA, WB	UNICEF

Source: WHO-UNFPA-UNICEF-World Bank Joint Country Support for Accelerated Implementation of Maternal and Newborn Continuum of Care, 22 July 2008.

for further streamlining and harmonization of aid and technical assistance.

Attention must also be paid to the need for sustainable, predictable, flexible resources to support the long-term recurrent costs of health provision, such as salaries, and for governments to create fiscal space for health in their budgets. Further, other sectors that have a direct impact on access to maternal and newborn health care – such as transportation – must also be given due consideration in initiatives to develop sustainable health systems.

These challenges are not insurmountable. But they will require commitment on behalf of all key partners to work together to meet obligations to mothers, newborns and children. A focus on evidence and results must drive efforts. The Millennium Development Goals provide a firm reference point for action in the coming years. Achieving the goals will require building firm links between all contributing partners – national governments, donors, global health partnerships and programmes, international agencies, civil society organizations, the private sector, and communities and families themselves. The marked progress already achieved in recent years in strengthening collaboration and focusing on results provides hope for greater gains in the years to 2015 and beyond.

Delivering for mothers and newborns

In examining the global situation of mothers and newborns, and the diverse and sometimes complex tasks for improving their survival and health, it is possible to lose sight of the human side of the equation: the millions of women who face labour and delivery with trepidation, given the fact that this or subsequent pregnancies may result in their death or lifelong disfigurement, and that without adequate primary care, their newborn is also very likely to face death or illness.

Looking at the situation of mothers since 1990 puts the toll of death into sharp focus. Assuming that roughly 500,000 women have died each year since the beginning of that period, around 10 million women in all have died from causes related to pregnancy and childbirth. The latest available estimates for newborn deaths place them at nearly 4 million a year. The tragedy is that most of these lives could have been saved with cost-effective, proven interventions.

This situation must not be allowed to continue. There is no need to wait for a scientific breakthrough or a new paradigm to illuminate the best way forward. The knowledge that can save millions of newborn and maternal lives is available; data and analysis are improving rapidly; the framework for action is set; the challenge of the Millennium Development Goals is clear.

The opportunity to save the lives of thousands of women and millions of children lies within reach. Efforts now must focus on ensuring that the human and financial resources, the political will, and the commitment and collaboration increasingly evident nationally and internationally all remain dedicated to the task of improving the health and survival of mothers and newborns.

Enhancing health information systems: The Health Metrics Network

Sound information is essential to public health decisions. It informs policy, programmes, budgets and evaluation and forms the basis of accountability for governments' commitments to their citizens. In many developing countries, however, underinvestment in health information systems has left gaps in data collection, dissemination and analysis. With health challenges on the rise, and the deadline for the health-related Millennium Development Goals drawing ever closer, fulfilling the demand for sound information is imperative.

The Health Metrics Network (HMN) is an international partnership between developing countries, international agencies, foundations, global health partnerships and technical experts that aims to strengthen health information systems. Such systems incorporate all the multiple subsystems and data sources that, taken together, contribute to generating health information: vital registration, censuses and surveys, disease surveillance and response, service statistics and health management information, financial data and resource tracking. In line with current trends in health-system development, HMN seeks to broaden the base of health information and statistical systems beyond specific diseases and to foster leadership in the production and use of health information at the national level. These objectives require enhanced coordination and cooperation between countries and international partners, and a harmonized plan to develop health information systems. A further aim of HMN is to focus donor participation on a unified, country-owned plan to develop health information systems, thereby reducing duplication, fragmentation and overlap.

Central to the harmonized plan is the development of the Framework and Standards for Country Health Information Systems – known as the HMN Framework – which the partnership intends to set as the universal paradigm for data collection, reporting and usage by 2011. At the core of the framework is the HMN tool, a standardized questionnaire with which country stakeholders assess the current status of the health information against specific criteria. The tool provides a gauge of baseline status, critical gaps in health information results, processes, context and resources, and an assessment of performance and achievements. Countries receiving technical and financial assistance from the partnership are required to undergo an assessment using the HMN tool.

The purpose of the HMN Framework is twofold: to target investment on the standardization of health information, and to enhance access and, by extension, usage of better health information at the national and international levels. Rather than seeking to replace existing guidelines on health systems information, the HMN framework seeks to build on appropriate standards and promote best practices. The process is envisaged as a dynamic one, which will evolve through the incorporation of better evidence and wider experience.

In addition to developing the dynamic framework, the HMN has two related objectives: to deepen health information systems through providing technical and catalytic financial support to implement the HMN Framework; and to broaden access, dissemination and usage of health information by stakeholders at all levels. The partnership is based on a single and sound premise: It is not because countries are poor that they cannot afford good health information; it is because they are poor that they cannot afford to be without it.

See References, page 112.

References

CHAPTER 1

1. Wessel, Hans, et al., 'Deaths among Women of Reproductive Age in Cape Verde: Causes and avoidability', *Acta Obstetricia et Gynecologica Scandinavica*, vol. 78, no. 3, March 1999, pp. 225–232; Bartlett, Linda A., et al., 'Where Giving Birth is a Forecast of Death: Maternal mortality in four districts of Afghanistan, 1999–2002', *The Lancet*, vol. 365, no. 9462, 5–11 March 2005, pp. 864–870; Kilpatrick, Sarah J., et al., 'Preventability of Maternal Deaths: Comparison between Zambian and American referral hospitals', *Obstetrics & Gynecology*, vol. 100, 2002, pp. 321–326.

2. World Health Organization, *Neonatal and Perinatal Mortality: Country, regional and global estimates 2004*, WHO, Geneva, 2006, p. 4.

3. Derived from UNICEF global databases, 2008; World Health Organization, United Nations Children's Fund, United Nations Population Fund and the World Bank, *Maternal Mortality in 2005: Estimates developed by WHO, UNICEF, UNFPA and the World Bank*, WHO, Geneva, 2007, p. 35.

4. Nanda, Geeta, Kimberly Switlick and Elizabeth Lule, *Accelerating Progress towards Achieving the MDG to Improve Maternal Health: A collection of promising approaches*, World Bank, Washington, D.C., April 2005, p. 4.

5. Fishman, Steven M., et al., 'Childhood and maternal underweight', Chapter 2 in *Comparative Quantification of Health Risks: Global and regional burden of disease attributable to selected major risk factors*, edited by Majid Ezzati et al., World Health Organization, Geneva, 2004, pp. 84–86.

6. Barlett, Linda A. et al., 'Where Giving Birth is a Forecast of Death: Maternal mortality in four districts of Afghanistan, 1999–2002', *The Lancet*, vol. 365, no. 9462, 5–11 March 2005, p. 868.

7. World Health Organization, United Nations Children's Fund, United Nations Population Fund and the World Bank, *Maternal Mortality in 2005: Estimates developed by WHO, UNICEF, UNFPA and the World Bank*, WHO, Geneva, 2007, pp. 3–8, 35.

8. Figures derived from United Nations Children's Fund, *Progress for Children: A report card on maternal mortality*, Number 7, UNICEF, New York, September 2008, pp. 42–45; World Health Organization, United Nations Children's Fund, United Nations Population Fund and the World Bank, *Maternal Mortality in 2005: Estimates developed by WHO, UNICEF, UNFPA and the World Bank*, WHO, Geneva, 2007, pp. 23–27, 35.

9. World Health Organization, *Neonatal and Perinatal Mortality: Country, regional and global estimates 2004*, WHO, Geneva, 2006, p. 2.

10. Lawn, Joy E., Simon Cousens and Jelka Zupan, '4 Million Neonatal Deaths: When? where? why?', *The Lancet*, vol. 365, no. 9462, 5 March 2005, pp. 891–892.

11. UNICEF estimates based on data from World Health Organization, *Neonatal and Perinatal Mortality: Country, regional and global estimates 2004*, WHO, Geneva, 2006.

12. Ronsmans, Carine, and Wendy J. Graham, 'Maternal Mortality: Who, when, where and why', *The Lancet*, vol. 368, no. 9542, 30 September 2006, p. 1193; Li, X.F., et al., 'The Postpartum Period: The key to maternal mortality', *International Journal of Gynecology & Obstetrics*, vol. 54, no. 1, 1996, pp. 1–10; World Health Organization, *World Health Report 2005: Make every mother and child count*, WHO, Geneva, 2005, pp. 10, 62.

13. Ronsmans, Carine, and Wendy J. Graham, 'Maternal Mortality: Who, when, where and why', *The Lancet*, vol. 368, no. 9542, 30 September 2006, p. 1195.

14. Black, Robert E., et al., 'Maternal and Child Undernutrition: Global and regional exposures and health consequences, *The Lancet*, vol. 371, no. 9608, 19 January 2008, pp. 243–244; World Health Organization, *Adolescent Pregnancy: Unmet needs and undone deeds – A review of the literature and programmes*, WHO, Geneva, 2007, pp. 19–20.

15. Center for Disease Control and Prevention, 'Trends in Wheat-Flour Fortification with Folic Acid and Iron – Worldwide, 2004 and 2007', *Morbidity and Mortality Weekly Report*, vol. 57, no. 1, 11 January 2008, pp. 8–10.

16. Allen, Lindsay H., and Stuart R. Gillespie, 'What Works? A Review of the Efficacy and Effectiveness of Nutrition Interventions', ACC/SCN Nutrition Policy Paper No. 19/ADB Nutrition and Development Series No. 5, Asian Development Bank with the UN Administrative Committee on Coordination Sub-Committee on Nutrition (ACC/SCN), Manila, 2001, pp. 56, 59.

17. World Health Organization, *The World Health Report 2005: Make every mother and child count*, WHO, Geneva, 2005, p. 44; United Nations Children's Fund, *Progress for Children: A report card on maternal mortality*, Number 7, UNICEF, New York, September 2008, p. 6.

18. Ronsmans, Carine, and Wendy J. Graham, 'Maternal Mortality: Who, when, where and why', *The Lancet*, vol. 368, no. 9542, 30 September 2006, pp. 1194–1195.

19. Brahmbhatt, Heena, et al., 'Association of HIV and Malaria with Mother-to-Child Transmission, Birth Outcomes, and Child Mortality', *Journal of Acquired Immune Deficiency Syndromes*, vol. 47, no. 4, 1 April 2008, p. 475.

20. United Nations Children's Fund, *Progress for Children: A report card on maternal mortality*, Number 7, UNICEF, New York, September 2008, p. 6; World Health Organization, *Adolescent Pregnancy: Unmet needs and undone deeds – A review of literature and programmes*, WHO, Geneva, 2007, pp. 19–20; Gunasekera, Prasanna, Junko Sazaki and Godfrey Walker, 'Pelvic Organ Prolapse: Don't forget developing countries', *The Lancet*, vol. 369, no. 9575, 26 May 2007, pp. 1789–1790.

21. Lawn, Joy E., Simon Cousens and Jelka Zupan, '4 Million Neonatal Deaths: When? Where? Why?', *The Lancet*, vol. 365, no. 9462, 5 March 2005, pp. 894–895; Desai, Meghna, et al., 'Epidemiology and Burden of Malaria in Pregnancy', *The Lancet Infectious Diseases*, vol. 7, no. 2, February 2007, pp. 96–97.

22. Bang, Abhay, M. H. Reddy and M. D. Deshmukh, 'Child Mortality in Maharashtra', *Economic and Political Weekly*, vol. 37, no. 49, 7 December 2002, pp. 4947–4965; Black, Robert E., et al., 'Maternal and Child Undernutrition: Global and regional exposures and health consequences, *The Lancet*, vol. 371, no. 9608, 19 January 2008, pp. 243–244.

23. Desai, Meghna, et al., 'Epidemiology and Burden of Malaria in Pregnancy', *The Lancet Infectious Diseases*, vol. 7, no. 2, February 2007, pp. 96–97.

24. Setty-Venugopal, Vidya, and Ushma D. Upadhyay, 'Birth Spacing: Three to five saves lives', *Population Reports*, Series L, no. 13, Johns Hopkins University Bloomberg School of Public Health, Population Information Program, Baltimore, 2002, p. 1.

25. World Health Organization, *World Health Report 2005: Make every mother and child count*, WHO, Geneva, 2005, p. 10; JHPIEGO, *Best Practices: Detecting and treating newborn asphyxia*, JHPIEGO, 2004, <http://www.mnh.jhpiego.org/best/detasphyxia.pdf>, accessed 31 August 2008.

26. Lawn, Joy E., Simon Cousens and Jelka Zupan, '4 Million Neonatal Deaths: When? where? why?', *The Lancet*, vol. 365, no. 9462, 5 March 2005, p. 896.

27. Lawn, Joy E., et al., 'Newborn Survival', Chapter 27 in *Disease Control Priorities in Developing Countries*, 2nd ed., edited by Dean T. Jamison, et al., Oxford University Press and the World Bank, Washington, D.C., 2006, p. 534.

28. Adapted from United Nations Children's Fund, *Progress for Children: A report card on maternal mortality*, Number 7, UNICEF, New York, September 2008, pp. 37–38; Kerber, Kate J., et al., 'Continuum of Care for Maternal, Newborn and Child Health: From slogan to service delivery', *The Lancet*, vol. 370, no. 9595, 13 October 2007, pp. 1358–1369; Bryce, Jennifer, and J. H. Requejo, *Tracking Progress in Maternal, Newborn & Child Survival: The 2008 report*, Countdown to 2015, United Nations Children's Fund, New York, 2008, pp. 41–48.

29. The World Bank's definition of fragile states covers low-income countries scoring 3.2 and below on the Country Policy and Institutional Assessment (CPIA). The list of fragile states is updated annually, based on the computation of the countries' individual CPIAs. For further details of the definition see, *Global Monitoring Report 2007: Confronting the challenges of gender equality and fragile states*, World Bank, Washington D.C., 2007, p. 40. For the countries and territories on the World Bank's International Development Association list for fiscal year 2007, see <http://web.worldbank.org/WBSITE/EXTERNAL/EXTABOUTUS/IDA/0,,contentMDK:21389974~pagePK:51236175~piPK:437394~theSitePK:73154,00.html>, accessed 30 August 2008.

30. United Nations Millennium Project, *Investing in Development: A practical plan to achieve the Millennium Development Goals*, Earthscan, London/Sterling, VA, 2005, pp. 113, 188.

CHAPTER 1 PANELS

Challenges in measuring maternal deaths
World Health Organization, United Nations Children's Fund, United Nations Population Fund and the World Bank, *Maternal Mortality in 2005: Estimates developed by WHO, UNICEF, UNFPA, and the World Bank*, WHO, Geneva, 2007, pp. 1–10.

Creating a supportive environment for mothers and newborns
Gill, Kirrin, Rohini Pande and Anju Malhotra, 'Women Deliver for Development: Executive Summary', Family Care International, New York, 2007, p. 1; United Nations, *The Millennium Development Goals Report 2007*, UN, New York, 2007, p. 17.

Maternal and newborn health in Nigeria: Developing strategies to accelerate progress
United Nations Population Fund/Engender Health, *Obstetric Fistula Needs Assessment Report: Findings from nine African countries*, UNFPA/Engender Health, New York, 2003, p. 57–58; World Health Organization, *Neonatal and Perinatal Mortality: Country, regional and global estimates 2004*, WHO, Geneva, 2006, p. 11; Wall, L. Lewis, 'Dead Mothers and Injured Wives: The social context of maternal morbidity and mortality among the Hausa of northern Nigeria', *Studies in Family Planning*, vol. 29, no. 4, December 1998, p. 350.

Expanding Millennium Development Goal 5: Universal access to reproductive health by 2015
Glasier, A., et al., 'Sexual and Reproductive Health: A matter of life and death', *The Lancet*, vol. 368, no. 9547, 4 November 2006, p. 1595; derived from United Nations Population Fund, *The State of World Population 2004: The Cairo consensus at ten – Population, reproductive health and the global effort to end poverty*, UNFPA, New York, 2004, pp. 4–7, 12.

Prioritizing maternal health in Sri Lanka
UNICEF Sri Lanka, *Annual Report 2007*, Colombo, 2008, pp.7–8; Padmanathan, Indra, et al., *Investing in Maternal Health: Learning from Malaysia and Sri Lanka*, Washington, D.C., World Bank, 2003, pp. 1–3, 107, 110, 114, 116–117, 122, 131.

The global food crisis and its potential impact on maternal and newborn health
Food and Agricultural Organization of the United Nations, *Soaring Food Prices: Facts, perspectives, impacts and actions required*, FAO, Rome, June 2008, pp. 2–4, 17; Young, Helen, et al., 'Public Nutrition in Complex Emergencies', *The Lancet*, vol. 364, no. 9448, 20 November 2004, p. 1899; United Nations High Commissioner for Refugees, United Nations Children's Fund, World Food Programme and World Health Organization, *Food and Nutrition Needs in Emergencies*, UNHCR/UNICEF/WFP/WHO, p. 21; Food and Agriculture Organization of the United Nations, *The Global Information and Early Warning System on Food and Agriculture*, <http://www.fao.org/giews/english/giews_en.pdf >, accessed 1 August 2008.

CHAPTER 2

[1] World Health Organization, *Ouagadougou Declaration on Primary Health Care and Health Systems in Africa: Achieving better health for Africa in the New Millennium*, WHO, Geneva, April 2008, p. 1.

[2] Kerber, Kate, et al., 'Continuum of Care for Maternal, Newborn and Child Health: From slogan to service delivery,' *The Lancet*, vol. 370, no. 9595, 13 October 2007, pp. 1358–1369.

[3] United Nations Children's Fund, *The State of the World's Children 2008*, UNICEF, New York, January 2008, pp. 39–41, 63–64.

[4] Lawn, Joy E., Simon Cousens and Jelka Zupan, '4 Million Neonatal Deaths: When? Where? Why?', *The Lancet*, vol. 365, no. 9462, 5 March 2005, pp. 894–895; Black, Robert E., et al., 'Maternal and Child Undernutrition: Global and regional exposures and health consequences, *The Lancet*, vol. 371, no. 9608, 19 January 2008, pp. 245–248.

[5] World Bank, *Education and Development*, World Bank, Washington, D.C., 2002, p. 20.

[6] United Nations, Universal Declaration of Human Rights, Article 26, UN, New York, 1948; United Nations, Convention on the Rights of the Child, Article 28, UN, New York, 1989.

[7] United Nations Children's Fund, Progress for Children: A World Fit for Children Statistical Review, Number 6, UNICEF, New York, December 2007, pp. 16, 35.

[8] Lloyd, Cynthia B., 'Schooling and Adolescent Reproductive Behavior in Developing Countries', background paper to *Public Choices, Private Decisions: Sexual and Reproductive Health and the Millennium Development Goals*, United Nations Millennium Project, New York, 2006.

[9] Rowbottom, Sara, *Giving Girls Today and Tomorrow: Breaking the cycle of adolescent pregnancy*, United Nations Population Fund, New York, 2007, p. 2.

[10] Ibid., p. 5.

[11] United Nations Population Fund, *The State of the World's Population 2005: The promise of equality, gender equity, reproductive health and the millennium development goals*, UNFPA, New York, 2005, pp. 34–38.

[12] Ibid.

[13] World Bank, *Education and Development*, World Bank, Washington D.C., 2002, p. 5.

[14] United Nations Children's Fund, Progress for Children: A World Fit for Children Statistical Review, Number 6, UNICEF, New York, December 2007, p. 45.

[15] Derived from Statistical Table 9, pp. 150.

[16] International Planned Parenthood Federation and the Forum on Marriage and the Rights of Women and Girls, *Ending Child Marriage: A guide for global policy action*, IPPF, London, September 2006, pp. 7, 11, 15.

[17] United Nations Children's Fund, Progress for Children: A World Fit for Children Statistical Review, Number 6, UNICEF, New York, 2007, p. 44.

[18] World Health Organization, *Female genital mutilation and obstetric outcome: WHO collaborative prospective study in six African countries*, WHO, Geneva, 2006, p. 6.

[19] World Health Organization, *Eliminating Female Genital Mutilation: An interagency statement – OHCHR, UNAIDS, UNDP, UNECA, UNESCO, UNFPA, UNHCR, UNICEF, UNIFEM, WHO*, WHO, Geneva, 2008, p. 11.

[20] TOSTAN, *2006 Annual Report*, pp. 12–16.

[21] World Health Organization, summary report, *WHO Multi-country Study on Women's Health and Domestic Violence against Women: Initial results on prevalence, health outcomes and women's responses*, WHO, Geneva, 2005, p. 22.

[22] Ganatra, B.R., K.J. Coyaji and V.N. Rao, ' Too far, too little, too late: A community-based case-control study of maternal mortality in rural west Maharashtra, India', *Bulletin of the World Health Organization*, vol. 76, no. 6, 1998, pp. 591–598.

[23] Vlachova, Marie, and Lea Biason, *Women in an Insecure World: Violence against women – Facts, figures and analysis*, Geneva Centre for the Democratic Control of Armed Forces, Geneva, 2005, pp. 15–16.

[24] United Nations Children's Fund, *Progress for Children: A report card on maternal mortality*, Number 7, UNICEF, New York, September 2008, p. 12; and United Nations, *In-depth Study on All Forms of Violence against Women: Report of the Secretary-General*, UN, New York, 2006, p. 49.

[25] Leung W.C., et al., 'Pregnancy outcome following domestic violence in a Chinese community', *International Journal of Gynecology and Obstetrics*, vol. 72, no. 1, January 2001, pp. 79–80; and Valladares, Eliette M., et al., 'Physical Partner Abuse During Pregnancy: A risk factor for low birth weight in Nicaragua', *Obstetrics & Gynecology*, vol. 100, no. 4, October 2002, pp. 700–705.

[26] United Nations, *In-depth Study on All Forms of Violence against Women: Report of the Secretary-General*, UN, New York, 2006, p. 49.

[27] Campbell, Jacquelyn C., 'Health consequences of intimate partner violence', *The Lancet,* vol. 359, no. 9314, April 2002, pp. 1331–1336.

[28] Åsling-Monemi, Kajsa, et al., 'Violence against Women Increases the Risk of Infant and Child Mortality: A case-referent study from Nicaragua', *Bulletin of the World Health Organization*, vol. 81, no. 1, 2003, pp. 10–16.

[29] United Nations Children's Fund, *The State of the World's Children 2007*, UNICEF, New York, 2006, pp. 17–18.

[30] Ibid, pp. 23–28.

[31] Desai, Sonalde, and Kiersten Johnson, 'Women's Decisionmaking and Child Health: Familial and social hierarchies', in Sunitor Kishor, ed., *A Focus on Gender: Collected papers on gender using DHS data*, ORC Macro and Measure DHS, Maryland, USA, 2005, p. 66.

[32] Smith, Lisa C., et al., *The Importance of Women's Status for Child Nutrition in Developing Countries*, research report 131, International Food Policy Research Institute, Washington, D.C., 2003, pp. xi–xii, 8–14.

[33] Quisumbing, Agnes R., ed., *Household Decisions, Gender, and Development: A synthesis of recent*

research, Johns Hopkins University Press for International Food Policy Research Institute, Washington, D.C., 2004, p. 118.

[34] Data drawn from the Inter-Parliamentary Union database on 'Women in National Parliaments', <www.ipu.org/wmn-e/world.htm>, accessed July 2008.

[35] Data drawn from United Cities and Local Governments database on women in local decision making, <www.cities-localgovernments.org/uclg/index.asp?pag=wldmstatistics.asp&type=&L=EN&pon=1>, accessed July 2008.

[36] United Nations Development Fund for Women, *Progress of Arab Women 2004*, UNIFEM Arab States Regional Office, Amman, 2004, p. 62.

[37] United Nations Children's Fund, 'National Situational Analysis of Children and Women', UNICEF Mozambique, 2006; United Nations Development Fund for Women, *Progress of Arab Women 2004*, UNIFEM Arab States Regional Office, Amman, p. 62.

[38] Cowan, Carolyn Pape, et al., 'Encouraging strong relationships between fathers and children', *Working Strategies*, vol. 8, no. 4, Summer 2005, p. 2.

CHAPTER 2 PANELS

Primary health care: 30 years since Alma-Ata
Chan, Margaret, 'Address to the 61st World Health Assembly', WHO, Geneva, 19 May 2008; International Declaration of Alma-Ata, 1978; United Nations, 'Resolutions adopted by the General Assembly during its Sixth Special Session', 9 April–2 May 1974, Supplement No. 1 (A/9559), pp. 3–5; Thieren, Michel, 'Background paper on the concept of universal access', prepared for the Technical Meeting for the Development of a Framework for Universal Access to HIV/AIDS Prevention, Treatment and Care in the Health Sector', WHO, Geneva, 18–20 October 2005; Haines, Andy, Richard Horton and Zulfiqar Bhutta, 'Primary Health Care Comes of Age: Looking forward to the 30th anniversary of Alma-Ata – A call for papers,' *The Lancet*, vol. 370, no. 9591, 15 September 2007, pp. 911–913.

Addressing the health worker shortage: A critical action for improving maternal and newborn health
World Health Organization, *World Health Report 2006: Working together for health*, WHO, Geneva, 2006, pp. 8–12, 24, 99–101; Koblinsky, Marge, et al., 'Going to scale with professional skilled care', *The Lancet*, vol. 368, no. 9544, pp. 1377–1386; Tawfik, Linda, 'The impact of HIV/AIDS on the health workforce in developing countries', background paper for the *World Health Report 2006: Working together for health*, WHO, Geneva, 2006, p. 8; Physicians for Human Rights, *An Action Plan to Prevent Brain Drain: Building Equitable Health Systems in Africa*, PHR, Boston, 2004; Shisana, Olive, et al., 'HIV/AIDS Prevalence Among South African Health Workers', *South African Medical Journal*, vol. 94, no. 10, 2004, pp. 846–850, cited in Freedman, Lynn P., et al., *Child Health and Maternal Health: Who's Got the Power? Transforming health systems for women and children*, Task Force on Child Health and Maternal Health, UN Millennium Project, UNDP, 2005, p. 122.

Towards greater equity in health for mothers and newborns
Gwatkin, Davidson R., et al., *Socio-Economic Differences in Health, Nutrition, and Population within Developing Countries: An overview*, Health, Nutrition and Population, World Bank, Washington, D.C., September 2007, pp. 123–124; Fotso, Jean-Christophe, 'Child Health Inequities in Developing Countries: Differences across urban and rural areas', *International Journal for Equity in Health*, vol. 5, no. 9, 2006; Countdown 2008 Equity Analysis Group et al., 'Mind the Gap: Equity and trends in coverage of maternal, newborn and child health services in 54 Countdown countries', *The Lancet*, vol. 371, no. 9620, 12 April 2008, pp. 1259–1269; Victora, Cesar G., et al., 'Explaining Trends in Inequities: Evidence from Brazilian child health studies', *The Lancet*, vol. 356, no. 9235, pp. 1093–1098; Kerber, Kate J., 'The Continuum of Care for Maternal, Newborn and Child Health: Coverage, co-coverage and equity analysis from Demographic and Health Surveys', Faculty of Health Sciences, University of Cape Town (unpublished), 2007, pp. 16, 23–40.

Adapting maternity services to the cultures of rural Peru
Countdown Coverage Writing Group et al., 'Countdown to 2015 for Maternal, Newborn and Child Survival: The 2008 report on tracking coverage of interventions', *The Lancet*, vol. 371, no. 9620, 12 April 2008, pp. 1254–1255; World Health Organization, Maternal Mortality in 2005: Estimates developed by WHO, UNICEF, UNFPA and the World Bank, WHO, Geneva, 2007, p. 26; Pan American Health Organization, *Gender, Health and Development in the Americas 2003*, PAHO and Population Reference Bureau, 2003; and information supplied by UNICEF Peru.

Southern Sudan: After the peace, a new battle against maternal mortality
Central Bureau of Statistics and Southern Sudan Commission for Census, Statistics and Evaluation, *Sudan Household Health Survey 2006*, CBS and SSCCSE, Khartoum, pp. 43, 161, 164, 178; United Nations Population Fund Sudan Country Office, *Annual Report 2006*, UNFPA Sudan, pp. 3–4; and information provided by UNICEF Sudan.

CHAPTER 3

[1] Kerber, Kate J., et al., 'Continuum of Care for Maternal, Newborn and Child Health: From slogan to service delivery', *The Lancet*, vol. 370, no. 9595, 13 October 2007, pp. 1358–1369.

[2] Glasier, Anna, et al., 'Sexual and Reproductive Health: A matter of life and death,' *The Lancet*, vol. 368, no. 9547, 4 November 2006, p. 1602.

[3] Joint United Nations Programme on HIV/AIDS, *Report on the Global AIDS Epidemic 2008*, UNAIDS, Geneva, 2008, p. 33.

[4] World Health Organization, *Reproductive Health Strategy to Accelerate Progress towards the Attainment of International Development Goals and Targets*, WHO, Geneva, 2004, pp. 26–30.

[5] Black, Robert E., et al., 'Maternal and Child Undernutrition: Global and regional exposures and health consequences', *The Lancet*, vol. 371, no. 9608, 19 January 2008, p. 244.

[6] Ibid., p. 249.

[7] Joint United Nations Programme on HIV/AIDS, *Report on the Global AIDS Epidemic 2008*, UNAIDS, Geneva, 2008, p. 30.

[8] Briand, Valérie, et al., 'Intermittent preventive treatment for the prevention of malaria during pregnancy in high transmission areas', *Malaria Journal*, vol. 6, no. 1, 2007, p. 160.

[9] World Health Organization and United Nations Children's Fund, *Antenatal Care in Developing Countries: Promises, achievements and missed opportunities – An analysis of trends, levels and differentials, 1990–2001*, WHO, Geneva, 2003, p. 2.

[10] United Nations Children's Fund, *Progress for Children: A report card on maternal mortality*, Number 7, UNICEF, New York, September 2008, p. 44.

[11] World Health Organization, *World Health Report 2005: Make every mother and child count*, WHO, Geneva, 2005, pp.10, 62.

[12] United Nations Children's Fund, *Progress for Children: A report card on maternal mortality*, Number 7, UNICEF, New York, September 2008, p. 44.

[13] Paul, Vinod K., 'Meeting MDG 5: Good news from India,' *The Lancet*, vol. 369, no. 9561, 17 February 2007, p. 558; Chatterjee, Patralekha, 'India addresses maternal deaths in rural areas', *The Lancet*, vol. 370, no. 9592, 22 September 2007, pp. 1023–1024.

[14] United Nations Children's Fund, *Progress for Children: A report card on maternal mortality*, Number 7, UNICEF, New York, September 2008, p. 9.

[15] World Health Organization, *Postpartum care of the mother and newborn: A practical guide*, WHO, Geneva, 1998, p. 17.

[16] United Nations Children's Fund, *Progress for Children: A report card on maternal mortality*, Number 7, UNICEF, New York, September 2008, pp. 11, 44.

[17] Olsen, Øystein Evjen, Sidney Ndeki and Ole Frithjof Norheim, 'Availability, distribution and use of emergency obstetric care in northern Tanzania', *Health Policy and Planning*, vol. 20, no. 3, 2005, pp. 171–173.

[18] World Health Organization, *Postpartum care of the mother and newborn: A practical guide*, WHO, Geneva, 1998, p. 2; World Health Organization, *World Health Report 2005: Make every mother and child count*, WHO, Geneva, 2005, pp. 62, 73–74.

[19] Kerber, Kate J., et al., 'Continuum of Care for Maternal, Newborn and Child Health: From slogan to service delivery', *The Lancet*, vol. 370, no. 9595, 13 October 2007, p. 1366.

[20] World Health Organization, *World Health Report 2005: Make every mother and child count*, WHO, Geneva, 2005, pp. 73–74.

[21] Prince, Martin, et al., 'No health without mental health', *The Lancet*, vol. 370, no. 9595, 8 September 2007, pp. 867–8.

22 Knippenberg, R., et al., 'Systematic scaling up of neonatal care in countries', *The Lancet*, vol. 365, no. 9464, 19 March 2005, pp. 1088–1089; Countdown Coverage Writing Group et al., 'Countdown to 2015 for Maternal, Newborn and Child Survival: The 2008 report on tracking coverage of interventions, *The Lancet,* vol. 371, no. 9620, 12 April 2008, p. 1256.

23 Derived from Statistical Table 8, page 149.

24 Declaration of Alma-Ata, articles 6–8, International Conference on Primary Health Care, Alma-Ata, USSR, 1978; Haines, Andy, et al., 'Achieving Child Survival Goals: Potential contribution of community health workers', *The Lancet*, vol. 369, no. 9579, 23 June 2007, p. 2121.

25 Haines, Andy, et al., 'Achieving child survival goals: Potential contribution of community health workers', *The Lancet*; vol. 369, no. 9579, 23 June 2007, p. 2123.

26 Freedman, Lynn P., et al., *Child Health and Maternal Health: Who's got the power? Transforming health systems for women and children*, Task Force on Child Health and Maternal Health, UN Millennium Project, UNDP, 2005, p. 65.

27 Kerber, Kate J., et al., 'Continuum of Care for Maternal, Newborn and Child Health: From slogan to service delivery', *The Lancet*, vol. 370, no. 9595, 13 October 2007, p. 1361.

28 Lawn, Joy, and Kate Kerber, eds., *Opportunities for Africa's Newborns: Practical data, policy and programmatic support for newborn care in Africa*, Partnership for Maternal, Newborn and Child Health, Cape Town, 2006, p. 32.

29 Kerber, Kate J., et al., 'Continuum of Care for Maternal, Newborn and Child Health: From slogan to service delivery', *The Lancet*, vol. 370, no. 9595, 13 October 2007, p. 1364.

30 Ibid.

31 Lawn, Joy, and Kate Kerber, eds., *Opportunities for Africa's Newborns: Practical data, policy and programmatic support for newborn care in Africa*, Partnership for Maternal, Newborn and Child Health, Cape Town, 2006, p. 33.

32 Bartlett, Linda A., et al., 'Where Giving Birth Is a Forecast of Death: Maternal mortality in four districts of Afghanistan, 1999–2002', *The Lancet*, vol. 365, no. 9462, 5 March 2005; pp. 864–870.

33 Paxton, A., et al., 'Global patterns in availability of emergency obstetric care', *International Journal of Gynecology & Obstetrics*, vol. 93, no. 3, 2006, pp. 300–307.

CHAPTER 3 PANELS

Eliminating maternal and neonatal tetanus
World Health Organization, *Weekly epidemiological record*, WHO, Geneva: nos. 20, 19 May 2006, pp. 198–208; 81, 31 March 2006, pp. 120–127; 44, 30 October 1987, pp. 332–335; 82, 29 June 2007, pp. 237–242; and 34, 22 August 2008, pp. 301–307; Roper, Martha H., Jos H. Vandelaer and François L. Gasse, 'Maternal and neonatal tetanus', *The Lancet*, vol. 370, no. 9603, 8 December 2007, pp. 1947–1959.

Hypertensive disorders; Common yet complex
Khan, Khalid S., et al., 'WHO Analysis of Causes of Maternal Death: A systematic review', *The Lancet*, vol. 367, no. 9516, 1 April 2006, p. 1073; Podymow, Tiina, and Phyllis August, 'Hypertension in pregnancy', *Advances in Chronic Kidney Disease*, vol. 14, no. 2 , April 2007, pp. 178–179, 181; Hofmeyr, G.J., A.N. Attalah and L. Duley, 'Calcium supplementation during pregnancy for preventing hypertensive disorders and related problems', *Cochrane Database of Systematic Reviews 2006*, vol. 3, article no. CD001059; Bhutta, Zulfiqar A., et al., 'What works? Interventions for maternal and child undernutrition and survival', *The Lancet*, vol. 371, no. 9610, 2 February 2008, p. 431; Dolea, Carmen, and Carla AbouZahr, 'Global burden of hypertensive disorders of pregnancy in the year 2000', *Global Burden of Disease 2000*, World Health Organization, Geneva, 2003.

The first 28 days of life
Lawn, Joy E., Simon Cousens and Jelka Zupan, '4 million neonatal deaths: When? Where? Why?', *The Lancet*, vol. 365, no. 9462, 5 March 2005, pp. 891–900; Lawn, Joy E., Kenji Shibuya and Claudia Stein, 'No Cry at Birth: Global estimates of intrapartum stillbirths and intrapartum-related neonatal deaths', *Bulletin of the World Health Organization*, vol. 83, no. 6, June 2005, pp. 409–17; Bang, Abhay T., et al., 'Effect of Home-based Neonatal Care and Management of Sepsis on Neonatal Mortality: Field trial in rural India,' *The Lancet*, vol. 354, no. 9194, 4 December 1999, pp. 1955–1961; Baqui, Abdullah H., et al., 'Effect of Community-based Newborn-care Intervention Package Implemented through Two Service-delivery Strategies in Sylhet District, Bangladesh: A cluster-randomized controlled trial', *The Lancet* , vol. 371, no. 9628, 7 June 2008, pp. 1936–1944; Manandhar, D.S., et al., 'Effect of a Participatory Intervention with Women's Groups on Birth Outcomes in Nepal: Cluster-randomized controlled trial, *The Lancet*, vol. 364, no. 9438, 11 September 2004, pp. 970–979; Kumar, V., et al., 'Effect of Community-based Behaviour Change Management on Neonatal Mortality in Shivgarh, Uttar Pradesh, India: A cluster-randomized controlled trial', *The Lancet*, vol. 372, no. 9644, 27 September 2008, pp. 1151–1162; Bhutta, Zulfiqar A., et al., 'Implementing Community-based Perinatal Care: Results from a pilot study in rural Pakistan, *Bulletin of the World Health Organization*, vol. 86, no. 6, June 2008, pp. 452–459; Kerber, Kate J., et al., 'Continuum of Care for Maternal, Newborn and Child Health: From slogan to service delivery', *The Lancet*, vol. 370, no. 9595, 13 October 2007, pp. 1358–1369; Bhutta, Zulfiqar A., et al., 'Interventions to Address Maternal, Newborn and Child Survival: What difference can integrated primary health care strategies make?', *The Lancet*, vol. 372, no. 9642, 13 September 2008, pp. 972–989; Bhutta, Zulfiqar A., et al., 'Community-based Interventions for Improving Perinatal and Neonatal Health Outcomes in Developing Countries: A review of the evidence', *Pediatrics*, vol. 115, no. 2, February 2005, pp. 519–617; Haws, Rachel A., et al., 'Impact of Packaged Interventions on Neonatal Health: A review of the evidence', Health Policy and Planning, vol. 22, no. 4, 25 May 2007, pp. 193–215.

Midwifery in Afghanistan
World Health Organization, United Nations Children's Fund, United Nations Population Fund and the World Bank, *Maternal Mortality in 2005: Estimates developed by WHO, UNICEF, UNFPA and The World Bank*, WHO, Geneva, 2007, p. 23; United Nations Children's Fund, *Progress for Children: A report card on maternal mortality*, Number 7, UNICEF, New York, September 2008, pp. 10, 43; UNICEF Regional Office for South Asia, *Maternal and Neonatal Health Review in South Asia Region*, 25 June 2008, pp. 67–68; Currie, Sheena, Pashtoon Azfar and Rebecca C. Fowler, 'A bold new beginning for *midwifery* in Afghanistan', Midwifery, vol. 23, no. 3, September 2007, pp. 226–234; Afghan Ministry of Public Health, *Maternal Mortality in Afghanistan: Magnitude, causes, risk factors and preventability*, Afghan Ministry of Public Health, Centers for Disease Control and Prevention and UNICEF, 6 November 2002, p. 4; and information supplied by UNICEF Afghanistan.

Kangaroo mother care in Ghana
Whitelaw, A., and K. Sleath, 'Myth of the Marsupial Mother: Home care of very low birthweight babies in Bogota, Colombia', *The Lancet*, vol. 1, no. 8439, 25 May 1985, pp. 1206–1208; Pattinson, Robert C., et al., 'Implementation of Kangaroo Mother Care: A randomized trial of two outreach strategies', *Acta Paediatrica*, vol. 94, no. 7, 2005, pp. 924–927; Bergh, A.-M., and Robert C. Pattinson, 'Development of a Conceptual Tool for the Implementation of Kangaroo Mother Care', *Acta Paediatrica*, vol. 92, no. 6, pp. 709–714; and information supplied by UNICEF Ghana.

HIV/malaria co-infection in pregnancy
Desai, Meghna, et al., 'Epidemiology and Burden of Malaria in Pregnancy', *The Lancet Infectious Diseases*, vol. 7, no. 2, February 2007, pp. 93–104; Ter Kuile, F.O., et al., 'The Burden of Co-infection with HIV Type I and Malaria in Pregnant Women in Sub-Saharan Africa', *American Journal of Tropical Medicine and Hygiene*, vol. 71, supplement 2, 2004, pp. 41–54; World Health Organization, 'Malaria and HIV Interactions and their Implications for Public Health Policy', WHO, Geneva, 2005, pp. 10–11; United Nations Children Fund, 'Malaria and HIV Factsheet', UNICEF Technical Note no. 6, February 2003, p. 2; World Health Organization, 'Technical Expert Group Meeting on Intermittent Preventive Treatment in pregnancy (IPTp)', Geneva, 2008, p. 4; World Health Organization, 'Assessment of the Safety of Artemisinin Compounds in Pregnancy', Geneva, 2003, p. 2.

The challenges faced by adolescent girls in Liberia.
Information supplied by UNICEF Liberia.

CHAPTER 4

1 Hill, K., et al., 'Interim Measures for Meeting Needs for Health Sector Data: Births, deaths and causes of death', *The Lancet*, vol. 370, no. 9600, 17 November 2007, pp. 1726–1735.

2 World Health Organization, *Beyond the Numbers*: *Reviewing maternal deaths and complications to make pregnancy safer*, WHO, Geneva, 2004, pp. 1–2.

3 Measure Evaluation, 'Measuring Maternal Mortality from a Census: Guidelines for potential users', <www.cpc.unc.edu/measure/publications>, accessed 30 September 2008; World Health Organization, *Verbal Autopsy: Ascertaining and attributing causes of death*, WHO, Geneva, 2007, p. 6.

4 Setel, P.W., et al., 'Sample Registration of Vital Events with Verbal Autopsy: A renewed commitment to measuring and monitoring vital statistics, *Bulletin of the World Health Organization*, vol. 83, no. 8, 2005, pp. 611–617; Measure Evaluation, 'Sample Registration of Vital Events with Verbal Autopsy', <www.cpc.unc.edu/measure/tools/monitoring-evaluation-systems/savvy>, accessed 30 September 2008.

5 World Health Organization, *Beyond the Numbers: Reviewing maternal deaths and complications to make pregnancy safer*, WHO, Geneva, 2004, pp. 106–107.

6 US Centers for Disease Control and Prevention, 'Updated Guidelines for Evaluating Public Health Surveillance Systems', *Morbidity and Mortality Weekly Report – Recommendations and Reports*, vol. 50, no. RR13, CDC, Washington, D.C., 27 July 2001, pp. 1–35.

7 United Nations Children's Fund, World Health Organization and United Nations Population Fund, *Guidelines for Monitoring the Availability and Use of Obstetric Services*, UNICEF, August 1997; Averting Maternal Death and Disability Program, *Averting Maternal Death and Disability Program Report, 1999–2005*, Mailman School of Public Health, Columbia University, New York, October 2006, pp. 2–4.

8 World Health Organization, *Beyond the Numbers: Reviewing maternal deaths and complications to make pregnancy safer*, WHO, Geneva, 2004, p. 4.

9 Granja, A.C., F. Machungo and S. Bergstrom, 'Avoidability of Maternal Death in Mozambique: Audit and retrospective risk assessment in 106 consecutive cases', *African Journal of Health Sciences*, vol. 7, no. 3–4, July–December 2000, pp. 83–7.

10 Blouse, A., P. Gomez and B. Kinzie, *Site Assessment and Strengthening for Maternal and Newborn Health Programmes*, JHPIEGO, Baltimore, 2004, pp. 1–42; EngenderHealth, *COPE for Maternal Health Services: A process and tools for improving the quality of maternal health services*, New York, 2001.

11 Byass, Peter, et al., 'Direct Data Capture Using Hand-held Computers in Rural Burkina Faso: Experienes, benefits and lessons learnt, *Tropical Medicine and International Health*, vol. 13, special issue 1, July 2008, p. 29.

12 World Health Organization, *World Health Report 2006: Working together for health*, WHO, Geneva, 2006, p. 12.

13 World Health Organization, *World Health Report 2005: Make every mother and child count*, WHO, Geneva, 2005, p. 96.

14 United Nations Population Fund, *Investing in People: National progress in implementing the ICPD Programme of Action 1994–2004*, UNFPA, New York, 2004, p. 45; World Health Organization, International Confederation of Midwives, and International Federation of Gynecology and Obstetrics, *Making Pregnancy Safer: The critical role of the skilled attendant – A joint statement by WHO, ICM and FIGO*, WHO, Geneva, 2004, p. 1; World Health Organization, Department of Reproductive Health and Research, 'Proportion of Births Attended by Skilled Health Workers', 2008 updates, WHO, Geneva, p. 3.

15 United Nations Children's Fund and World Health Organization, *Management of Sick Children by Community Health Workers*, UNICEF/WHO, New York, January 2006, p. 7.

16 Ibid.

17 Derived from United Nations Children's Fund, *The State of the World's Children 2008: Child survival*, UNICEF, New York, January 2008, p. 77.

18 UNICEF Regional Office for South Asia, *Maternal and Neonatal Health Review in the South Asia Region*, 25 June 2008, p. 152.

19 Dambisya, Ysowa, 'A Review of Non-financial Incentives for Health Worker Retention in Eastern and Southern Africa', Regional Network for Equity in Health in East and Southern Africa, Discussion Paper no. 44, May 2007, p. 49.

20 Lawn, Joy E., and Kate J. Kerber, eds., *Opportunities for Africa's Newborns: Practical data, policy and programmatic support for newborn care in Africa*, Partnership for Maternal, Newborn and Child Health, Cape Town, 2006, p. 73.

21 Vivar, Susana Camacho, 'Ecuador Addresses Cultural Issues for Pregnant Women', *The Lancet*, vol. 370, no. 9595, 13 October 2007, p. 1302.

22 Lawoyin, Taiwo, O, O.C Olushevi, and David A. Adewole, 'Men's Perception of Maternal Mortality in Nigeria', *Journal of Public Health Policy*, vol. 28, no. 3, 2007, pp. 299–318.

23 Lawn, Joy E., and Kate J. Kerber, eds., *Opportunities for Africa's Newborns: Practical data, policy and programmatic support for newborn care in Africa*, Partnership for Maternal, Newborn and Child Health, Cape Town, 2006, p. 87.

24 Bryce, Jennifer, and J.H. Requejo, *Tracking Progress in Maternal, Newborn & Child Survival: The 2008 report*, Countdown to 2015, United Nations Children's Fund, New York, 2008, p. 44.

25 Data prepared by the Health Policies and Systems Development Unit, Health Systems Strengthening Area, Pan American Health Organization.

26 United Nations Economic and Social Commission, United Nations Economic Commission for Africa, African Union Commission, 'Meeting Africa's New Development Challenges in the 21st Century: Issues paper', Addis Ababa, 21 March 2008, p. 13.

27 Borghi, J.O., et al., 'Mobilizing Financial Resources for Maternal Health', *The Lancet*, vol. 368, no. 21, October 2006, pp. 1457–1465.

28 Witter, Sophie, et al., 'The Experience of Ghana in Implementing a User Fee Exemption Policy to Provide Free Delivery Care', *Reproductive Health Matters*, vol. 15, no. 30, 2007, pp. 61–71; Borghi, J.O., et al., 'Mobilizing Financial Resources for Health', *The Lancet*, vol. 368, no. 21, October 2006, pp. 1457–1465.

29 Gilson, Lucy, and Di McIntyre, 'Removing Fees for Primary Care in Africa: The need for careful action', *British Medical Journal*, vol. 331, 2005, pp. 331, 762–765.

30 Borghi, J.O., et al., 'Mobilizing Financial Resources for Health', *The Lancet*, vol. 368, no. 21, October 2006, pp. 1457–1465; Deininger, K., and P. Mpuga, *Economic and Welfare Effects of the Abolition of Health User Fees: Evidence from Uganda*, World Bank policy research working paper no. 3276, Washington, D.C., 2004; Nabyonga, J., et al., 'Abolition of Cost-sharing Is Pro-poor: Evidence from Uganda', *Health Policy Plan*, vol. 20, pp. 100–108.

31 Borghi, J.O., et al., 'Mobilizing Financial Resources for Health', *The Lancet*, vol. 368, no. 21, October 2006, pp. 1457–1465; Gilson, Lucy, and Di McIntyre, 'Removing User Fees for Primary Care in Africa: The need for careful action', *British Medical Journal*, vol. 331, 1 October 2005, pp. 762–765.

32 Gilson, Lucy, and Di McIntyre, 'Removing User Fees for Primary Care in Africa: The need for careful action, *British Medical Journal*, vol. 331, 1 October 2005, pp. 762–765.

33 Dmytraczenko, T., et al., *Evaluacion del Seguro Nacional de Maternidad y Ninez en Bolivia*, Partnerships for Health Reform, Abt Associates, Bethesda, Maryland, 1998; Borghi, J.O., et al., 'Mobilizing Financial Resources for Maternal Health', *The Lancet*, vol. 368, no. 9545, 21 October 2006, pp. 1457–1465.

34 Schneider, P., et al., *Utilization, Cost and Financing of District Health Services in Rwanda*, Partnerships for Health Reform, Abt Associates, Bethesda, Maryland, March 2001; Fox-Rushby, J.A., 'Cost-effectiveness Analysis of a Mobile Maternal Health Care Service in West Kiang, The Gambia', *World Health Stat Quarterly*, vol. 48, no. 1, 1995; pp. 23–27.

35 Richard, F., et al., 'Reducing Financial Barriers to Emergency Obstetric Care: Experience of cost-sharing mechanism in a district hospital in Burkina Faso', *Tropical Medicine and International Health*, vol. 12, no. 8, August 2007, pp. 972–981.

36 Gertler, P., and S. Boyce, *An Experiment in Incentive-based Welfare: The impact of Progresa on health in Mexico*, University of California, Berkeley, 2001; Morris, S.S., et al., 'Monetary Incentives in Primary Health Care and Effects on Use and Coverage of Preventive Health Care Interventions in Rural Honduras: A cluster randomized trial, *The Lancet*, vol. 364, no. 9450, 4 December 2004; pp. 30–37.

37 Peters, David H., Gita G. Mirchandani and Peter M. Hansen, 'Strategies for Engaging the Private Sector in Sexual and Reproductive Health: How effective are they?', *Health Policy and Planning*, vol. 19, supplement 1, pp. 5–21.

38 Bhatia, Jagdish, and John Cleland, 'Health Care of Female Outpatients in South-central India: Comparing public and private sector provision', *Health Policy and Planning*, vol. 19, no. 6, pp. 402–409; Barber, Sarah L., 'Public and Private

Prenatal Care Providers in Urban Mexico: How does their quality compare?', *International Journal for Quality in Health Care*, 4 May 2006, pp. 1–8; Barber, SL, PJ Gertler, and P Hasrimurti, 'Differences in access to high-quality outpatient care in Indonesia', *Health Affairs*, vol 26, no 3 May–June 2007, pp 352-366.

[39] World Health Organization, *World Health Statistics 2008*, WHO, Geneva, 2008, pp. 82–83.

[40] Mbonye, A.K., et al., 'Declining Maternal Mortality Ratio in Uganda: Priority interventions to achieve the MDG, *International Journal of Gynecology and Obstetrics*, vol. 98, no. 3, September 2007, p. 287.

[41] World Health Organization, International Planned Parenthood Foundation, John Snow, Inc., PATH, Population Services International, United Nations Population Fund, World Bank, *The Interagency List of Essential Medicines for Reproductive Health*, WHO, Geneva, 2006.

[42] Barker, Carol, et al., 'Support to the Safe Motherhood Programme in Nepal: An integrated approach', *Reproductive Health Matters*, vol. 15, no. 30, November 2007, p. 5.

[43] Pan American Health Organization, *Neonatal Health in the Context of Maternal, Newborn and Child Health for the Attainment of the Millennium Development Goals of the UN Millennium Declaration*, PAHO, Washington D.C., 2006, p. 19.

[43] Ganatra, B.R., K.J. Coyaji and V.N. Rao, 'Too Far, Too Little, Too Late: A community-based, case-control study of maternal mortality in rural west Maharashtra, India', *Bulletin of the World Health Organization*, 1988, vol. 76, no. 6, pp. 591–598; George, Asha, 'Persistence of High Maternal Mortality in Koppal District, Karnataka, India: Observed service delivery constraints', *Reproductive Health Matters*, vol. 15, no. 30, 2007, pp. 91–102; Murray, Susan F., and Stephen C. Pearson, 'Maternity Referral Systems in Developing Countries: Current knowledge and future research needs', *Social Science and Medicine*, vol. 62, 2006, pp. 2205–2215.

[44] Pittrof, Rudiger, Oona Campbell and Veronique Filippi, 'What Is Quality in Maternity Care? An international perspective', *Acta Obstetricia et Gynecologica Scandinavica*, vol. 81, no. 4, April 2002, p. 278.

[45] Delvaux, Therese, et al., 'Quality of Antenatal and Delivery Care Before and After the Implementation of a Prevention of Mother-to-child HIV Transmission Programme in Cote d'Ivoire', *Tropical Medicine and International Health*, vol.13, no. 8, August 2008, p. 974.

[46] Kayongo, M., et al., 'Strengthening Emergency Obstetric Care in Ayacucho, Peru', *International Journal of Gynaecology and Obstetrics*, vol. 92 , no. 3, March 2006, pp. 299–307; Otchere, S.A., and H.T. Binh, 'Strengthening Emergency Obstetrics in Thanh Hoah and Quang Tri provinces in Vietnam', *International Journal of Gynaecology and Obstetrics*, vol. 99, no. 3, September 2007, pp. 165–172; Otchere, S.A., and A. Kayo, 'The Challenges of Improving Emergency Obstetric Care in Two Rural Districts in Mali', *International Journal of Gynaecology and Obstetrics*, vol. 99, August 2007, pp. 173–182.

[47] Thomas, Lena Susan, et al., 'Making Systems Work: The hard part of improving maternal health services in South Africa', *Reproductive Health Matters*, vol. 15, no. 30, September 2007, pp. 45–48.

CHAPTER 4 PANELS

Using critical link methodology in health-care systems to prevent maternal deaths
Núñez Urquiza, Rosa María, et al., 'Más Allá de las Cifras: Detección de eslabones críticos en los procesos de atención para prevenir muertes maternas', *Género y Salud en Cifras*, vol. 3, nos. 2/3, May–December 2005, pp. 5–15.

New directions in maternal health
Starrs, Ann M., 'Delivering for Women', *The Lancet*, vol. 370, no. 9595, 13 October 2007, p. 1285; World Health Organization, United Nations Children's Fund, United Nations Population Fund and World Bank, *Maternal Mortality in 2005: Estimates developed by WHO, UNICEF, UNFPA and the World Bank*, WHO, Geneva, 2005; World Health Organization, *World Health Report 2005: Make every mother and child count*, WHO, Geneva, 2005; Braveman, Paula, and Eleuther Tarimo, 'Social Inequalities in Health within Countries: Not only an issue for affluent nations', *Social Science & Medicine*, vol. 54, no. 11, 2002, pp. 1621–1635; Marmot, Michael, 'Social Determinants of Health Inequalities', *The Lancet*, vol. 365, no. 9464, 19 March 2005, pp. 1099–1104; Hill, Kenneth, et al., 'Estimates of Maternal Mortality Worldwide between 1990 and 2005: An assessment of available data', *Obstetric Anesthesia Digest*, vol. 28, no. 2, June 2008, pp. 94–95; Bryce, Jennifer, and J. H. Requejo, *Tracking Progress in Maternal, Newborn & Child Survival: The 2008 report*, Countdown to 2015, United Nations Children's Fund, New York, 2008; Sedgh, Gilda, et al., 'Induced Abortion: Rates and trends worldwide', *The Lancet*, vol. 370, no 9595, 13 October 2007, pp. 1338–1345; Gülmezoglu, A. Metin, et al., 'WHO Systematic Review of Maternal Mortality and Morbidity: Methodological issues and challenges', *BMC Medical Research Methodology*, vol. 4, no. 16, 2004, p. 16; Filippi, V., et al., 'Health of Women after Severe Obstetric Complications in Burkina Faso: A longitudinal study', *The Lancet*, vol. 370, no. 9595, 13 October 2007, pp. 1329–1337; Bhutta, Zulfiqar A., et al., 'What Works? Interventions for maternal and child undernutrition and survival, *The Lancet*, vol. 371, no. 9610, 2 February 2008, pp. 417–440; Shankar, A.H., et al., 'Effect of Maternal Multiple Micronutrient Supplementation on Fetal Loss and Infant Death in Indonesia: A double-blind cluster-randomized trial', *The Lancet*, vol. 371, no. 9608, 19 January 2008, pp. 215–227; Campbell, O.M., and W.J. Graham, 'Strategies for Reducing Maternal Mortality: Getting on with what works', *The Lancet*, vol. 368, no. 9543, 7 October 2006, pp. 1284–1299; Villar, J., et al., 'World Health Organization randomized trial of calcium supplementation among low calcium intake pregnant women', American Journal of Obstetrics & Gynecology, vol. 193, no. 6S2, February 2006, pp. 639–649; Altman, D., et al., 'Do women with pre-eclampsia, and their babies, benefit from magnesium sulphate? The Magpie Trial: A randomized placebo-controlled trial', *The Lancet*, vol. 359, no. 9321, 1 June 2002, pp. 1877–1890; Althabe, Fernando, et al., 'A behavioral intervention to improve obstetrical care', *New England Journal of Medicine*, vol. 358, no. 18, 1 May 2008, pp. 1929–1940; Villar, J., et al., 'WHO Antenatal Care Randomized Trial for the Evaluation of a New Model of Routine Antenatal Care', *The Lancet*, vol. 357, no. 9268, 19 May 2001, pp. 1551–1564; United Nations Children's Fund, Malaria & Children: Progress in intervention coverage, UNICEF, New York, 2007; Kerber, Kate J., et al., 'Continuum of Care for Maternal, Newborn, and Child Health: From slogan to service delivery', *The Lancet*, vol. 370; no. 9595, 13 October 2007, pp. 1358–1369.

Strengthening the health system in the Lao People's Democratic Republic
Economist Intelligence Unit, Country Report Laos, January 2008, EIU, London, 2008, pp. 7, 12; United Nations Children's Fund, The State of Asia-Pacific's Children 2008, UNICEF, New York, May 2008, p. 38; United Nations Population Fund, Maternal and Neonatal Health in East and Southeast Asia, UNFPA, New York, 18 May 2008, p. 1; Perks, Carol, Michael J. Toole and Khamla Phouthonsy, 'District Health Programmes and Health-sector Reform: Case study in the Lao People's Democratic Republic', Bulletin of the World Health Organization, vol. 84, no. 2, February 2006, pp. 133–135; UNICEF Lao People's Democratic Republic, Annual Report 2007, pp.3–4, 9.

Saving mothers and newborn lives – the crucial first days after birth
Lawn, Joy E., Simon Cousens and Jelka Zupan, '4 Million Neonatal Deaths: When? where? why?', *The Lancet*, vol. 365, no. 9462, 5 March 2005, pp. 891–900; Baqui, A.H., et al., 'Effect of Timing of First Postnatal Care Home Visit on Neonatal Mortality in Bangladesh: An observational study', 2008 (unpublished); Darmstadt, G.L., et al., 'Evidence-based, Cost-effective Interventions: How many newborn babies can we save?', *The Lancet*, vol. 365, no. 9463, 12 March 2005, pp. 977–988; Bhutta, Zulfiqar A., et al., 'What Works? Interventions for maternal and child undernutrition and survival', *The Lancet*, vol. 371, no. 9610, 2 February 2008, pp. 417–440; Dearden, Kirk, et al., 'The Impact of Mother-to-mother Support on Optimal Breast-feeding: A controlled community intervention trial in peri-urban Guatemala City, Guatemala', *Pan American Journal of Public Health*, vol. 12, no. 3, September 2002, pp. 193–201; Kerber, Kate J., et al., 'Continuum of Care for Maternal, Newborn and Child Health: From slogan to service delivery', *The Lancet*, vol. 370, no. 9595, 13 October 2007, pp. 1358–1369; Bryce, J., et al., 'Countdown to 2015 for Maternal, Newborn and Child Survival: The 2008 report on tracking coverage of interventions', *The Lancet*, vol. 371, no. 9620, 12 April 2008, pp. 1247–1258; Tinker, Anne, et al., 'A Continuum of Care to Save Newborn Lives', *The Lancet*, vol. 365, no. 9462, 5 March 2005, pp. 822–825; Lawn, Joy E., and Kerber, Kate J., eds., *Opportunities for Africa's Newborns: Practical data, policy and programmatic support for newborn care in Africa*, Partnership on Maternal, Newborn and Child Health, Cape Town, 2006, p.84; Peterson, S., et al., 'Coping with Paediatric Referral: Ugandan parents' experience', *The Lancet*, vol. 363, no. 9425, 12 June 2004, pp. 1955–1956; Bang, A.T., et al., 'Effect of Home-based Neonatal Care and Management of Sepsis on Neonatal Mortality: Field trial in rural India, *The Lancet*, vol. 354, no. 9194, 4 December 1999, pp. 1955–1961; Baqui, Abdullah H., et al., 'Effect of Community-based Newborn-care Intervention Package Implemented through Two Service-delivery Strategies in Sylhet District, Bangladesh:

A cluster-randomized controlled trial', *The Lancet*, vol. 371, no. 9628, 7 June 2008, pp. 1936–1944.

Burundi: Government commitment to maternal and child health care
Economist Intelligence Unit, *Country Report Burundi, May 2008*, EIU, London, 2008; United Nations Development Programme, *Human Development Report 2007/2008: Fighting Climate Change – Human solidarity in a divided world*, UNDP, New York, 2007, p. 240; United Nations Children's Fund, *The State of the World's Children 2008: Child survival*, UNICEF, New York, January 2008, pp. 114, 118, 126, 142; Philips, Mit, et al., 'Burundi: A population deprived of basic health care', *British Journal of General Practice*, vol. 54, no. 505, 1 August 2004, p. 634; *Human Rights Watch*, 'A High Price to Pay: Detention of poor patients in Burundian hospitals, Human Rights Watch, vol. 18, no. 8(A), September 2006, pp. 7, 21, 27; United Nations Children's Fund, *Annual Report 2007*, UNICEF, New York, 2008, pp. 11, 25–26; International Health Partnership; *Scaling-Up for Better Health (IHP+) Update*, no. 1, WHO, 1 November 2007, p. 1, , <www.who.int/healthsystems/ihp/en/index.html>, accessed 30 July 2008.

Integrating maternal and newborn health care in India
United Nations Children's Fund, The State of Asia-Pacific's Children 2008, UNICEF, New York, May 2008, pp. 20, 53; United Nations Children's Fund, The State of the World's Children 2008: Child survival, UNICEF, New York, January 2008, pp. 115, 143; Maternal and Neonatal Health Review in the South Asian Region, 25 June 2008, pp. 16, 103; United Nations Children's Fund, Annual Report 2007, UNICEF, New York, 2008, p. 4; Government of India, Ministry of Health & Family Welfare, Janani Suraksha Yojana: Guidelines for implementation, September 2006, p. 5; Sharma, Ramakant, 'Janani Suraksha Yojana: A study of the implementation status in selected districts of Rajasthan', Population Research Centre, Mohanlal Sukhadia University, 2007–2008; United Nations Population Fund, 'Rapid Assessment of Chiranjeevi Yojana in Gujarat 2006', UNFPA India, pp. v, 23; Bhat, Ramesh, Dale Huntington and Sunil Maheshwari, 'Public-Private Partnerships: Managing contracting arrangements to strengthen the Reproductive and Child Health Programme in India – Lessons and implications from three case studies', World Health Organization, 2007, p. 12–13; UNICEF India Country Office, 'Assessment of Chiranjeevi Performance', February 2008, <http://gujhealth.gov.in/Chiranjeevi%20Yojana/M_index.htm>, accessed August 4, 2008.

CHAPTER 5

[1] World Health Organization, 'Progress in Global Measles Control and Mortality Reduction, 2000–2006', *Morbidity and Mortality Weekly Report*, vol. 82, no. 48, 30 November 2007, p. 422.

[2] Joint United Nations Monitoring Programme on HIV/AIDS, United Nations Children's Fund and World Health Organization, *Towards Universal Access: Scaling up HIV services for women and children in the health sector – Progress Report 2008*, UNAIDS/UNICEF/WHO, pp. 88–89,98.

[3] Overseas Development Institute, 'Global Health: Making partnerships work', Briefing paper no. 15, ODI, London, January 2007, p. 1

[4] International Health Partnership, 'Informal Meeting of Global Health Leaders', Outcome Document, July 2007, <www.internationalhealthpartnership.net/ihp_plus_about_agencies.html>, accessed 30 September 2008.

[5] International Health Partnership, <http://www.internationalhealthpartnership.net>, accessed 15 September 2008.

[6] High Level Forum on Aid Effectiveness, 'Paris Declaration on Aid Effectiveness: Ownership, harmonisation, alignment, results and mutual accountability', Paris, 28 February–2 March 2005; 3rd High Level Forum on Aid Effectiveness, 'Accra Agenda for Action', Accra, 2–4 September 2008.

[7] Canadian International Development Agency, Office of Economic Cooperation and Development and the World Bank, *Building a New Aid Relationship: The Paris Declaration on Aid Effectiveness*, 3rd High Level Forum on Aid Effectiveness, Accra, 2–4 September 2008, p. 26.

[8] Partnership for Maternal, Newborn and Child Health, 'A Global Call for G8 Leaders and Other Donors to Champion Maternal, Newborn and Child Health', World Health Organization, Geneva, April 2008, pp. 1–4.

[9] Toyako Framework for Action on Global Health: Report of the G8 Health Experts Group, Tokyo, 8 July 2008, pp. 1–10.

[10] Greco, Giulia, et al., 'Countdown to 2015: Assessment of donor assistance to maternal, newborn and child health between 2003 and 2006', *The Lancet*, vol. 371, no. 9620, 12 April 2008, pp. 1268–1275.

CHAPTER 5 PANELS

Working together for maternal and newborn health
World Health Organization: *The Health of the People: The African regional health report 2006*, WHO Regional Office for Africa, Brazzaville, 2006, p. 19; The White Ribbon Alliance for Safe Motherhood, *Annual Report 2007*; Graham, Wendy J., 'How Japan Reduced Maternal Mortality in One Generation', brief published by the Partnership for Maternal, Newborn and Child Health, <www.who.int/pmnch/topics/maternal/japanexample/en/print.html>, accessed 30 September 2008.

Key global partnerships for maternal and newborn health
Information derived from partnerships websites, accessed 30 August 2008.

Partnering for mothers and newborns in the Central African Republic
Information supplied by UNICEF CAR.

UN agencies strengthen their collaboration in support of maternal and newborn health
World Health Organization, 'Accelerating Efforts to Save the Lives of Women and Newborns', joint statement on behalf of UNICEF, United Nations Population Fund, the World Bank and WHO, 25 September 2008; *WHO-UNFPA-UNICEF-World Bank Joint Country Support for Accelerated Implementation of Maternal and Newborn Continuum of Care*, <www.who.int/mediacentre/news/statements/2008/who_unfpa_unicef_joint_country_support.pdf>, accessed 28 October 2008.

Enhancing health systems: The Health Metrics Network
World Health Organization, *Health Metrics Network, Framework and Standards for Country Health Information Systems*, 2nd edition, WHO, Geneva, 2008, pp. 5–8; Health Metrics Network website, <www.who.int/healthmetric/about/en>, accessed 30 September 2008.

STATISTICAL TABLES

Economic and social statistics on the countries and territories of the world, with particular reference to children's well-being.

General note on the data ....page 114
Explanation of symbols ....page 116
Under-five mortality rankings..page 117
Summary indicators..page 152
Measuring human development:
  An introduction to Table 10 ....page 153

TABLES

1 Basic indicators...page 118
2 Nutrition ....page 122
3 Health ....page 126
4 HIV/AIDS ....page 130
5 Education ....page 134
6 Demographic indicators ....page 138
7 Economic indicators ....page 142
8 Women ....page 146
9 Child protection ....page 150
10 The rate of progress ....page 154

STATISTICAL TABLES

Economic and social statistics on the countries and territories of the world, with particular reference to children's well-being.

General note on the data

The data presented in the following statistical tables are derived from the UNICEF Global Databases, which include only internationally comparable and statistically sound data; these data are accompanied by definitions, sources and explanations of symbols. Data from the responsible United Nations organization have been used wherever possible. In the absence of such internationally standardized estimates, the tables draw on other sources, particularly data drawn from nationally representative household surveys. Data presented in this year's report reflect information available as of 1 July 2008. More detailed information on methodology and the data sources is available at <www.childinfo.org>.

Several of the indicators, such as the data for life expectancy, total fertility rates and crude birth and death rates, are part of the regular work on estimates and projections undertaken by the United Nations Population Division. These and other internationally produced estimates are revised periodically, which explains why some data will differ from earlier UNICEF publications. This report includes the latest estimates and projections from the World Population Prospects 2006.

Data quality is likely to be adversely affected for countries that have recently suffered human-caused or natural disasters. This is particularly true where basic country infrastructure has been fragmented or major population movements have occurred.

Mortality estimates

Each year, UNICEF includes in *The State of the World's Children* mortality estimates, such as the infant mortality rate, under-five mortality rate and under-five deaths, for at least two reference years, if possible. These figures represent the best estimates available at the time the report is produced and are based on the work of the Inter-agency Group for Child Mortality Estimation, which includes UNICEF, the World Health Organization (WHO), the World Bank and the United Nations Population Division. This group updates these estimates every year, undertaking a detailed review of all newly available data points. At times, this review will result in adjustments to previously reported estimates. Therefore, estimates published in consecutive editions of *The State of the World's Children* may not be comparable and should not be used for analysing mortality trends over time. It is important to note that comparable under-five mortality estimates for the periods 1970, 1990 and the latest year are available in Table 10. In addition, the full time series for all countries is published at <www.childinfo.org> and <www.childmortality.org>, the website of the Inter-agency Group for Child Mortality Estimation. This time series is based on the most recent estimates produced by the Inter-agency Group for Child Mortality Estimation.

Multiple Indicator Cluster Surveys (MICS)

For more than a decade, UNICEF has supported countries in collecting statistically sound and internationally comparable data through the Multiple Indicator Cluster Surveys (MICS). Since 1995, nearly 200 surveys have been conducted in approximately 100 countries, and the latest round of MICS surveys was conducted in more than 50 countries during 2005–2006, allowing for a new and more comprehensive assessment of the situation of children and women globally. The next round of MICS surveys is planned for 2009–2010.

The UNICEF-supported MICS, along with the Demographic and Health Surveys, are among the largest sources of data for monitoring progress towards the Millennium Development Goals and may be used for reporting on 21 of the 53 MDG indicators. These data are also used for monitoring other internationally agreed commitments, such as the 'World Fit for Children Plan of Action' and the global goals on AIDS and malaria. They have been incorporated into the statistical tables appearing in this report and have also been used to inform the report's analyses. More information on these data is available at <www.childinfo.org>.

Revisions

The following revisions have been made to indicators included in this year's statistical tables.

Table 1. Basic Indicators: Table 1 presents estimates of child mortality as developed by the Inter-agency Group for Child Mortality Estimation. Note that the neonatal mortality rates for the year 2004, as presented in this table, are produced by WHO and have not been formally assessed by the Inter-agency Group for Child Mortality Estimation. These estimates, therefore, may not necessarily be consistent with the age structure of child mortality implicit in the infant and under-five mortality estimates for 2007. In addition, child mortality estimates for 12 countries in Eastern and Southern Africa (Botswana, Lesotho, Malawi, Mozambique, Namibia, Rwanda, South Africa, Swaziland, Uganda, the United Republic of Tanzania, Zambia and Zimbabwe) were revised to reflect UNAIDS estimates of child deaths due to AIDS. These UNAIDS estimates are produced based on information related not only to the prevalence of HIV but also to recent efforts in HIV and AIDS prevention and treatment. A more detailed explanation of these estimation methods is available at <www.childmortality.org>.

Table 2. Nutrition: Prevalence of underweight, stunting and wasting among children under five years of age is estimated by comparing actual measurements to an international standard reference population. In April 2006, the World Health Organization released the 'WHO Child Growth Standards' to replace the widely used National Center for Health Statistics/WHO reference population, which was based on a limited sample of children from the United States. The new standards are the result of an intensive study project involving more than 8,000 children from Brazil, Ghana, India, Norway, Oman and the United States. Overcoming the technical and biological drawbacks of the old reference, the new standards confirm that children born anywhere in the world and given the optimum start in life have the potential to develop to within the same range of height and weight, i.e., differences in children's growth to age five are more influenced by nutrition, feeding practices, environment and health care than genetics or ethnicity.

This is the first year that Table 2 includes underweight estimates according to the new 'WHO Child Growth Standards'. It should be noted that due to the differences between the old reference population and the new standards, prevalence estimates of child anthropometry indicators based on these two references are not readily comparable.

Table 4. HIV and AIDS: In August 2008, the Joint United Nations Programme on HIV/AIDS (UNAIDS) and WHO released new global HIV and AIDS estimates for 2007 that were derived from a more refined methodology and reflect the availability of more reliable data from population-based surveys and expanded national sentinel surveillance systems in a number of countries.

Differences between the new UNAIDS and WHO estimates for adult HIV prevalence, adults and children living with HIV and children orphaned by AIDS for 2007 are, for the most part, less marked than estimates published in previous reports. Figures published in this report are not comparable to previous estimates and therefore do not reflect trends over time. UNAIDS has published comparable estimates by applying the new methods to earlier HIV and AIDS estimates, which can be accessed at <www.unaids.org>.

Table 5. Education: The survival rate to grade 5 (percentage of primary school entrants reaching grade 5) was replaced by the survival rate to the last grade of primary school (percentage of children entering the first grade of primary school who are expected to reach the last grade). The survival rate to the last grade replaced the survival rate to grade 5 and became an official indicator for Millennium Development Goal 2 (universal primary education) in January 2008.

Table 7. Economics: The World Bank recently announced a new poverty line that is based on revised estimates of purchasing power parity (PPP) price levels around the world. Table 7 reflects this updated poverty line, and thus reports on the proportion of the population living below US$1.25 per day at 2005 prices, adjusted for purchasing power parity. The new poverty threshold reflects revisions to purchasing power parity exchange rates based on the results of the 2005 International Comparison Program. The revisions reveal that the cost of living is higher across the developing world than previously estimated. As a result of these revisions, poverty rates for individual countries cannot be compared with poverty rates reported in previous editions. More detailed information on the definition, methodology and sources of the data presented is available at <www.worldbank.org>.

Table 8. Women: In addition to presenting the proportion of women who were attended at least once during pregnancy by skilled health personnel, this year's table presents the proportion attended at least four times by any provider. The two antenatal care indicators are part of a revised monitoring framework for MDG 5 that went into

STATISTICAL TABLES

Economic and social statistics on the countries and territories of the world, with particular reference to children's well-being.

General note on the data (continued)

effect in January 2008 under a new target: achieving universal access to reproductive health.

Table 9. Child Protection: Data on child disability are derived from household surveys, and the indicator is defined as the proportion of children aged 2–9 years who screened positive for at least one type of disability (e.g., cognitive, motor, seizure, vision or hearing). Questions on child disability are addressed to the parent or caretaker of the child, who is asked to provide a personal assessment of the child's physical and mental development and functioning. As of June 2008, the methodology used to calculate these estimates from MICS surveys changed. Previously, the estimates were calculated based on 9 of the 10 MICS questions on disability. In this year's report and going forward, the data will be based on all 10 questions.

Explanation of symbols

Because the aim of these statistical tables is to provide a broad picture of the situation of children and women worldwide, detailed data qualifications and footnotes are seen as more appropriate for inclusion elsewhere. Sources and years for specific data points included in the statistical tables are available at <www.childinfo.org>.

Symbols specific to a particular table are included in the table footnotes. The following symbols are common across all tables:

–   Data are not available.

x   Data refer to years or periods other than those specified in the column heading, differ from the standard definition or refer to only part of a country. Such data are not included in the calculation of regional and global averages.

y   Data refer to years or periods other than those specified in the column heading, differ from the standard definition or refer to only part of a country. Such data are included in the calculation of regional and global averages.

*   Data refer to the most recent year available during the period specified in the column heading.

§   Includes territories as well as countries within each category or regional group. Countries and territories in each country category or regional group are listed on page 152.

Under-five mortality rankings

The following list ranks countries and territories in descending order of their estimated 2007 under-five mortality rate (U5MR), a critical indicator of the well-being of children. Countries and territories are listed alphabetically in the tables on the following pages.

	Under-5 mortality rate (2007)	
	Value	Rank
Sierra Leone	262	1
Afghanistan	257	2
Chad	209	3
Equatorial Guinea	206	4
Guinea-Bissau	198	5
Mali	196	6
Burkina Faso	191	7
Nigeria	189	8
Rwanda	181	9
Burundi	180	10
Niger	176	11
Central African Republic	172	12
Zambia	170	13
Mozambique	168	14
Democratic Republic of the Congo	161	15
Angola	158	16
Guinea	150	17
Cameroon	148	18
Somalia	142	19
Liberia	133	20
Uganda	130	21
Côte d'Ivoire	127	22
Djibouti	127	22
Congo	125	24
Benin	123	25
Kenya	121	26
Ethiopia	119	27
Mauritania	119	27
United Republic of Tanzania	116	29
Ghana	115	30
Senegal	114	31
Madagascar	112	32
Malawi	111	33
Gambia	109	34
Sudan	109	34
Myanmar	103	36
Togo	100	37
Sao Tome and Principe	99	38
Timor-Leste	97	39
Cambodia	91	40
Gabon	91	40
Swaziland	91	40
Pakistan	90	43
Zimbabwe	90	43
Bhutan	84	45
Lesotho	84	45
Haiti	76	47
Yemen	73	48
India	72	49
Eritrea	70	50
Lao People's Democratic Republic	70	50
Solomon Islands	70	50
Namibia	68	53
Tajikistan	67	54
Comoros	66	55
Papua New Guinea	65	56
Kiribati	63	57
Bangladesh	61	58
Guyana	60	59
South Africa	59	60
Bolivia	57	61
Democratic People's Republic of Korea	55	62
Nepal	55	62
Marshall Islands	54	64
Turkmenistan	50	65
Iraq	44	66
Mongolia	43	67
Uzbekistan	41	68
Botswana	40	69
Micronesia (Federated States of)	40	69
Azerbaijan	39	71
Guatemala	39	71
Dominican Republic	38	73
Kyrgyzstan	38	73
Algeria	37	75
Tuvalu	37	75
Egypt	36	77
Mexico	35	78
Nicaragua	35	78
Trinidad and Tobago	35	78
Morocco	34	81
Vanuatu	34	81
Iran (Islamic Republic of)	33	83
Cape Verde	32	84
Kazakhstan	32	84
Indonesia	31	86
Jamaica	31	86
Georgia	30	88
Maldives	30	88
Nauru	30	88
Lebanon	29	91
Paraguay	29	91
Suriname	29	91
Philippines	28	94
Occupied Palestinian Territory	27	95
Samoa	27	95
Belize	25	97
Saudi Arabia	25	97
Armenia	24	99
El Salvador	24	99
Honduras	24	99
Jordan	24	99
Ukraine	24	99
Panama	23	104
Tonga	23	104
Turkey	23	104
Brazil	22	107
China	22	107
Ecuador	22	107
Sri Lanka	21	110
Tunisia	21	110
Colombia	20	112
Peru	20	112
Grenada	19	114
Saint Vincent and the Grenadines	19	114
Venezuela (Bolivarian Republic of)	19	114
Cook Islands	18	117
Fiji	18	117
Libyan Arab Jamahiriya	18	117
Moldova	18	117
Saint Kitts and Nevis	18	117
Saint Lucia	18	117
Syrian Arab Republic	17	123
The former Yugoslav Republic of Macedonia	17	123
Argentina	16	125
Albania	15	126
Mauritius	15	126
Qatar	15	126
Romania	15	126
Russian Federation	15	126
Viet Nam	15	126
Bosnia and Herzegovina	14	132
Uruguay	14	132
Bahamas	13	134
Belarus	13	134
Seychelles	13	134
Barbados	12	137
Bulgaria	12	137
Oman	12	137
Antigua and Barbuda	11	140
Costa Rica	11	140
Dominica	11	140
Kuwait	11	140
Malaysia	11	140
Bahrain	10	145
Montenegro	10	145
Palau	10	145
Brunei Darussalam	9	148
Chile	9	148
Latvia	9	148
Lithuania	8	151
Serbia	8	151
Slovakia	8	151
United Arab Emirates	8	151
United States	8	151
Cuba	7	156
Hungary	7	156
Poland	7	156
Thailand	7	156
Australia	6	160
Canada	6	160
Croatia	6	160
Estonia	6	160
New Zealand	6	160
United Kingdom	6	160
Belgium	5	166
Cyprus	5	166
Israel	5	166
Republic of Korea	5	166
Malta	5	166
Netherlands	5	166
Switzerland	5	166
Austria	4	173
Czech Republic	4	173
Denmark	4	173
Finland	4	173
France	4	173
Germany	4	173
Greece	4	173
Ireland	4	173
Italy	4	173
Japan	4	173
Monaco	4	173
Norway	4	173
Portugal	4	173
San Marino	4	173
Slovenia	4	173
Spain	4	173
Andorra	3	189
Iceland	3	189
Liechtenstein	3	189
Luxembourg	3	189
Singapore	3	189
Sweden	3	189
Holy See	–	
Niue	–	

TABLE 1. BASIC INDICATORS

Countries and territories	Under-5 mortality rank	Under-5 mortality rate		Infant mortality rate (under 1)		Neonatal mortality rate 2004	Total population (thousands) 2007	Annual no. of births (thousands) 2007	Annual no. of under-5 deaths (thousands) 2007	GNI per capita (US$) 2007	Life expectancy at birth (years) 2007	Total adult literacy rate (%) 2000–2007*	Primary school net enrolment/ attendance (%) 2000–2007*	% share of household income 1995–2005*	
		1990	2007	1990	2007									lowest 40%	highest 20%
Afghanistan	2	260	257	168	165	60	27145	1314	338	250x	44	28	61	–	–
Albania	126	46	15	37	13	9	3190	52	1	3290	76	99	94	21	40
Algeria	75	69	37	54	33	22	33858	704	26	3620	72	75	95	19	43
Andorra	189	6	3	5	3	2	75	0	0	d	–	–	83	–	–
Angola	16	258	158	150	116	54	17024	810	128	2560	42	67	58s	–	–
Antigua and Barbuda	140	–	11	–	10	8	85	0	0	11520	–	–	–	–	–
Argentina	125	29	16	25	15	10	39531	693	11	6050	75	98	99	11	55
Armenia	99	56	24	48	22	18	3002	37	1	2640	72	100	99s	21	43
Australia	160	9	6	8	5	3	20743	256	2	35960	81	–	96	18x	41x
Austria	173	9	4	8	4	3	8361	77	0	42700	80	–	97	22	38
Azerbaijan	71	98	39	78	34	35	8467	134	5	2550	67	99	73s	19	45
Bahamas	134	29	13	22	12	5	331	6	0	15730x	73	–	88	–	–
Bahrain	145	19	10	15	9	4	753	13	0	19350	76	89	98	–	–
Bangladesh	58	151	61	105	47	36	158665	3998	244	470	64	54	81s	21	43
Barbados	137	17	12	15	11	8	294	3	0	d	77	–	96	–	–
Belarus	134	24	13	20	12	3	9689	91	1	4220	69	100	89	23	37
Belgium	166	10	5	9	4	2	10457	109	1	40710	79	–	97	22	41
Belize	97	43	25	35	22	17	288	7	0	3800	76	–	97	–	–
Benin	25	184	123	111	78	36	9033	365	45	570	56	41	67s	19	45
Bhutan	45	148	84	91	56	30	658	12	1	1770	66	56	70s	–	–
Bolivia	61	125	57	89	48	24	9525	263	15	1260	65	90	78s	7	63
Bosnia and Herzegovina	132	22	14	18	13	10	3935	34	0	3580	75	97	91s	19	43
Botswana	69	57	40	45	33	46	1882	47	2	5840	50	83	84	9x	65x
Brazil	107	58	22	49	20	13	191791	3706	82	5910	72	91	94	9	61
Brunei Darussalam	148	11	9	10	8	4	390	8	0	26930x	77	95	94	–	–
Bulgaria	137	18	12	15	10	7	7639	68	1	4590	73	98	92	22	38
Burkina Faso	7	206	191	112	104	32	14784	654	125	430	52	29	47	18	47
Burundi	10	189	180	113	108	41	8508	399	72	110	49	59	75	15	48
Cambodia	40	119	91	87	70	48	14444	382	35	540	59	76	90	17	50
Cameroon	18	139	148	85	87	30	18549	649	96	1050	50	68	84s	15	51
Canada	160	8	6	7	5	3	32876	340	2	39420	81	–	100	20	40
Cape Verde	84	60	32	45	24	9	530	15	0	2430	72	84	88	–	–
Central African Republic	12	171	172	113	113	52	4343	158	27	380	44	49	59s	7x	65x
Chad	3	201	209	120	124	42	10781	492	103	540	51	26	36s	–	–
Chile	148	21	9	18	8	5	16635	250	2	8350	79	97	–	11	60
China	107	45	22	36	19	18	1328630	17374	382	2360	73	93	99	13	52
Colombia	112	35	20	28	17	13	46156	876	18	3250	73	94	89	10	61
Comoros	55	120	66	88	49	25	839	28	2	680	65	75	73	–	–
Congo	24	104	125	67	79	30	3768	133	17	1540	55	87	86s	–	–
Cook Islands	117	32	18	26	16	10	13	0	0	–	–	–	74	–	–
Costa Rica	140	18	11	16	10	8	4468	80	1	5560	79	96	92	13	53
Côte d'Ivoire	22	151	127	104	89	64	19262	687	87	910	48	49	62s	14	51
Croatia	160	13	6	11	5	5	4555	41	0	10460	76	99	90	22	38
Cuba	156	13	7	11	5	4	11268	118	1	c	78	100	97	–	–
Cyprus	166	11	5	9	3	2	855	10	0	24940	79	98	99	–	–
Czech Republic	173	12	4	10	3	2	10186	93	0	14450	76	–	93	25	36
Democratic People's Republic of Korea	62	55	55	42	42	22	23790	317	17	a	67	–	–	–	–
Democratic Republic of the Congo	15	200	161	127	108	47	62636	3118	502	140	46	67	52s	–	–
Denmark	173	9	4	7	4	3	5442	62	0	54910	78	–	96	23	36
Djibouti	22	175	127	116	84	45	833	24	3	1090	55	–	79s	–	–
Dominica	140	18	11	14	9	10	67	0	0	4250	–	–	77	–	–
Dominican Republic	73	66	38	53	31	18	9760	231	9	3550	72	89	78	12	55
Ecuador	107	57	22	43	20	13	13341	283	6	3080	75	93	97	11	58
Egypt	77	93	36	68	30	17	75498	1840	66	1580	71	72	96	22	42
El Salvador	99	60	24	47	21	12	6857	158	4	2850	72	86	94	10	56
Equatorial Guinea	4	170	206	103	124	47	507	20	4	12860	51	87	61s	–	–
Eritrea	50	147	70	88	46	21	4851	191	13	230	58	–	47	–	–
Estonia	160	18	6	14	4	4	1335	14	0	13200	71	100	94	19	43
Ethiopia	27	204	119	122	75	41	83099	3201	381	220	53	36	45s	22	39
Fiji	117	22	18	19	16	10	839	18	0	3800	69	–	91	–	–
Finland	173	7	4	6	3	2	5277	58	0	44400	79	–	97	24	37

THE STATE OF THE WORLD'S CHILDREN 2009

...TABLE 1

	Under-5 mortality rank	Under-5 mortality rate		Infant mortality rate (under 1)		Neonatal mortality rate 2004	Total population (thousands) 2007	Annual no. of births (thousands) 2007	Annual no. of under-5 deaths (thousands) 2007	GNI per capita (US$) 2007	Life expectancy at birth (years) 2007	Total adult literacy rate (%) 2000–2007*	Primary school net enrolment/ attendance (%) 2000–2007*	% share of household income 1995–2005*	
		1990	2007	1990	2007									lowest 40%	highest 20%
France	173	9	4	7	4	2	61647	758	3	38500	81	–	99	20	40
Gabon	40	92	91	60	60	31	1331	34	3	6670	57	86	94s	–	–
Gambia	34	153	109	104	82	44	1709	60	7	320	59	–	62	14	53
Georgia	88	47	30	41	27	25	4395	48	1	2120	71	–	95s	16	47
Germany	173	9	4	7	4	3	82599	678	3	38860	79	–	98	22	37
Ghana	30	120	115	76	73	43	23478	703	81	590	60	65	72	16	47
Greece	173	11	4	9	4	3	11147	103	0	29630	79	97	100	19	42
Grenada	114	37	19	30	15	11	106	2	0	4670	69	–	84	–	–
Guatemala	71	82	39	60	29	19	13354	449	18	2440	70	73	94	12	54
Guinea	17	231	150	137	93	39	9370	377	57	400	56	30	51s	18	46
Guinea-Bissau	5	240	198	142	118	47	1695	84	17	200	46	65	54s	14x	53x
Guyana	59	88	60	64	45	22	738	13	1	1300	66	–	96s	–	–
Haiti	47	152	76	105	57	32	9598	270	21	560	61	62	50s	9	63
Holy See	–	–	–	–	–	–	1	–	–	–	–	–	–	–	–
Honduras	99	58	24	45	20	17	7106	200	5	1600	70	83	79s	11	58
Hungary	156	17	7	15	6	5	10030	93	1	11570	73	99	88	22	39
Iceland	189	7	3	5	2	1	301	4	0	54100	82	–	98	–	–
India	49	117	72	83	54	39	1169016	27119	1953	950	64	66	83s	19	45
Indonesia	86	91	31	60	25	17	231627	4386	136	1650	70	91	96	18	47
Iran (Islamic Republic of)	83	72	33	54	29	19	71208	1441	48	3470	71	85	94	17	45
Iraq	66	53	44	42	36	63	28993	935	41	2170x	59	74	89	–	–
Ireland	173	9	4	8	4	4	4301	67	0	48140	79	–	95	20	42
Israel	166	12	5	10	4	3	6928	137	1	21900	81	–	97	16	45
Italy	173	10	4	8	3	3	58877	539	2	33540	81	99	99	19	42
Jamaica	86	33	31	28	26	10	2714	55	2	3710	72	86	97s	15	52
Japan	173	6	4	5	3	1	127967	1070	4	37670	83	–	100	25x	36x
Jordan	99	40	24	33	21	16	5924	154	4	2850	72	93	90	18	46
Kazakhstan	84	60	32	51	28	32	15422	297	10	5060	67	100	98s	19	42
Kenya	26	97	121	64	80	34	37538	1479	179	680	53	74	76	16	49
Kiribati	57	88	63	65	46	25	95	0	0	1170	–	–	97	–	–
Kuwait	140	15	11	13	9	7	2851	51	1	31640	78	94	84	–	–
Kyrgyzstan	73	74	38	62	34	30	5317	115	4	590	66	99	92s	22	39
Lao People's Democratic Republic	50	163	70	120	56	30	5859	157	11	580	64	73	84	20	43
Latvia	148	17	9	13	7	6	2277	21	0	9930	73	100	90	19	43
Lebanon	91	37	29	32	26	19	4099	74	2	5770	72	–	82	–	–
Lesotho	45	102	84	81	68	52	2008	59	5	1000	42	82	85s	6	67
Liberia	20	205	133	138	93	66	3750	189	25	150	45	56	40	–	–
Libyan Arab Jamahiriya	117	41	18	35	17	11	6160	145	3	9010	74	87	–	–	–
Liechtenstein	189	10	3	9	2	–	35	0	0	d	–	–	88	–	–
Lithuania	151	16	8	12	7	5	3390	30	0	9920	73	100	89	19	43
Luxembourg	189	9	3	8	2	3	467	5	0	75880	79	–	97	–	–
Madagascar	32	168	112	103	70	41	19683	722	81	320	59	71	76s	13	54
Malawi	33	209	111	124	71	26	13925	573	64	250	48	72	91	18	47
Malaysia	140	22	11	16	10	5	26572	555	6	6540	74	92	100	13	54
Maldives	88	111	30	79	26	24	306	7	0	3200	68	97	97	–	–
Mali	6	250	196	148	117	54	12337	595	117	500	54	23	61	16	47
Malta	166	11	5	10	4	3	407	4	0	15310	79	92	91	–	–
Marshall Islands	64	92	54	63	49	24	59	0	0	3070	–	–	66	–	–
Mauritania	27	130	119	81	75	40	3124	102	12	840	64	56	57s	17	46
Mauritius	126	24	15	21	13	9	1262	19	0	5450	73	87	95	–	–
Mexico	78	52	35	42	29	11	106535	2088	73	8340	76	92	98	13	55
Micronesia (Federated States of)	69	58	40	45	33	11	111	3	0	2470	68	–	92	–	–
Moldova	117	37	18	30	16	12	3794	43	1	1260	69	99	88	20	41
Monaco	173	9	4	7	3	2	33	0	0	d	–	–	–	–	–
Mongolia	67	98	43	71	35	18	2629	49	2	1290	67	97	97s	20	41
Montenegro	145	16	10	14	9	9	598	8	0	5180	74	–	97s	–	–
Morocco	81	89	34	69	32	24	31224	641	22	2250	71	56	88	17	47
Mozambique	14	201	168	135	115	35	21397	855	144	320	42	44	60s	15	54
Myanmar	36	130	103	91	74	49	48798	891	92	220x	62	90	84s	–	–
Namibia	53	87	68	57	47	20	2074	53	4	3360	52	88	91s	4x	79x
Nauru	88	–	30	–	25	14	10	0	0	–	–	–	60	–	–

STATISTICAL TABLES 119

TABLE 1. BASIC INDICATORS

	Under-5 mortality rank	Under-5 mortality rate		Infant mortality rate (under 1)		Neonatal mortality rate 2004	Total population (thousands) 2007	Annual no. of births (thousands) 2007	Annual no. of under-5 deaths (thousands) 2007	GNI per capita (US$) 2007	Life expectancy at birth (years) 2007	Total adult literacy rate (%) 2000–2007*	Primary school net enrolment/ attendance (%) 2000–2007*	% share of household income 1995–2005*	
		1990	2007	1990	2007									lowest 40%	highest 20%
Nepal	62	142	55	99	43	32	28196	796	44	340	64	57	84s	15	55
Netherlands	166	8	5	7	4	3	16419	184	1	45820	80	–	98	21	39
New Zealand	160	11	6	9	5	3	4179	57	0	28780	80	–	99	18	44
Nicaragua	78	68	35	52	28	16	5603	140	5	980	73	81	90	15	49
Niger	11	304	176	143	83	41	14226	701	123	280	57	30	38s	10	53
Nigeria	8	230	189	120	97	47	148093	5959	1126	930	47	72	63	15	49
Niue	–	–	–	–	–	16	2	0	–	–	–	–	90	–	–
Norway	173	9	4	7	3	2	4698	56	0	76450	80	–	98	24	37
Occupied Palestinian Territory	95	38	27	33	24	–	4017	145	4	1230	73	93	76	–	–
Oman	137	32	12	25	11	5	2595	58	1	11120	76	84	74	–	–
Pakistan	43	132	90	102	73	53	163902	4446	400	870	65	55	56s	22	41
Palau	145	21	10	18	9	13	20	0	0	8210	–	–	96	–	–
Panama	104	34	23	27	18	11	3343	70	2	5510	75	93	99	9	60
Papua New Guinea	56	94	65	69	50	32	6331	190	12	850	57	58	–	12	57
Paraguay	91	41	29	34	24	12	6127	153	4	1670	72	94	94	9	62
Peru	112	78	20	58	17	11	27903	584	12	3450	71	91	96	11	57
Philippines	94	62	28	43	23	15	87960	2295	64	1620	72	93	91	15	51
Poland	156	17	7	15	6	5	38082	360	3	9840	76	99	96	19	43
Portugal	173	15	4	11	3	3	10623	112	0	18950	78	95	98	17	46
Qatar	126	26	15	20	12	4	841	14	0	12000x	76	90	94	–	–
Republic of Korea	166	9	5	8	4	4	48224	448	2	19690	79	–	98	22	38
Romania	126	32	15	25	13	10	21438	211	3	6150	72	98	93	21	40
Russian Federation	126	27	15	23	13	7	142499	1515	23	7560	65	100	91	17	47
Rwanda	9	195	181	117	109	48	9725	435	79	320	46	65	86s	14	53
Saint Kitts and Nevis	117	36	18	30	16	11	50	1	0	9630	–	–	71	–	–
Saint Lucia	117	21	18	16	14	11	165	3	0	5530	74	–	98	–	–
Saint Vincent and the Grenadines	114	22	19	18	17	13	120	2	0	4210	71	–	90	–	–
Samoa	95	50	27	40	22	14	187	5	0	2430	71	99	90	–	–
San Marino	173	13	4	12	4	2	31	0	0	45130	–	–	–	–	–
Sao Tome and Principe	38	101	99	65	64	38	158	5	0	870	65	88	98	–	–
Saudi Arabia	97	44	25	35	20	11	24735	618	15	15440	73	85	–	–	–
Senegal	31	149	114	72	59	35	12379	439	50	820	63	43	58s	17	48
Serbia	151	–	8	–	7	9	9858	127	1	4730	74	–	95	21	38
Seychelles	134	19	13	17	12	7	87	3	0	8960	–	92	99	–	–
Sierra Leone	1	290	262	169	155	56	5866	268	70	260	42	38	69s	17	47
Singapore	189	8	3	6	2	1	4436	37	0	32470	80	94	–	14	49
Slovakia	151	15	8	13	7	4	5390	53	0	11730	75	–	92	24	35
Slovenia	173	11	4	9	3	2	2002	18	0	20960	78	100	95	21	40
Solomon Islands	50	121	70	86	53	23	496	15	1	730	63	–	62	–	–
Somalia	19	203	142	121	88	49	8699	377	54	140x	48	–	22s	–	–
South Africa	60	64	59	49	46	17	48577	1092	64	5760	50	88	88	10	62
Spain	173	9	4	7	4	2	44279	476	2	29450	81	97	100	19	42
Sri Lanka	110	32	21	26	17	8	19299	292	6	1540	72	92	98	18	48
Sudan	34	125	109	79	69	27	38560	1230	134	960	58	61	54s	–	–
Suriname	91	51	29	41	27	17	458	9	0	4730	70	90	96	–	–
Swaziland	40	96	91	70	66	40	1141	33	3	2580	40	80	84s	13	56
Sweden	189	7	3	6	3	2	9119	102	0	46060	81	–	95	23	37
Switzerland	166	8	5	7	4	3	7484	69	0	59880	82	–	89	20	41
Syrian Arab Republic	123	37	17	30	15	7	19929	535	9	1760	74	83	95	–	–
Tajikistan	54	117	67	91	57	38	6736	186	12	460	67	100	89s	20	42
Thailand	156	31	7	26	6	9	63884	932	7	3400	70	94	94	16	49
The former Yugoslav Republic of Macedonia	123	38	17	33	15	9	2038	22	0	3460	74	97	92	17	46
Timor-Leste	39	184	97	138	77	29	1155	48	5	1510	61	–	75s	–	–
Togo	37	150	100	89	65	39	6585	245	25	360	58	53	80	–	–
Tonga	104	32	23	26	19	12	100	3	0	2320	73	99	96	–	–
Trinidad and Tobago	78	34	35	30	31	10	1333	20	1	14100	70	99	98s	17x	45x
Tunisia	110	52	21	41	18	13	10327	173	4	3200	74	78	96	16	47
Turkey	104	82	23	67	21	16	74877	1381	32	8020	72	89	91	15	50
Turkmenistan	65	99	50	81	45	37	4965	109	5	b	63	100	99s	16	48
Tuvalu	75	53	37	42	30	21	11	0	0	–	–	–	100	–	–
Uganda	21	175	130	106	82	30	30884	1445	188	340	51	74	82s	15	53
Ukraine	99	25	24	22	20	7	46205	419	10	2550	68	100	97s	23	37
United Arab Emirates	151	15	8	13	7	4	4380	71	1	26210x	79	90	88	–	–

120   THE STATE OF THE WORLD'S CHILDREN 2009

...TABLE 1

	Under-5 mortality rank	Under-5 mortality rate		Infant mortality rate (under 1)		Neonatal mortality rate 2004	Total population (thousands) 2007	Annual no. of births (thousands) 2007	Annual no. of under-5 deaths (thousands) 2007	GNI per capita (US$) 2007	Life expectancy at birth (years) 2007	Total adult literacy rate (%) 2000–2007*	Primary school net enrolment/ attendance (%) 2000–2007*	% share of household income 1995–2005*	
		1990	2007	1990	2007									lowest 40%	highest 20%
United Kingdom	160	9	6	8	5	3	60769	722	4	42740	79	–	98	18	44
United Republic of Tanzania	29	157	116	96	73	35	40454	1600	186	400	52	72	73s	19	42
United States	151	11	8	9	7	4	305826	4281	34	46040	78	–	92	16	46
Uruguay	132	25	14	21	12	7	3340	51	1	6380	76	98	100	14	51
Uzbekistan	68	74	41	61	36	26	27372	623	26	730	67	97	100s	19	45
Vanuatu	81	62	34	48	28	18	226	7	0	1840	70	78	87	–	–
Venezuela (Bolivarian Republic of)	114	32	19	27	17	11	27657	597	11	7320	74	93	91	12	52
Viet Nam	126	56	15	40	13	12	87375	1653	25	790	74	90x	95	18	45
Yemen	48	127	73	90	55	41	22389	860	63	870	62	59	75	19	45
Zambia	13	163	170	99	103	40	11922	473	80	800	42	68x	57s	12	55
Zimbabwe	43	95	90	62	59	36	13349	373	34	340	43	91	88	13	56

SUMMARY INDICATORS

Sub-Saharan Africa		186	148	109	89	41	767218	30323	4480	965	50	62	64	13	54
Eastern and Southern Africa		165	123	101	80	36	378926	14268	1761	1245	50	65	68	12	58
West and Central Africa		206	169	116	97	45	388292	16056	2719	698	50	60	60	16	48
Middle East and North Africa		79	46	58	36	25	389176	9726	445	3666	69	75	86	18	45
South Asia		125	78	89	59	41	1567187	37986	2985	889	64	63	80	19	46
East Asia and Pacific		56	27	42	22	18	1984273	29773	799	2742	72	93	97	16	46
Latin America and Caribbean		55	26	44	22	13	566646	11381	302	5628	73	91	93	11	56
CEE/CIS		53	25	44	22	16	405992	5560	138	5686	68	97	93	20	42
Industrialized countries§		10	6	8	5	3	974913	11021	66	38579	79	–	96	20	40
Developing countries§		103	74	71	51	31	5432837	122266	9109	2405	67	79	83	15	50
Least developed countries§		179	130	112	84	40	804450	29076	3775	491	55	57	65	15	50
World		93	68	64	47	28	6655406	135770	9216	7952	68	81	85	19	42

§ Also includes territories within each country category or regional group. Countries and territories in each country category or regional group are listed on page 152.

DEFINITIONS OF THE INDICATORS

Under-five mortality rate – Probability of dying between birth and exactly five years of age, expressed per 1,000 live births.

Infant mortality rate – Probability of dying between birth and exactly one year of age, expressed per 1,000 live births.

Neonatal mortality rate – Probability of dying during the first 28 completed days of life, expressed per 1,000 live births.

GNI per capita – Gross national income (GNI) is the sum of value added by all resident producers, plus any product taxes (less subsidies) not included in the valuation of output, plus net receipts of primary income (compensation of employees and property income) from abroad. GNI per capita is gross national income divided by midyear population. GNI per capita in US dollars is converted using the World Bank Atlas method.

Life expectancy at birth – Number of years newborn children would live if subject to the mortality risks prevailing for the cross section of population at the time of their birth.

Adult literacy rate – Number of literate persons aged 15 and above, expressed as a percentage of the total population in that age group.

Primary school net enrolment/attendance ratios – Number of children enrolled in or attending primary school, expressed as a percentage of the total number of children of primary school age. The indicator is either the primary school net enrolment ratio or the primary school net attendance ratio. In general, if both indicators are available, the primary school net enrolment ratio is preferred unless the data for primary school attendance is considered to be of superior quality. Definitions for both the primary school net enrolment ratio and the primary school net attendance ratio are given in Table 5, p. 134.

Income share – Percentage of income received by the 20 per cent of households with the highest income and by the 40 per cent of households with the lowest income.

MAIN DATA SOURCES

Under-five and infant mortality rates – UNICEF, World Health Organization, United Nations Population Division and United Nations Statistics Division.

Neonatal mortality rate – World Health Organization using vital registration systems and household surveys.

Total population – United Nations Population Division.

Births – United Nations Population Division.

Under-five deaths – UNICEF.

GNI per capita – World Bank.

Life expectancy – United Nations Population Division.

Adult literacy – UNESCO Institute for Statistics (UIS), including the Education for All 2000 Assessment.

School enrolment/attendance – UIS, Multiple Indicator Cluster Surveys (MICS) and Demographic and Health Surveys (DHS).

Household income – World Bank.

NOTES

a: low income ($935 or less).
b: lower-middle income ($936 to $3,705).
c: upper-middle income ($3,706 to $11,455).
d: high income ($11,456 or more).

– Data not available.
x Data refer to years or periods other than those specified in the column heading, differ from the standard definition or refer to only part of a country. Such data are not included in the calculation of regional and global averages.
s National household survey data.
* Data refer to the most recent year available during the period specified in the column heading.

TABLE 2. NUTRITION

Countries and territories	% of infants with low birthweight 2000–2007*	% of children (2000–2007*) who are:			% of under-fives (2000–2007*) suffering from:					Vitamin A supplementation coverage rate (6–59 months) 2007		% of households consuming iodized salt 2000–2007*
		exclusively breastfed (<6 months)	breastfed with complementary food (6–9 months)	still breastfeeding (20–23 months)	underweight† (WHO ref. pop.) moderate & severe	underweight† (NCHS/WHO) moderate & severe	underweight† (NCHS/WHO) severe	wasting‡ (NCHS/WHO) moderate & severe	stunting‡ (NCHS/WHO) moderate & severe	at least one dose‡ (%)	full coverageΔ (%)	
Afghanistan	–	–	29	54	33y	39y	12y	7y	54y	94	92	28
Albania	7	40	69	22	6	8	1	7	22	–	–	60
Algeria	6	7	39	22	3	4	1	3	11	–	–	61
Andorra	–	–	–	–	–	–	–	–	–	–	–	–
Angola	12	11	77	37	26	31	8	6	45	36	36	35
Antigua and Barbuda	5	–	–	–	–	–	–	–	–	–	–	–
Argentina	7	–	–	28	2y	4y	–	1y	4y	–	–	90x
Armenia	8	33	57	15	4	4	0	5	13	–	–	97
Australia	7	–	–	–	–	–	–	–	–	–	–	–
Austria	7	–	–	–	–	–	–	–	–	–	–	–
Azerbaijan	12	12	44	16	8	10	2	5	21	95	95w	54
Bahamas	7x	–	–	–	–	–	–	–	–	–	–	–
Bahrain	8x	34x	65x	41x	–	9x	2x	5x	10x	–	–	–
Bangladesh	22	37	52	89	41	46	–	16	36	95	94	84
Barbados	14	–	–	–	–	–	–	–	–	–	–	–
Belarus	4	9	38	4	1	1	0	1	3	–	–	55
Belgium	8x	–	–	–	–	–	–	–	–	–	–	–
Belize	8	10	–	27	–	6	1	1	18	–	–	90x
Benin	15	43	72	57	18	23	5	7	38	73	73	55
Bhutan	15x	–	–	–	14x	19x	3x	3x	40x	48	48	96
Bolivia	7	54	74	46	5	8	1	1	27	–	–	90
Bosnia and Herzegovina	5	18	29	10	1	2	0	3	7	–	–	62
Botswana	10	34	57	11	11	13	2	5	23	–	–	66
Brazil	8	–	30x	17x	4	5	–	–	–	–	–	88
Brunei Darussalam	10x	–	–	–	–	–	–	–	–	–	–	–
Bulgaria	10	–	–	–	–	–	–	–	–	–	–	100
Burkina Faso	16	7	50	85	32	37	14	23	35	95	73	34
Burundi	11	45	88	–	35	39	14	7	53	83	83	98
Cambodia	14	60	82	54	28	36	7	7	37	76	76	73
Cameroon	11	21	64	21	16	19	5	6	30	–	–	49
Canada	6	–	–	–	–	–	–	–	–	–	–	–
Cape Verde	13x	57x	64x	13x	–	–	–	–	–	–	–	0x
Central African Republic	13	23	55	47	24	29	8	10	38	78	78	62
Chad	22	2	77	65	–	37	14	14	41	54	54	56
Chile	6	85k	–	–	–	1y	–	0y	1y	–	–	100x
China	2	51	32	15	6	7	–	–	11	–	–	94
Colombia	9	47	65	32	5y	7y	1y	1y	12y	–	–	92x
Comoros	25	21	34	45	–	25	–	8	44	93	0	82
Congo	13	19	78	21	11	14	3	7	26	95	79	82
Cook Islands	3	19x	–	–	–	10x	–	–	–	–	–	–
Costa Rica	7	35x	47x	12x	–	5x	0x	2x	6x	–	–	92x
Côte d'Ivoire	17	4	54	37	16	20	4	7	34	63	4	84
Croatia	5	23x	–	–	–	1x	–	1x	1x	–	–	90x
Cuba	5	26	47	16	–	4	0	2	5	–	–	88
Cyprus	–	–	–	–	–	–	–	–	–	–	–	–
Czech Republic	7	–	–	–	–	–	–	–	–	–	–	–
Democratic People's Republic of Korea	7	65	31	37	18y	23y	8y	7y	37y	95	95	40
Democratic Republic of the Congo	12	36	82	64	28	31	9	13	38	79	79	72
Denmark	5	–	–	–	–	–	–	–	–	–	–	–
Djibouti	10	1	23	18	24	29	10	21	33	95	94	0
Dominica	9	–	–	–	–	–	–	–	–	–	–	–
Dominican Republic	11	4	36	15	–	5	1	1	7	–	–	19
Ecuador	16x	40	77	23	6	9	1	2	23	–	–	99x
Egypt	14	38	67	37	5	6	1	4	18	87	87w	78
El Salvador	7	24	76	43	6y	10y	1y	1y	19y	20	13	62
Equatorial Guinea	13	24	–	–	–	19	4	7	39	–	–	33
Eritrea	14	52	43	62	35	40	12	13	38	51	50	68
Estonia	4	–	–	–	–	–	–	–	–	–	–	–
Ethiopia	20	49	54	–	33	38	11	11	47	88	86	20

...TABLE 2

	% of infants with low birthweight 2000–2007*	% of children (2000–2007*) who are:			% of under-fives (2000–2007*) suffering from:					Vitamin A supplementation coverage rate (6–59 months) 2007		% of households consuming iodized salt 2000–2007*
		exclusively breastfed (<6 months)	breastfed with complementary food (6–9 months)	still breastfeeding (20–23 months)	underweight† (WHO ref. pop.) moderate & severe	underweight† (NCHS/WHO) moderate & severe	severe	wasting‡ (NCHS/WHO) moderate & severe	stunting‡ (NCHS/WHO) moderate & severe	at least one dose‡ (%)	full coverageΔ (%)	
Fiji	10x	47x	–	–	–	–	–	–	–	–	–	31x
Finland	4	–	–	–	–	–	–	–	–	–	–	–
France	7x	–	–	–	–	–	–	–	–	–	–	–
Gabon	14	6	62	9	8	12	2	3	21	90	0	36
Gambia	20	41	44	53	16	20	4	6	22	93	82	7
Georgia	5	11	35	20	2	2	0	2	10	–	–	87
Germany	7x	–	–	–	–	–	–	–	–	–	–	–
Ghana	9	54	58	56	13	18	3	5	22	95	77	32
Greece	8x	–	–	–	–	–	–	–	–	–	–	–
Grenada	9	39x	–	–	–	–	–	–	–	–	–	–
Guatemala	12	51	67	47	18y	23y	4y	2y	49y	33	29	40
Guinea	12	27	41	71	22	26	7	9	35	95	94	51
Guinea-Bissau	24	16	35	61	15	19	4	7	41	66	64	1
Guyana	13	11	42	31	10	12	2	8	14	–	–	–
Haiti	25	41	87	35	18	22	6	9	24	–	–	3
Holy See	–	–	–	–	–	–	–	–	–	–	–	–
Honduras	10	30	69	48	8	11	1	1	25	–	–	80x
Hungary	9	–	–	–	–	–	–	–	–	–	–	–
Iceland	4	–	–	–	–	–	–	–	–	–	–	–
India	28	46	57	77	43	46	–	19	38	53	33	51
Indonesia	9	40	75	59	23	28	9	–	–	87	87	73
Iran (Islamic Republic of)	7x	23	68	58	–	11x	2x	5x	15x	–	–	99
Iraq	15	25	51	36	6	8	1	5	21	–	–	28
Ireland	6x	–	–	–	–	–	–	–	–	–	–	–
Israel	8	–	–	–	–	–	–	–	–	–	–	–
Italy	6x	–	–	–	–	–	–	–	–	–	–	–
Jamaica	12	15	36	24	3	4	–	4	3	–	–	100x
Japan	8	–	–	–	–	–	–	–	–	–	–	–
Jordan	12	22	66	11	–	4	1	2	9	–	–	88
Kazakhstan	6	17	39	16	4	4	1	4	13	–	–	92
Kenya	10	13	84	57	16	20	4	6	30	22	15	91
Kiribati	5x	80x	–	–	–	13x	–	–	–	–	–	–
Kuwait	7x	12x	26x	9x	–	10x	3x	11x	24x	–	–	–
Kyrgyzstan	5	32	49	26	2	3	0	4	14	95	95	76
Lao People's Democratic Republic	14	23	10	47	31	37	9	7	40	83	69	75
Latvia	5	–	–	–	–	–	–	–	–	–	–	–
Lebanon	6	27	35	11	–	4	–	5	11	–	–	92
Lesotho	13	36	79	60	–	20	4	4	38	85	38	91
Liberia	–	35	70	45	23	26	8	6	39	85	85	–
Libyan Arab Jamahiriya	7x	–	–	23x	4x	5x	1x	3x	15x	–	–	90x
Liechtenstein	–	–	–	–	–	–	–	–	–	–	–	–
Lithuania	4	–	–	–	–	–	–	–	–	–	–	–
Luxembourg	8	–	–	–	–	–	–	–	–	–	–	–
Madagascar	17	67	78	64	36	42	11	13	48	95	95	75
Malawi	14	57	89	72	15	21	4	4	46	90	90	50
Malaysia	9	29x	–	12x	–	8	1	–	–	–	–	–
Maldives	22	10	85	–	–	30	7	13	25	62	62	44
Mali	19	38	30	56	27	32	10	13	34	95	89	79
Malta	6	–	–	–	–	–	–	–	–	–	–	–
Marshall Islands	12x	63x	–	–	–	–	–	–	–	39	39	–
Mauritania	–	20	78	57	–	32	10	13	35	95	89	2
Mauritius	14	21	–	–	–	15x	2x	14x	10x	–	–	0x
Mexico	8	38x	36x	21x	3	5	–	2	13	–	–	91
Micronesia (Federated States of)	18	60x	–	–	–	15x	–	–	–	–	–	–
Moldova	6	46	18	2	–	4	1	4	8	–	–	60
Monaco	–	–	–	–	–	–	–	–	–	–	–	–
Mongolia	6	57	57	65	5	6	1	2	21	95	94	83
Montenegro	4	19	35	13	2	3	1	3	5	–	–	71
Morocco	15	31	66	15	9	10	2	9	18	–	–	21
Mozambique	15	30	80	65	20	24	6	4	41	48	42	54
Myanmar	15	15	66	67	–	32	7	9	32	94	93	60
Namibia	14	24	72	28	–	24	5	9	24	–	–	63
Nauru	–	–	–	–	–	–	–	–	–	–	–	–

STATISTICAL TABLES 123

TABLE 2. NUTRITION

Countries and territories	% of infants with low birthweight 2000–2007*	% of children (2000–2007*) who are:			% of under-fives (2000–2007*) suffering from:					Vitamin A supplementation coverage rate (6–59 months) 2007		% of households consuming iodized salt 2000–2007*
		exclusively breastfed (<6 months)	breastfed with complementary food (6–9 months)	still breastfeeding (20–23 months)	underweight† (WHO ref. pop.) moderate & severe	underweight† (NCHS/WHO) moderate & severe	severe	wasting‡ (NCHS/WHO) moderate & severe	stunting‡ (NCHS/WHO) moderate & severe	at least one dose‡ (%)	full coverageΔ (%)	
Nepal	21	53	75	95	39	45	10	12	43	95	95	63
Netherlands	–	–	–	–	–	–	–	–	–	–	–	–
New Zealand	6	–	–	–	–	–	–	–	–	–	–	83x
Nicaragua	12	31	83	43	–	7	1	1	17	95	–	97
Niger	27	9	73	–	39	44	15	10	50	95	95	46
Nigeria	14	17	64	34	24	29	9	9	38	77	55	97
Niue	0	–	–	–	–	–	–	–	–	–	–	–
Norway	5	–	–	–	–	–	–	–	–	–	–	–
Occupied Palestinian Territory	7	27	–	–	–	3	0	1	10	–	–	86
Oman	9	–	91	73	13x	18x	1x	7x	10x	–	–	61x
Pakistan	19x	37	36	55	31	38	13	13	37	95	95	17
Palau	9x	59x	–	–	–	–	–	–	–	–	–	–
Panama	10	25x	38x	21x	6x	8x	1x	1x	18x	–	–	95x
Papua New Guinea	11x	59x	74x	66x	–	–	–	–	–	7	7	–
Paraguay	9	22	60	–	3	4	–	1	14	–	–	94
Peru	10	63	82	47	6	5	1	1	30	–	–	91
Philippines	20	34	58	32	21	28	–	6	30	83	83	45
Poland	6	–	–	–	–	–	–	–	–	–	–	–
Portugal	8	–	–	–	–	–	–	–	–	–	–	–
Qatar	10x	12x	48x	21x	–	6x	–	2x	8x	–	–	–
Republic of Korea	4	–	–	–	–	–	–	–	–	–	–	–
Romania	8	16	41	–	4	3	0	2	10	–	–	74
Russian Federation	6	–	–	–	–	3x	1x	4x	13x	–	–	35
Rwanda	6	88	69	77	18	23	4	4	45	89	76	88
Saint Kitts and Nevis	9	56x	–	–	–	–	–	–	–	–	–	100
Saint Lucia	11	–	–	–	–	–	–	–	–	–	–	–
Saint Vincent and the Grenadines	8	–	–	–	–	–	–	–	–	–	–	–
Samoa	4x	–	–	–	–	–	–	–	–	–	–	–
San Marino	–	–	–	–	–	–	–	–	–	–	–	–
Sao Tome and Principe	8	60	60	18	7	9	1	8	23	55	48	37
Saudi Arabia	11x	31x	60x	30x	–	14x	3x	11x	20x	–	–	–
Senegal	19	34	61	42	14	17	3	8	16	94	94	41
Serbia	5	15	39	8	1	2	0	3	6	–	–	73
Seychelles	–	–	–	–	–	–	–	–	–	–	–	–
Sierra Leone	24	8	52	57	25	30	8	9	40	95	86	45
Singapore	8	–	–	–	3	3	0	2	2	–	–	–
Slovakia	7	–	–	–	–	–	–	–	–	–	–	–
Slovenia	6	–	–	–	–	–	–	–	–	–	–	–
Solomon Islands	13x	65	–	–	16x	21x	–	–	–	–	–	–
Somalia	–	9	15	35	32	36	12	11	38	89	4	1
South Africa	15x	7	46	–	10x	12x	2x	3x	25x	–	–	62x
Spain	6x	–	–	–	–	–	–	–	–	–	–	–
Sri Lanka	22	53	–	73	23y	29y	–	14y	14y	–	–	94
Sudan	31x	16	47	40	–	41	15	16	43	90	90	1
Suriname	13	9	25	11	7	10	1	5	8	–	–	–
Swaziland	9	32	77	31	5	7	–	2	24	–	–	80
Sweden	4x	–	–	–	–	–	–	–	–	–	–	–
Switzerland	6x	–	–	–	–	–	–	–	–	–	–	–
Syrian Arab Republic	9	29	37	16	9	10	2	9	22	–	–	79
Tajikistan	10	25	15	34	14	17	4	7	27	92	92	46
Thailand	9	5	43	19	7	9	0	4	12	–	–	47
The former Yugoslav Republic of Macedonia	6	37x	8x	10x	2	2	0	2	9	–	–	94
Timor-Leste	12	31	82	35	–	49	15	25	54	57	50	60
Togo	12	28	35	44	22	26	7	14	24	95	64	25
Tonga	3	62x	–	–	–	–	–	–	–	–	–	–
Trinidad and Tobago	19	13	43	22	–	6	1	4	4	–	–	28
Tunisia	7	47	–	22	–	4	1	2	12	–	–	97
Turkey	16x	21	38	24	–	4	1	1	12	–	–	64
Turkmenistan	4	11	54	37	8	11	2	6	15	–	–	87
Tuvalu	5	–	–	–	–	–	–	–	–	–	–	–
Uganda	14	60	80	54	16	20	5	5	32	64	–	96

THE STATE OF THE WORLD'S CHILDREN 2009

...TABLE 2

	% of infants with low birthweight 2000–2007*	% of children (2000–2007*) who are:			% of under-fives (2000–2007*) suffering from:					Vitamin A supplementation coverage rate (6–59 months) 2007		% of households consuming iodized salt 2000–2007*
		exclusively breastfed (<6 months)	breastfed with complementary food (6–9 months)	still breastfeeding (20–23 months)	underweight† (WHO ref. pop.) moderate & severe	underweight† (NCHS/WHO) moderate & severe	underweight† (NCHS/WHO) severe	wasting‡ (NCHS/WHO) moderate & severe	stunting‡ (NCHS/WHO) moderate & severe	at least one dose‡ (%)	full coverageΔ (%)	
Ukraine	4	6	49	11	–	1y	0y	0y	3y	–	–	18
United Arab Emirates	15x	34x	52x	29x	–	14x	3x	15x	17x	–	–	–
United Kingdom	8	–	–	–	–	–	–	–	–	–	–	–
United Republic of Tanzania	10	41	91	55	17	22	4	3	38	93	93	43
United States	8	–	–	–	1y	2y	0y	0y	1y	–	–	–
Uruguay	8	54	32	31	–	5	1	2	11	–	–	–
Uzbekistan	5	26	45	38	4	5	1	3	15	84	84	53
Vanuatu	6	50x	–	–	–	–	–	–	–	–	–	–
Venezuela (Bolivarian Republic of)	9	7x	50x	31x	–	5	–	4	12	–	–	90x
Viet Nam	7	17	70	23	–	20	5	8	36	95	95w	93
Yemen	32x	–	–	–	42	46	15	12	53	47	47w	30
Zambia	12	61	93	42	15	19	3	5	39	95	95	77
Zimbabwe	11	22	79	–	12	17	3	6	29	83	83	91

SUMMARY INDICATORS

Sub-Saharan Africa	15	31	68	51	24	28	8	9	38	77	67	64
Eastern and Southern Africa	14	40	71	56	23	28	7	7	40	73	68	56
West and Central Africa	15	23	65	47	24	28	9	10	36	81	67	72
Middle East and North Africa	12	26	57	36	11	17	5	8	26	–	–	60
South Asia	27	44	53	75	41	45	–	18	38	64	50	51
East Asia and Pacific	6	43	45	27	11	14	–	–	16	86	86**	86
Latin America and Caribbean	9	–	–	–	5	6	–	2	16	–	–	83
CEE/CIS	6	20	41	23	–	5	1	2	12	–	–	50
Industrialized countries§	7	–	–	–	–	–	–	–	–	–	–	–
Developing countries§	15	39	55	51	24	26	–	11	30	72	62**	70
Least developed countries§	17	37	64	64	30	34	9	11	40	84	82	55
World	14	38	55	50	23	25	–	11	28	72	62**	68

§ Also includes territories within each country category or regional group. Countries and territories in each country category or regional group are listed on page 152.

DEFINITIONS OF THE INDICATORS

Low birthweight – Percentage of infants weighing less than 2,500 grams at birth.

Underweight (WHO ref. pop.) – Moderate and severe: Percentage of children aged 0–59 months who are below minus two standard deviations from median weight for age of the WHO Child Growth Standards published in 2006.

Underweight (NCHS/WHO) – Moderate and severe: Percentage of children aged 0–59 months who are below minus two standard deviations from median weight for age of the National Center for Health Statistics (NCHS)/WHO reference population; Severe: Percentage of children aged 0–59 months who are below minus three standard deviations from median weight for age of the NCHS/WHO reference population.

Wasting (NCHS/WHO) – Moderate and severe: Percentage of children aged 0–59 months who are below minus two standard deviations from median weight for height of the NCHS/WHO reference population.

Stunting (NCHS/WHO) – Moderate and severe: Percentage of children aged 0–59 months who are below minus two standard deviations from median height for age of the NCHS/WHO reference population.

Vitamin A – Percentage of children aged 6–59 months who received vitamin A supplements in 2007.

Iodized salt consumption – Percentage of households consuming adequately iodized salt (15 parts per million or more).

MAIN DATA SOURCES

Low birthweight – Demographic and Health Surveys (DHS), Multiple Indicator Cluster Surveys (MICS), other national household surveys, data from routine reporting systems, UNICEF and WHO.

Breastfeeding – DHS, MICS, other national household surveys and UNICEF.

Underweight, wasting and stunting – DHS, MICS, other national household surveys, WHO and UNICEF.

Vitamin A – UNICEF.

Salt iodization – DHS, MICS, other national household surveys and UNICEF.

NOTES

- – Data not available.
- x Data refer to years or periods other than those specified in the column heading, differ from the standard definition or refer to only part of a country. Such data are not included in the calculation of regional and global averages.
- y Data refer to years or periods other than those specified in the column heading, differ from the standard definition or refer to only part of a country. Such data are included in the calculation of regional and global averages.
- k Refers to exclusive breastfeeding for less than four months.
- w Identifies countries with national vitamin A supplementation programmes targeted towards a reduced age range. Coverage figure is reported as targeted.
- † In this year's report, the 'underweight' statistics apply the same indicators to two different reference populations. Due to this difference, the data presented here are not strictly comparable with each other or with previous editions of this report. The WHO Child Growth Standards are gradually replacing the widely used NCHS/WHO reference population. For a more detailed description of this transition, please see the *General note on the data* on page 114.
- ‡ The data for 'wasting' and 'stunting' refer to the same reference populations and are therefore comparable with each other and with data published in previous editions of this report.
- ‡ Refers to the percentage of children who received at least one dose in 2007 (the most recent coverage point at the time of reporting).
- Δ The percentage of children reached with two doses in 2007 is reported as the lower percentage of two coverage points. '0' (zero) indicates that only one dose was delivered in 2007.
- * Data refer to the most recent year available during the period specified in the column heading.
- ** Excludes China.

TABLE 3. HEALTH

Countries and territories	% of population using improved drinking-water sources 2006			% of population using improved sanitation facilities 2006			% of routine EPI vaccines financed by government 2007	Immunization 2007 1-year-old children immunized against:							% new-borns protected against tetanus	% under-fives with suspected pneumonia taken to an appropriate health-care provider	% under-fives with suspected pneumonia receiving antibiotics	% under-fives with diarrhoea receiving oral rehydration and continued feeding	Malaria 2003–2007*		
								TB	DPT		Polio	Measles	HepB	Hib					% under-fives sleeping under a mosquito net	% under-fives sleeping under a treated mosquito net	% under-fives with fever receiving anti-malarial drugs
	total	urban	rural	total	urban	rural	total	BCG	DPT1β	DPT3β	polio3	measles	HepB3	Hib3		2000–2007*		2000–2007*			
Afghanistan	22	37	17	30	45	25	0	77	93	83	83	70	83	–	73	28	–	48	–	–	–
Albania	97	97	97	97	98	97	100	98	98	98	99	97	98	–	87	45	38	50	–	–	–
Algeria	85	87	81	94	98	87	100	99	98	95	95	92	90	–	70	53	59	24	–	–	–
Andorra	100	100	100	100	100	100	–	–	98	96	96	94	91	95	–	–	–	–	–	–	–
Angola	51	62	39	50	79	16	18	88	99	83	83	88	83	83	81	58	–	32	21	18	29
Antigua and Barbuda	–	95	–	–	98	–	–	–	99	99	98	99	97	99	–	–	–	–	–	–	–
Argentina	96	98	80	91	92	83	–	99	94	96	94	99	92	96	–	–	–	–	–	–	–
Armenia	98	99	96	91	96	81	33	94	96	88	90	92	85	–	–	36	11	59	–	–	–
Australia	100	100	100	100	100	100	88	–	97	92	92	94	94	94	–	–	–	–	–	–	–
Austria	100	100	100	100	100	100	–	–	95	85	85	79	85	85	–	–	–	–	–	–	–
Azerbaijan	78	95	59	80	90	70	72	98	97	95	95	97	97	–	–	36	–	45	12x	1x	1x
Bahamas	–	98	–	100	100	100	100	–	99	95	95	96	93	95	93	–	–	–	–	–	–
Bahrain	–	100	–	–	100	–	100	–	97	97	97	99	97	97	66	–	–	–	–	–	–
Bangladesh	80	85	78	36	48	32	60	97	97	90	96	88	90	–	91	30	22	49	–	–	–
Barbados	100	100	100	99	99	100	–	–	93	93	93	75	93	93	–	–	–	–	–	–	–
Belarus	100	100	99	93	91	97	100	98	99	99	99	99	91	–	–	90	67	54	–	–	–
Belgium	–	100	–	–	–	–	–	–	99	99	99	92	94	98	–	–	–	–	–	–	–
Belize	–	100	–	–	–	–	100	99	98	96	97	96	96	96	85	71	44	–	–	–	–
Benin	65	78	57	30	59	11	11	88	84	67	64	61	67	67	93	36	–	42	47	20	54
Bhutan	81	98	79	52	71	50	0	94	92	95	93	95	95	–	86	–	–	–	–	–	–
Bolivia	86	96	69	43	54	22	100	93	94	81	79	81	81	81	71	52	–	54	–	–	–
Bosnia and Herzegovina	99	100	98	95	99	92	95	98	95	95	95	96	94	95	–	91	73	53	–	–	–
Botswana	96	100	90	47	60	30	100	99	98	97	97	90	85	–	78	14	–	7	–	–	–
Brazil	91	97	58	77	84	37	–	99	98	99	99	99	95	98	93	46x	15x	28x	–	–	–
Brunei Darussalam	–	–	–	–	–	–	–	96	99	99	99	97	99	99	65	–	–	–	–	–	–
Bulgaria	99	100	97	99	100	96	100	98	96	95	95	96	95	–	–	–	–	–	–	–	–
Burkina Faso	72	97	66	13	41	6	23	99	99	99	99	94	99	99	80	39	15	42	18	10	48
Burundi	71	84	70	41	44	41	–	84	86	74	64	75	74	74	78	38	26	23	13	8	30
Cambodia	65	80	61	28	62	19	17	90	87	82	82	79	82	–	87	48	–	50	88	4	0
Cameroon	70	88	47	51	58	42	40	81	90	82	81	74	82	–	81	35	38	22	27	13	58
Canada	100	100	99	100	100	99	–	–	97	94	90	94	14	94	–	–	–	–	–	–	–
Cape Verde	–	–	–	–	–	–	90	86	83	81	81	74	79	–	77	51	–	–	–	–	–
Central African Republic	66	90	51	31	40	25	1	74	65	54	47	62	–	–	54	32	39	47	33	15	57
Chad	48	71	40	9	23	4	80	40	45	20	36	23	–	–	60	12	–	27	27x	1x	53x
Chile	95	98	72	94	97	74	–	98	95	94	94	91	94	94	–	–	–	–	–	–	–
China	88	98	81	65	74	59	–	94	94	93	94	94	92	–	–	–	–	–	–	–	–
Colombia	93	99	77	78	85	58	100	93	97	93	93	95	93	93	78	62	–	39	24x	–	–
Comoros	85	91	81	35	49	26	0	77	79	75	75	65	75	–	89	49	–	31	36x	9x	63x
Congo	71	95	35	20	19	21	100	86	80	80	80	67	80	–	90	48	–	39	68	6	48
Cook Islands	95	98	88	100	100	100	100	99	99	99	99	98	99	–	–	–	–	–	–	–	–
Costa Rica	98	99	96	96	96	95	–	91	90	89	89	90	89	88	–	–	–	–	–	–	–
Côte d'Ivoire	81	98	66	24	38	12	31	94	DPT 93	76	75	67	76	–	76	35	19	45	17	3	36
Croatia	99	100	98	99	99	98	100	99	98	96	96	96	95	96	–	–	–	–	–	–	–
Cuba	91	95	78	98	99	95	99	99	97	93	99	99	93	97	–	–	–	–	–	–	–
Cyprus	100	100	100	100	100	100	36	–	99	97	97	87	93	90	–	–	–	–	–	–	–
Czech Republic	100	100	100	99	100	98	100	99	98	99	99	97	99	99	–	–	–	–	–	–	–
Democratic People's Republic of Korea	100	100	100	–	–	–	–	96	93	92	99	99	92	–	91	93	–	–	–	–	–
Democratic Republic of the Congo	46	82	29	31	42	25	0	94	96	87	87	79	87	–	81	42	–	17	19	6	30
Denmark	100	100	100	100	100	100	100	–	97	75	75	89	–	75	–	–	–	–	–	–	–
Djibouti	92	98	54	67	76	11	0	90	92	88	88	74	25	25	77	62	43	33	9	1	10
Dominica	–	100	–	–	–	–	100	90	93	96	93	96	93	93	–	–	–	–	–	–	–
Dominican Republic	95	97	91	79	81	74	–	92	87	79	83	96	70	59	85	64	–	42	–	–	–
Ecuador	95	98	91	84	91	72	–	99	99	99	99	99	99	99	67	–	–	–	–	–	–
Egypt	98	99	98	66	85	52	100	98	98	98	98	97	98	–	85	63	–	27	–	–	–
El Salvador	84	94	68	86	90	80	100	93	98	96	96	98	96	96	87	62	–	–	–	–	–
Equatorial Guinea	43	45	42	51	60	46	100	73	65	33	39	51	–	–	62	–	–	36	15x	1x	49x
Eritrea	60	74	57	5	14	3	–	99	99	97	96	95	97	–	80	44	–	54	12x	4x	4x
Estonia	100	100	99	95	96	94	100	98	98	95	95	96	95	95	–	–	–	–	–	–	–
Ethiopia	42	96	31	11	27	8	0	72	81	73	71	65	73	73	85	19	5	15	35	33	10
Fiji	47	43	51	71	87	55	100	90	82	83	84	81	84	83	94	–	–	–	–	–	–
Finland	100	100	100	100	100	100	100	97	99	99	97	98	–	97	–	–	–	–	–	–	–

...TABLE 3

	% of population using improved drinking-water sources 2006			% of population using improved sanitation facilities 2006			% of routine EPI vaccines financed by government 2007	Immunization 2007							% new-borns protected against tetanus^λ	% under-fives with suspected pneumonia taken to an appropriate health-care provider	% under-fives with suspected pneumonia receiving antibiotics	% under-fives with diarrhoea receiving oral rehy-dration and continued feeding	Malaria 2003–2007*		
								TB	DPT		Polio	Measles	HepB	Hib					% under-fives sleeping under a mosquito net	% under-fives sleeping under a treated mosquito net	% under-fives with fever receiving anti-malarial drugs
								\	1-year-old children immunized against:												
									corresponding vaccines:												
	total	urban	rural	total	urban	rural	total	BCG	DPT1^β	DPT3^β	polio3	measles	HepB3	Hib3		2000–2007*		2000–2007*			
France	100	100	100	–	–	–	10	84	98	98	98	87	29	87	–	–	–	–	–	–	–
Gabon	87	95	47	36	37	30	100	89	69	38	31	55	38	–	67	48	–	44	–	–	–
Gambia	86	91	81	52	50	55	8	95	90	90	85	85	90	90	90	69	61	38	63	49	63
Georgia	99	100	97	93	94	92	43	96	99	98	88	97	94	–	–	74	56	37	–	–	–
Germany	100	100	100	100	100	100	–	–	98	97	97	94	87	94	–	–	–	–	–	–	–
Ghana	80	90	71	10	15	6	54	99	96	94	94	95	94	94	88	34	33	29	33	22	61
Greece	100	100	99	98	99	97	–	88	96	88	87	88	88	88	–	–	–	–	–	–	–
Grenada	–	97	–	97	96	97	100	–	91	99	99	98	99	99	–	–	–	–	–	–	–
Guatemala	96	99	94	84	90	79	–	97	94	82	82	93	82	82	80	64	–	22x	6x	1x	–
Guinea	70	91	59	19	33	12	70	91	96	75	62	71	83	–	95	42	–	38	12	1	44
Guinea-Bissau	57	82	47	33	48	26	0	89	83	63	64	76	–	–	92	57	42	25	73	39	46
Guyana	93	98	91	81	85	80	100	97	96	94	94	96	94	94	91	64	20	40	–	–	–
Haiti	58	70	51	19	29	12	0	75	83	53	52	58	–	–	43	31	3	43	–	–	5
Holy See	–	–	–	–	–	–	–	–	–	–	–	–	–	–	–	56	54	49	–	–	–
Honduras	84	95	74	66	78	55	100	91	95	86	86	89	86	86	94	–	–	–	–	–	1
Hungary	100	100	100	100	100	100	100	99	99	99	99	99	–	99	–	–	–	–	–	–	–
Iceland	100	100	100	100	100	100	–	–	97	97	97	95	–	97	–	–	–	–	–	–	–
India	89	96	86	28	52	18	100	85	81	62	62	67	6	–	86	69	13	33	–	–	8
Indonesia	80	89	71	52	67	37	92	91	91	75	83	80	74	–	83	61	–	56	32x	0x	1x
Iran (Islamic Republic of)	–	99	–	–	–	–	100	99	99	99	98	97	97	–	83	93	–	–	–	–	–
Iraq	77	88	56	76	80	69	100	92	84	62	66	69	58	–	69	82	82	64	7x	0x	1x
Ireland	–	100	–	–	–	–	–	93	97	92	92	87	–	92	–	–	–	–	–	–	–
Israel	100	100	100	–	100	–	–	–	98	96	95	97	99	95	–	–	–	–	–	–	–
Italy	–	100	–	–	–	–	–	–	98	96	96	87	96	95	–	–	–	–	–	–	–
Jamaica	93	97	88	83	82	84	100	87	85	85	85	76	85	85	54	75	52	39	–	–	–
Japan	100	100	100	100	100	100	–	–	99	98	95	98	–	–	–	–	–	–	–	–	–
Jordan	98	99	91	85	88	71	100	90	99	98	98	95	98	98	87	75	87	44	–	–	–
Kazakhstan	96	99	91	97	97	98	–	99	97	93	94	99	94	–	–	71	32	48	–	–	–
Kenya	57	85	49	42	19	48	–	92	89	81	76	80	81	81	74	49	–	33	15	6	27
Kiribati	65	77	53	33	46	20	100	90	99	94	93	93	96	–	–	–	–	–	–	–	–
Kuwait	–	–	–	–	–	–	–	–	99	99	99	99	99	99	83	–	–	–	–	–	–
Kyrgyzstan	89	99	83	93	94	93	50	98	98	94	94	99	94	–	–	62	45	22	–	–	–
Lao People's Democratic Republic	60	86	53	48	87	38	13	56	59	50	46	40	50	–	47	36	–	37	82x	18x	9x
Latvia	99	100	96	78	82	71	100	99	98	98	98	97	97	97	–	–	–	–	–	–	–
Lebanon	100	100	100	–	100	–	100	–	90	74	74	53	74	74	–	74	–	–	–	–	–
Lesotho	78	93	74	36	43	34	1	96	95	83	80	85	85	–	76	59	–	53	–	–	–
Liberia	64	72	52	32	49	7	1	86	99	88	84	95	–	–	89	70	–	–	–	–	59
Libyan Arab Jamahiriya	–	–	–	97	97	96	100	99	98	98	98	98	98	56	–	–	–	–	–	–	–
Liechtenstein	–	–	–	–	–	–	–	–	–	–	–	–	–	–	–	–	–	–	–	–	–
Lithuania	–	–	–	–	–	–	100	99	98	95	95	97	96	95	–	–	–	–	–	–	–
Luxembourg	100	100	100	100	100	100	100	–	99	99	99	96	87	99	–	–	–	–	–	–	–
Madagascar	47	76	36	12	18	10	26	94	92^β	82^β	81	81	82	–	72	48	–	47	30x	0x	34x
Malawi	76	96	72	60	51	62	33	95	96	87	88	83	87	87	86	52	30	27	31	25	25
Malaysia	99	100	96	94	95	93	–	99	88	96	96	90	87	89	89	–	–	–	–	–	–
Maldives	83	98	76	59	100	42	100	99	99	98	98	97	98	–	94	22	–	–	–	–	–
Mali	60	86	48	45	59	39	100	77	83	68	62	68	68	44	89	38	–	38	41	27	32
Malta	100	100	100	–	100	–	80	–	84	74	76	79	82	72	–	–	–	–	–	–	–
Marshall Islands	–	–	–	–	–	–	3	92	99	93	91	94	93	83	–	–	–	–	–	–	–
Mauritania	60	70	54	24	44	10	100	92	92	75	75	67	74	–	60	45	24	9	43	–	21
Mauritius	100	100	100	94	95	94	100	98	97	97	96	98	97	96	86	–	–	–	–	–	–
Mexico	95	98	85	81	91	48	–	99	99	98	98	96	98	98	87	–	–	–	–	–	–
Micronesia (Federated States of)	94	95	94	25	61	14	5	82	92	79	79	92	90	79	–	–	–	–	–	–	–
Moldova	90	96	85	79	85	73	–	98	95	92	94	96	95	–	–	60	–	48	–	–	–
Monaco	–	100	–	–	100	–	–	90	99	99	99	99	99	99	–	–	–	–	–	–	–
Mongolia	72	90	48	50	64	31	19	99	95	95	99	98	98	78	–	63	71	47	–	–	–
Montenegro	98	100	96	91	96	86	100	98	98	92	92	90	89	–	–	89	57	64	–	–	–
Morocco	83	100	58	72	85	54	100	96	98	95	95	95	95	90	85	38	–	46	–	–	–
Mozambique	42	71	26	31	53	19	–	87	88	72	70	77	72	–	82	55	–	47	10	–	15
Myanmar	80	80	80	82	85	81	–	89	89	86	84	81	85	–	91	66	–	65	–	–	–
Namibia	93	99	90	35	66	18	100	95	88	86	81	69	–	–	82	72	14	39	12	11	10
Nauru	–	–	–	–	–	–	100	99	99	99	99	99	99	–	–	–	–	–	–	–	–

STATISTICAL TABLES

TABLE 3. HEALTH

	% of population using improved drinking-water sources 2006			% of population using improved sanitation facilities 2006			% of routine EPI vaccines financed by government 2007	Immunization 2007 1-year-old children immunized against:							% newborns protected against tetanus^	% under-fives with suspected pneumonia taken to an appropriate health-care provider	% under-fives with suspected pneumonia receiving antibiotics	% under-fives with diarrhoea receiving oral rehydration and continued feeding	Malaria 2003–2007*		
								TB	DPT		Polio	Measles	HepB	Hib					% under-fives sleeping under a mosquito net	% under-fives sleeping under a treated mosquito net	% under-fives with fever receiving anti-malarial drugs
									corresponding vaccines:												
	total	urban	rural	total	urban	rural	total	BCG	DPT1§	DPT3§	polio3	measles	HepB3	Hib3		2000–2007*		2000–2007*			
Nepal	89	94	88	27	45	24	29	89	85	82	82	81	82	–	83	43	25	37	–	–	0
Netherlands	100	100	100	100	100	100	–	–	98	96	96	96	–	96	–	–	–	–	–	–	–
New Zealand	–	100	–	–	–	–	100	–	91	88	88	79	88	78	–	–	–	–	–	–	–
Nicaragua	79	90	63	48	57	34	49	99	94	87	88	99	87	87	94	57	–	49	–	–	2x
Niger	42	91	32	7	27	3	0	64	58	39	55	47	–	–	72	47	–	34	15	7	33
Nigeria	47	65	30	30	35	25	–	69	72	54	61	62	41	–	53	33	–	28	6	1	34
Niue	100	100	100	100	100	100	–	99	99	99	99	99	99	99	–	–	–	–	–	–	–
Norway	100	100	100	–	–	–	60	–	97	93	93	92	–	95	–	–	–	–	–	–	–
Occupied Palestinian Territory	89	90	88	80	84	69	–	99	99	99	99	99	99	99	–	65	–	–	–	–	–
Oman	–	–	–	–	97	–	–	99	99	99	97	97	99	99	95	–	–	–	–	–	–
Pakistan	90	95	87	58	90	40	31	89	90	83	83	80	83	–	81	69	50	37	2	–	3
Palau	89	79	94	67	96	52	0	–	99	94	94	91	91	95	–	–	–	–	–	–	–
Panama	92	96	81	74	78	63	–	99	88	88	88	89	88	88	–	–	–	–	–	–	–
Papua New Guinea	40	88	32	45	67	41	100	67	76	60	61	58	59	–	60	75x	–	–	–	–	–
Paraguay	77	94	52	70	89	42	–	68	86	66	65	80	66	66	81	51x	29x	–	–	–	–
Peru	84	92	63	72	85	36	–	97	90	80	95	99	80	80	82	67	–	57	–	–	–
Philippines	93	96	88	78	81	72	100	90	90	87	87	92	88	–	65	55	–	76	–	–	0
Poland	–	100	–	–	–	–	–	93	99	99	99	98	98	88	–	–	–	–	–	–	–
Portugal	99	99	100	99	99	98	–	98	94	97	96	95	97	97	–	–	–	–	–	–	–
Qatar	100	100	100	100	100	100	8	96	96	94	97	92	94	94	–	–	–	–	–	–	–
Republic of Korea	–	97	–	–	–	–	–	96	95	91	91	92	91	–	–	–	–	–	–	–	–
Romania	88	99	76	72	88	54	–	99	98	97	96	97	99	–	–	–	–	–	–	–	–
Russian Federation	97	100	88	87	93	70	–	96	98	98	99	99	98	–	–	–	–	–	–	–	–
Rwanda	65	82	61	23	34	20	24	89	96	97	98	99	97	96	82	28	–	24	16	13	12
Saint Kitts and Nevis	99	99	99	96	96	96	–	97	99	99	99	99	99	99	–	–	–	–	–	–	–
Saint Lucia	98	98	98	–	–	–	100	99	99	99	99	94	99	99	–	–	–	–	–	–	–
Saint Vincent and the Grenadines	–	–	–	–	–	96	100	99	99	99	99	99	99	99	–	–	–	–	–	–	–
Samoa	88	90	87	100	100	100	–	91	85	71	71	63	69	–	5	–	–	–	–	–	–
San Marino	–	–	–	–	–	–	–	–	92	92	92	92	92	92	–	–	–	–	–	–	–
Sao Tome and Principe	86	88	83	24	29	18	50	98	99	97	98	86	99	–	–	47	–	63	53	42	25
Saudi Arabia	–	97	–	–	100	–	100	96	97	96	96	96	96	96	–	–	–	–	–	–	–
Senegal	77	93	65	28	54	9	31	99	99	94	93	84	94	94	86	47	–	43	28	16	22
Serbia	99	99	98	92	96	88	100	98	97	94	93	95	99	89	–	93	57	71	–	–	–
Seychelles	–	100	–	–	–	100	100	99	99	99	99	99	–	–	–	–	–	–	–	–	–
Sierra Leone	53	83	32	11	20	5	0	82	77	64	64	67	64	64	94	48	21	31	20	5	52
Singapore	–	100	–	–	100	–	–	98	97	96	96	95	95	–	–	–	–	–	–	–	–
Slovakia	100	100	100	100	100	99	100	98	99	99	99	99	99	99	–	–	–	–	–	–	–
Slovenia	–	–	–	–	–	–	60	–	98	97	98	96	–	98	–	–	–	–	–	–	–
Solomon Islands	70	94	65	32	98	18	0	84	84	79	77	78	79	–	84	–	–	–	–	–	–
Somalia	29	63	10	23	51	7	–	52	58	39	39	34	–	–	68	13	32	7	18	11	8
South Africa	93	100	82	59	66	49	100	99	99	97	97	83	97	97	72	75x	–	37x	–	–	–
Spain	100	100	100	100	100	100	100	–	98	96	96	97	96	96	–	–	–	–	–	–	–
Sri Lanka	82	98	79	86	89	86	31	99	99	98	98	98	98	–	91	58	–	–	62	3	0
Sudan	70	78	64	35	50	24	0	83	95	84	84	79	78	–	72	57	–	38	23x	0x	50x
Suriname	92	97	79	82	89	60	100	–	96	84	84	85	84	84	93	74	37	28	–	–	–
Swaziland	60	87	51	50	64	46	100	99	97	95	95	91	95	–	86	73	24	22	1	1	1
Sweden	100	100	100	100	100	100	–	18	99	99	99	96	4	99	–	–	–	–	–	–	–
Switzerland	100	100	100	100	100	100	5	–	97	93	94	86	–	92	–	–	–	–	–	–	–
Syrian Arab Republic	89	95	83	92	96	88	100	99	99	99	99	98	98	99	92	77	71	34	–	–	–
Tajikistan	67	93	58	92	95	91	10	83	88	86	85	85	84	–	–	64	41	22	2	1	2
Thailand	98	99	97	96	95	96	–	99	98	98	98	96	96	–	89	84	65	46	–	–	–
The former Yugoslav Republic of Macedonia	100	100	99	89	92	81	100	95	98	95	96	96	96	–	–	93	74	45	–	–	–
Timor-Leste	62	77	56	41	64	32	–	74	76	70	70	63	–	–	59	24	–	–	48x	8x	47x
Togo	59	86	40	12	24	3	97	91	94	88	78	80	–	–	82	23	26	22	41	38	48
Tonga	100	100	100	96	98	96	56	99	99	99	99	99	99	99	–	–	–	–	–	–	–
Trinidad and Tobago	94	97	93	92	92	92	–	–	90	88	90	91	89	88	–	74	34	32	–	–	–
Tunisia	94	99	84	85	96	64	100	99	99	98	98	98	98	–	96	43	–	–	–	–	–
Turkey	97	98	95	88	96	72	100	94	98	96	96	96	96	76	69	41	–	19x	–	–	–
Turkmenistan	–	–	–	–	–	–	77	99	99	98	98	99	98	–	–	83	50	25	–	–	–
Tuvalu	93	94	92	89	93	84	10	99	99	97	97	95	97	–	–	–	–	–	–	–	–
Uganda	64	90	60	33	29	34	15	90	90	64	59	68	68	68	85	73	47	39	22	10	61

...TABLE 3

	% of population using improved drinking-water sources 2006			% of population using improved sanitation facilities 2006			% of routine EPI vaccines financed by government 2007	Immunization 2007							% newborns protected against tetanus^λ	% under-fives with suspected pneumonia taken to an appropriate health-care provider	% under-fives with suspected pneumonia receiving antibiotics	% under-fives with diarrhoea receiving oral rehydration and continued feeding	Malaria 2003–2007*		
								1-year-old children immunized against:													
								TB	DPT		Polio	Measles	HepB	Hib					% under-fives sleeping under a mosquito net	% under-fives sleeping under a treated mosquito net	% under-fives with fever receiving anti-malarial drugs
									corresponding vaccines:												
	total	urban	rural	total	urban	rural	total	BCG	DPT1^β	DPT3^β	polio3	measles	HepB3	Hib3		2000–2007*		2000–2007*			
Ukraine	97	97	97	93	97	83	–	97	98	98	99	98	96	11	–	–	–	–	–	–	–
United Arab Emirates	100	100	100	97	98	95	–	98	97	92	94	92	92	92	–	–	–	–	–	–	–
United Kingdom	100	100	100	–	–	–	100	–	97	92	92	86	–	92	–	–	–	–	–	–	–
United Republic of Tanzania	55	81	46	33	31	34	75	89	89	83	88	90	83	–	88	59	–	53	31	16	58
United States	99	100	94	100	100	99	–	–	99	96	92	93	92	94	–	–	–	–	–	–	–
Uruguay	100	100	100	100	100	99	100	99	98	94	94	96	94	94	–	–	–	–	–	–	–
Uzbekistan	88	98	82	96	97	95	64	99	94	96	98	99	98	–	–	68	56	28	–	–	–
Vanuatu	–	–	–	–	–	–	100	82	79	76	76	65	76	–	88	–	–	–	–	–	–
Venezuela (Bolivarian Republic of)	–	–	–	–	–	–	–	83	78	71	73	55	71	71	51	72	–	51	–	–	–
Viet Nam	92	98	90	65	88	56	87	94	92	92	92	83	67	–	86	83	55	65	95	5	3
Yemen	66	68	65	46	88	30	31	64	94	87	87	74	87	87	52	–	38	48	–	–	–
Zambia	58	90	41	52	55	51	24	92	92	80	77	85	80	80	89	68	–	48	34	29	38
Zimbabwe	81	98	72	46	63	37	0	76	77	62	66	66	62	–	78	25	8	47	7	3	5

SUMMARY INDICATORS

Sub-Saharan Africa	58	81	45	30	42	24	31	83	85	73	74	73	67	34	76	40	–	31	21	12	34
Eastern and Southern Africa	59	88	48	34	48	28	32	86	88	78	77	77	77	55	81	45	–	33	24	19	29
West and Central Africa	56	77	41	27	37	20	30	80	82	69	71	69	58	16	71	37	–	29	18	8	38
Middle East and North Africa	87	94	78	73	87	53	81	92	96	91	92	89	89	32	77	68	–	39	–	–	–
South Asia	87	94	84	33	57	23	83	87	84	69	69	71	29	–	85	63	18	35	–	–	–
East Asia and Pacific	88	96	81	66	75	59	–	93	93	89	91	90	87	2	–	65**	–	61**	–	–	–
Latin America and Caribbean	92	97	73	79	86	52	–	96	95	92	93	93	89	90	83	–	–	–	–	–	–
CEE/CIS	94	99	86	89	94	81	81	96	97	96	97	97	96	23	–	57	–	–	–	–	–
Industrialized countries§	100	100	98	100	100	99	–	–	98	96	94	93	65	84	–	–	–	–	–	–	–
Developing countries§	84	94	76	53	71	39	70	89	89	80	81	81	65	21	81	57**	–	38**	–	–	–
Least developed countries§	62	81	55	33	49	27	28	85	89	79	79	76	75	28	81	42	–	37	–	–	–
World	87	96	78	62	79	45	71	89	90	81	82	82	65	26	81	57**	–	38**	–	–	–

§ Also includes territories within each country category or regional group. Countries and territories in each country category or regional group are listed on page 152.

DEFINITIONS OF THE INDICATORS

Government funding of vaccines – Percentage of vaccines that are routinely administered in a country to protect children and are financed by the national government (including loans).

EPI – Expanded programme on immunization: The immunizations in this programme include those against tuberculosis (TB); diphtheria, pertussis (whooping cough) and tetanus (DPT); polio; and measles, as well as vaccination of pregnant women to protect babies against neonatal tetanus. Other vaccines, e.g., against hepatitis B (HepB), *Haemophilus influenzae* type b (Hib) or yellow fever, may be included in the programme in some countries.

BCG – Percentage of infants who received bacille Calmette-Guérin (vaccine against tuberculosis).

DPT1 – Percentage of infants who received their first dose of diphtheria, pertussis and tetanus vaccine.

DPT3 – Percentage of infants who received three doses of diphtheria, pertussis and tetanus vaccine.

HepB3 – Percentage of infants who received three doses of hepatitis B vaccine.

Hib3 – Percentage of infants who received three doses of *Haemophilus influenzae* type b vaccine.

% under-fives with suspected pneumonia taken to an appropriate health-care provider – Percentage of children (aged 0–4) with suspected pneumonia in the two weeks preceding the survey who were taken to an appropriate health-care provider.

% under-fives with suspected pneumonia receiving antibiotics – Percentage of children (aged 0–4) with suspected pneumonia in the two weeks preceding the survey who are receiving antibiotics.

% under-fives with diarrhoea receiving oral rehydration and continued feeding – Percentage of children (aged 0–4) with diarrhoea in the two weeks preceding the survey who received either oral rehydration therapy (oral rehydration solutions or recommended home-made fluids) or increased fluids and continued feeding.

Malaria:

% under-fives sleeping under a mosquito net – Percentage of children (aged 0–4) who slept under a mosquito net.

% under-fives sleeping under a treated mosquito net – Percentage of children (aged 0–4) who slept under an insecticide-treated mosquito net.

% under-fives with fever receiving antimalarial drugs – Percentage of children (aged 0–4) who were ill with fever in the two weeks preceding the survey and received any appropriate (locally defined) antimalarial drugs.

MAIN DATA SOURCES

Use of improved drinking-water sources and improved sanitation facilities – UNICEF and World Health Organization (WHO), Joint Monitoring Programme.

Government funding of vaccines – UNICEF and WHO.

Immunization – UNICEF and WHO.

Suspected pneumonia – Demographic and Health Surveys (DHS), Multiple Indicator Cluster Surveys (MICS) and other national household surveys.

Oral rehydration – DHS and MICS.

Malaria – DHS and MICS.

NOTES

– Data not available.

x Data refer to years or periods other than those specified in the column heading, differ from the standard definition or refer to only part of a country. Such data are not included in the calculation of regional and global averages.

β Coverage for DPT1 should be at least as high as DPT3. Discrepancies where DPT1 coverage is less than DPT3 reflect deficiencies in the data collection and reporting process. UNICEF and WHO are working with national and territorial systems to eliminate these discrepancies.

λ WHO and UNICEF have employed a model to calculate the percentage of births that can be considered as protected against tetanus because pregnant women were given two doses or more of tetanus toxoid (TT) vaccine. The model aims to improve the accuracy of this indicator by capturing or including other potential scenarios where women might be protected (e.g., women who receive doses of TT in supplemental immunization activities). A fuller explanation of the methodology can be found in the *General note on the data*, page 114.

* Data refer to the most recent year available during the period specified in the column heading.

** Excludes China.

TABLE 4. HIV/AIDS

Countries and territories	Estimated adult HIV prevalence rate (aged 15–49), 2007	Estimated number of people (all ages) living with HIV, 2007 (thousands) estimate	low estimate–high estimate	Mother-to-child transmission Estimated number of women (aged 15+) living with HIV, 2007 (thousands)	Paediatric infections Estimated number of children (aged 0–14) living with HIV, 2007 (thousands)	HIV prevalence among young people (aged 15–24), 2007 male	female	% who have comprehensive knowledge of HIV, 2002–2007* male	female	% who used condom at last higher-risk sex, 2002–2007* male	female	Orphans Children (aged 0–17) orphaned by AIDS, 2007 estimate (thousands)	orphaned due to all causes, 2007 estimate (thousands)	Orphan school attendance ratio 2002–2007*
Afghanistan	–	–	–	–	–	–	–	–	–	–	–	–	2100	–
Albania	–	–	<1.0	–	–	–	–	–	6	–	–	–	–	–
Algeria	0.1	21	11–43	6.0	–	0.1	0.1	–	13	–	–	–	570	–
Andorra	–	–	–	–	–	–	–	–	–	–	–	–	–	–
Angola	2.1	190	150–240	110	17	0.2	0.3	–	–	–	–	50	1200	90x
Antigua and Barbuda	–	–	–	–	–	–	–	–	–	–	–	–	–	–
Argentina	0.5	120	90–150	32	–	0.6	0.3	–	–	–	–	–	610	–
Armenia	0.1	2.4	1.8–3.5	<1.0	–	0.2	0.1	15	23	86	–	–	50	–
Australia	0.2	18	11–36	1.2	–	0.2	<0.1	–	–	–	–	–	140	–
Austria	0.2	9.8	7.6–13	2.9	–	0.2	0.1	–	–	–	–	–	52	–
Azerbaijan	0.2	7.8	4.7–16	1.3	–	0.3	0.1	5	5	31	–	–	190	–
Bahamas	3.0	6.2	4.0–8.7	1.6	<0.2	3.2	1.5	–	–	–	–	–	7	–
Bahrain	–	–	–	–	–	–	–	–	–	–	–	–	–	–
Bangladesh	–	12	7.7–19	2.0	–	–	–	–	16	–	–	–	5000	84
Barbados	1.2	2.2	1.5–3.2	<1.0	–	1.3	0.6	–	–	–	–	–	3	–
Belarus	0.2	13	10–19	3.9	–	0.3	0.1	–	34	–	–	–	190	–
Belgium	0.2	15	8.9–29	4.1	–	0.2	0.1	–	–	–	–	–	78	–
Belize	2.1	3.6	2.2–5.3	2.0	<0.2	0.5	1.5	–	40	–	–	–	6	–
Benin	1.2	64	58–73	37	5.4	0.3	0.9	35	16	45	28	29	340	90
Bhutan	0.1	<0.5	<1.0	<0.1	–	0.1	<0.1	–	–	–	–	–	22	–
Bolivia	0.2	8.1	6.5–11	2.2	–	0.2	0.1	18	15	37	20	–	300	74p
Bosnia and Herzegovina	<0.1	<0.5	<1.0	–	–	–	–	–	48	–	71	–	–	–
Botswana	23.9	300	280–310	170	15	5.1	15.3	33x	40x	88x	75x	95	130	99x
Brazil	0.6	730	600–890	240	–	1.0	0.6	–	–	71	58	–	3200	–
Brunei Darussalam	–	–	–	–	–	–	–	–	–	–	–	–	–	–
Bulgaria	–	–	–	–	–	–	–	15	17	70	57	–	95	–
Burkina Faso	1.6	130	110–160	61	10	0.5	0.9	–	19	–	64	100	690	61p
Burundi	2.0	110	78–130	53	15	0.4	1.3	–	30	–	25	120	600	85
Cambodia	0.8	75	67–84	20	4.4	0.8	0.3	45	50	84	–	–	600	83
Cameroon	5.1	540	430–640	300	45	1.2	4.3	–	32	–	62	300	1100	91
Canada	0.4	73	43–110	20	–	0.4	0.2	–	–	–	–	–	180	–
Cape Verde	–	–	–	–	–	–	–	36	36	79	56	–	–	–
Central African Republic	6.3	160	150–170	91	14	1.1	5.5	27	17	–	41	72	280	96
Chad	3.5	200	130–240	110	19	2.0	2.8	20	8	25	17	85	540	105
Chile	0.3	31	23–39	8.7	–	0.3	0.2	–	–	–	–	–	160	–
China	0.1	700	450–1000	200	–	0.1	0.1	–	–	–	–	–	17000	–
Colombia	0.6	170	110–230	47	–	0.7	0.3	–	–	–	36	–	790	85
Comoros	<0.1	<0.2	<1.0	<0.1	–	0.1	<0.1	–	10x	–	–	<0.1	27	–
Congo	3.5	79	65–94	43	6.6	0.8	2.3	35	26	36	16	69	210	88
Cook Islands	–	–	–	–	–	–	–	–	–	–	–	–	–	–
Costa Rica	0.4	9.7	6.1–15	2.7	–	0.4	0.2	–	–	–	–	–	36	–
Côte d'Ivoire	3.9	480	400–550	250	52	0.8	2.4	28	18	53	39	420	1200	83
Croatia	<0.1	<0.5	<1.0	–	–	–	–	–	–	–	–	–	–	–
Cuba	0.1	6.2	3.6–12	1.8	–	0.1	0.1	–	52	–	–	–	99	–
Cyprus	–	–	–	–	–	–	–	–	–	–	–	–	–	–
Czech Republic	–	1.5	<1.0–2.8	<0.5	–	<0.1	–	–	–	–	–	–	94	–
Democratic People's Republic of Korea	–	–	<0.1	–	–	–	–	–	–	–	–	–	530	–
Democratic Republic of the Congo	–	–	400–500	–	–	–	–	21	15	26	17	–	4500	77
Denmark	0.2	4.8	3.7–6.9	1.1	–	0.2	0.1	–	–	–	–	–	53	–
Djibouti	3.1	16	12–19	8.7	1.1	0.7	2.1	–	18	51	26	5	42	–
Dominica	–	–	–	–	–	–	–	–	–	–	–	–	–	–
Dominican Republic	1.1	62	52–71	30	2.7	0.3	0.6	34	41	70	44	–	170	96
Ecuador	0.3	26	15–40	7.1	–	0.4	0.2	–	–	–	–	–	200	–
Egypt	–	9.2	7.2–13	2.6	–	–	–	–	4y	–	–	–	1400	–
El Salvador	0.8	35	24–72	9.7	–	0.9	0.5	–	–	–	–	–	130	–
Equatorial Guinea	3.4	11	8.2–14	5.9	<1.0	0.8	2.5	–	4x	–	–	5	32	95x
Eritrea	1.3	38	25–58	21	3.1	0.3	0.9	–	37	–	–	18	280	83
Estonia	1.3	9.9	5.4–19	2.4	–	1.6	0.7	–	–	–	–	–	20	–
Ethiopia	2.1	980	880–1100	530	92	0.5	1.5	33	20	50	28	650	5000	90
Fiji	0.1	–	<0.5	–	–	0.1	–	–	–	–	–	–	22	–
Finland	0.1	2.4	1.4–4.4	<1.0	–	0.1	<0.1	–	–	–	–	–	48	–

...TABLE 4

	Estimated adult HIV prevalence rate (aged 15–49), 2007	Estimated number of people (all ages) living with HIV, 2007 (thousands)		Mother-to-child transmission Estimated number of women (aged 15+) living with HIV, 2007 (thousands)	Paediatric infections Estimated number of children (aged 0–14) living with HIV, 2007 (thousands)	Prevention among young people						Orphans		
						HIV prevalence among young people (aged 15–24), 2007		% who have comprehensive knowledge of HIV, 2002–2007*		% who used condom at last higher-risk sex, 2002–2007*		Children (aged 0–17)		Orphan school attendance ratio 2002–2007*
		estimate	low estimate–high estimate			male	female	male	female	male	female	orphaned by AIDS, 2007 estimate (thousands)	orphaned due to all causes, 2007 estimate (thousands)	
France	0.4	140	78–240	38	–	0.4	0.2	–	–	–	–	–	420	–
Gabon	5.9	49	37–68	27	2.3	1.3	3.9	22x	24x	48x	33x	18	67	98x
Gambia	0.9	8.2	3.7–13	4.5	<1.0	0.2	0.6	–	39	–	54	3	48	87
Georgia	0.1	2.7	1.5–6.1	<1.0	–	0.1	0.1	–	15	–	–	–	72	–
Germany	0.1	53	31–97	15	–	0.1	0.1	–	–	–	–	–	540	–
Ghana	1.9	260	230–290	150	17	0.4	1.3	33	25	56	42	160	1100	104p
Greece	0.2	11	6.1–19	3.0	–	0.2	0.1	–	–	–	–	–	73	–
Grenada	–	–	–	–	–	–	–	–	–	–	–	–	–	–
Guatemala	0.8	59	41–84	52	–	–	1.5	–	–	–	–	–	360	–
Guinea	1.6	87	73–110	48	6.3	0.4	1.2	23	17	37	26	25	380	73
Guinea-Bissau	1.8	16	11–23	8.7	1.5	0.4	1.2	–	18	–	39	6	110	97
Guyana	2.5	13	7.6–18	7.1	<1.0	0.5	1.7	–	50	68	62	–	23	–
Haiti	2.2	120	100–140	58	6.8	0.6	1.4	40	34	43	29	–	380	86
Holy See	–	–	–	–	–	–	–	–	–	–	–	–	–	–
Honduras	0.7	28	18–44	7.4	1.6	0.7	0.4	–	30	–	24	–	170	108
Hungary	0.1	3.3	2.0–5.9	<1.0	–	0.1	<0.1	–	–	–	–	–	130	–
Iceland	0.2	<0.5	<1.0	<0.2	–	0.2	0.1	–	–	–	–	–	2	–
India	0.3	2400	1800–3200	880	–	0.3	0.3	36	20	37	22	–	25000	72
Indonesia	0.2	270	190–400	54	–	0.3	0.1	0y	1	–	–	–	4400	82y
Iran (Islamic Republic of)	0.2	86	68–110	24	–	0.2	0.1	–	–	–	–	–	1300	–
Iraq	–	–	–	–	–	–	–	–	3	–	–	–	–	84
Ireland	0.2	5.5	4.1–7.7	1.5	–	0.2	0.1	–	–	–	–	–	38	–
Israel	0.1	5.1	2.5–12	2.9	–	<0.1	0.1	–	–	–	–	–	44	–
Italy	0.4	150	110–210	41	–	0.4	0.2	–	–	–	–	–	320	–
Jamaica	1.6	27	19–36	7.6	–	1.7	0.9	–	60	–	–	–	53	–
Japan	–	9.6	7.9–10	2.3	–	–	–	–	–	–	–	–	520	–
Jordan	–	<1.0	<2.0	–	–	–	–	–	3y	–	–	–	–	–
Kazakhstan	0.1	12	7.0–29	3.3	–	0.2	0.1	–	22	65x	32x	–	470	–
Kenya	–	–	1500–2000	–	–	–	–	47	34	47	25	–	2500	95
Kiribati	–	–	–	–	–	–	–	–	–	–	–	–	–	–
Kuwait	–	<1.0	<2.0	–	–	–	–	–	–	–	–	–	–	–
Kyrgyzstan	0.1	4.2	2.3–7.7	1.1	–	0.2	0.1	–	20	–	56	–	140	–
Lao People's Democratic Republic	0.2	5.5	3.3–13	1.3	–	0.2	0.1	–	–	–	–	–	210	–
Latvia	0.8	10	7.4–15	2.7	–	0.9	0.5	–	–	–	–	–	33	–
Lebanon	0.1	3.0	1.7–7.2	<1.0	–	0.1	0.1	–	–	–	–	–	71	–
Lesotho	23.2	270	260–290	150	12	5.9	14.9	18	26	53	53	110	160	95
Liberia	1.7	35	29–41	19	3.1	0.4	1.3	27	21	22	14	15	270	–
Libyan Arab Jamahiriya	–	–	–	–	–	–	–	–	–	–	–	–	–	–
Liechtenstein	–	–	–	–	–	–	–	–	–	–	–	–	–	–
Lithuania	0.1	2.2	1.2–4.6	<1.0	–	0.1	0.1	–	–	–	–	–	51	–
Luxembourg	0.2	–	<1.0	<0.2	–	0.2	0.1	–	–	–	–	–	4	–
Madagascar	0.1	14	9.1–23	3.4	<0.5	0.2	0.1	16	19	12	5	3	840	75
Malawi	11.9	930	860–1000	490	91	2.4	8.4	42	42	58	40	550	1100	97
Malaysia	0.5	80	52–120	21	–	0.6	0.3	–	–	–	–	–	410	–
Maldives	–	–	<0.1	–	–	–	–	–	–	–	–	–	9	–
Mali	1.5	100	88–120	56	9.4	0.4	1.1	22	18	36	17	44	550	87
Malta	0.1	<0.5	<1.0	–	–	0.1	0.1	–	–	–	–	–	3	–
Marshall Islands	–	–	–	–	–	–	–	39	27	–	–	–	–	–
Mauritania	0.8	14	8.3–26	3.9	<0.5	0.9	0.5	–	–	–	–	3	83	–
Mauritius	1.7	13	7.5–28	3.8	<0.1	1.8	1.0	–	–	–	–	<0.5	21	–
Mexico	0.3	200	150–310	57	–	0.3	0.2	–	–	–	–	–	1400	–
Micronesia (Federated States of)	–	–	–	–	–	–	–	–	–	–	–	–	–	–
Moldova	0.4	8.9	6.0–15	2.6	–	0.4	0.2	54y	42y	63	44	–	74	–
Monaco	–	–	–	–	–	–	–	–	–	–	–	–	–	–
Mongolia	0.1	<1.0	1.5	<0.2	–	0.1	–	–	35	–	–	–	64	96p
Montenegro	–	–	–	–	–	–	–	–	30	–	66	–	–	–
Morocco	0.1	21	15–31	5.9	–	0.1	0.1	–	12	–	–	–	630	–
Mozambique	12.5	1500	1300–1700	810	100	2.9	8.5	33	20	33	29	400	1400	80
Myanmar	0.7	240	160–370	100	–	0.7	0.6	–	–	–	–	–	1600	–
Namibia	15.3	200	160–230	110	14	3.4	10.3	62	65	81	64	66	110	100
Nauru	–	–	–	–	–	–	–	–	–	–	–	–	–	–
Nepal	0.5	70	50–99	17	–	0.5	0.3	44	28	78	–	–	990	–
Netherlands	0.2	18	10–32	4.9	–	0.2	0.1	–	–	–	–	–	110	–

STATISTICAL TABLES

TABLE 4. HIV/AIDS

	Estimated adult HIV prevalence rate (aged 15–49), 2007	Estimated number of people (all ages) living with HIV, 2007 (thousands)		Mother-to-child transmission Estimated number of women (aged 15+) living with HIV, 2007 (thousands)	Paediatric infections Estimated number of children (aged 0–14) living with HIV, 2007 (thousands)	Prevention among young people						Orphans Children (aged 0–17)		Orphan school attendance ratio
						HIV prevalence among young people (aged 15–24), 2007		% who have comprehensive knowledge of HIV, 2002–2007*		% who used condom at last higher-risk sex, 2002–2007*		orphaned by AIDS, 2007 estimate (thousands)	orphaned due to all causes, 2007 estimate (thousands)	2002–2007*
		estimate	low estimate–high estimate			male	female	male	female	male	female			
New Zealand	0.1	1.4	<1.0–2.6	<0.5	–	0.1	–	–	–	–	–	–	34	–
Nicaragua	0.2	7.7	5.3–15	2.1	–	0.3	0.1	–	22x	–	17x	–	110	106x
Niger	0.8	60	44–85	17	3.2	0.9	0.5	16	13	37y	18y	25	570	67
Nigeria	3.1	2600	2000–3200	1400	220	0.8	2.3	21	18	46	24	1200	9700	64p
Niue	–	–	–	–	–	–	–	–	–	–	–	–	–	–
Norway	0.1	3.0	1.7–5.0	<1.0	–	0.1	0.1	–	–	–	–	–	37	–
Occupied Palestinian Territory	–	–	–	–	–	–	–	–	–	–	–	–	–	–
Oman	–	–	–	–	–	–	–	–	–	–	–	–	–	–
Pakistan	0.1	96	69–150	27	–	0.1	0.1	–	3	–	–	–	3900	–
Palau	–	–	–	–	–	–	–	–	–	–	–	–	–	–
Panama	1.0	20	16–26	5.5	–	1.1	0.6	–	–	–	–	–	48	–
Papua New Guinea	1.5	54	53–55	21	1.1	0.6	0.7	–	–	–	–	–	330	–
Paraguay	0.6	21	12–38	5.8	–	0.7	0.3	–	–	–	–	–	130	–
Peru	0.5	76	57–97	21	–	0.5	0.3	–	19	–	32	–	570	85x
Philippines	–	8.3	6.0–11	2.2	–	–	–	18	12	25	11	–	1800	–
Poland	0.1	20	11–34	5.5	–	0.1	0.1	–	–	–	–	–	440	–
Portugal	0.5	34	20–63	9.4	–	0.5	0.3	–	–	–	–	–	82	–
Qatar	–	–	–	–	–	–	–	–	–	–	–	–	–	–
Republic of Korea	<0.1	13	7.5–42	3.6	–	<0.1	<0.1	–	–	–	–	–	360	–
Romania	0.1	15	12–16	7.0	–	0.2	0.2	1y	3y	–	–	–	300	–
Russian Federation	1.1	940	630–1300	240	5.2	1.3	0.6	–	–	–	–	–	4000	–
Rwanda	2.8	150	130–170	78	19	0.5	1.4	54	51	40	26	220	860	82
Saint Kitts and Nevis	–	–	–	–	–	–	–	–	–	–	–	–	–	–
Saint Lucia	–	–	–	–	–	–	–	–	–	–	–	–	–	–
Saint Vincent and the Grenadines	–	–	–	–	–	–	–	–	–	–	–	–	–	–
Samoa	–	–	–	–	–	–	–	–	–	–	–	–	–	–
San Marino	–	–	–	–	–	–	–	–	–	–	–	–	–	–
Sao Tome and Principe	–	–	–	–	–	–	–	–	44	–	56	–	–	–
Saudi Arabia	–	–	–	–	–	–	–	–	–	–	–	–	–	–
Senegal	1.0	67	47–96	38	3.1	0.3	0.8	24	19	52	36	8	350	83
Serbia	0.1	6.4	3.9–12	1.8	–	0.1	0.1	–	42	–	74	–	130	–
Seychelles	–	–	–	–	–	–	–	–	–	–	–	–	–	–
Sierra Leone	1.7	55	42–76	30	4.0	0.4	1.3	–	17	–	20	16	350	83
Singapore	0.2	4.2	2.6–7.3	1.2	–	0.2	0.1	–	–	–	–	–	24	–
Slovakia	<0.1	<0.5	<1.0	–	–	–	–	–	–	–	–	–	–	–
Slovenia	<0.1	<0.5	<1.0	–	–	–	–	–	–	–	–	–	–	–
Solomon Islands	–	–	–	–	–	–	–	–	–	–	–	–	–	–
Somalia	0.5	24	13–45	6.7	<1.0	0.6	0.3	–	4	–	–	9	590	78
South Africa	18.1	5700	4900–6600	3200	280	4.0	12.7	–	–	–	–	1400	2500	–
Spain	0.5	140	80–230	28	–	0.6	0.2	–	–	–	–	–	210	–
Sri Lanka	–	3.8	2.8–5.1	1.4	–	<0.1	–	–	–	–	–	–	330	–
Sudan	1.4	320	220–440	170	25	0.3	1.0	–	–	–	–	–	1800	96x
Suriname	2.4	6.8	4.2–12	1.9	<0.2	2.7	1.4	–	41	–	49	–	9	–
Swaziland	26.1	190	180–200	100	15	5.8	22.6	52	52	70	54	56	96	97
Sweden	0.1	6.2	3.5–11	2.9	–	0.1	0.1	–	–	–	–	–	66	–
Switzerland	0.6	25	14–43	9.2	–	0.4	0.5	–	–	–	–	–	39	–
Syrian Arab Republic	–	–	–	–	–	–	–	–	7	–	–	–	–	–
Tajikistan	0.3	10	5.0–23	2.1	<0.1	0.4	0.1	–	2	–	–	–	210	–
Thailand	1.4	610	410–880	250	14	1.2	1.2	–	46	–	–	–	1300	93
The former Yugoslav Republic of Macedonia	<0.1	<0.5	<1.0	–	–	–	–	–	27	–	70	–	–	–
Timor-Leste	–	–	–	–	–	–	–	–	–	–	–	–	48	–
Togo	3.3	130	110–150	69	10	0.8	2.4	–	28	–	50	68	260	94
Tonga	–	–	–	–	–	–	–	–	–	–	–	–	–	–
Trinidad and Tobago	1.5	14	9.5–19	7.7	–	0.3	1.0	–	54	–	51	–	20	–
Tunisia	0.1	3.7	2.7–5.4	1.0	–	0.1	<0.1	–	–	–	–	–	130	–
Turkey	–	<2.0	<5.0	–	–	–	–	–	–	–	–	–	–	–
Turkmenistan	<0.1	<0.5	<1.0	–	–	–	–	–	5	–	–	–	–	–
Tuvalu	–	–	–	–	–	–	–	–	–	–	–	–	–	–
Uganda	5.4	940	870–1000	480	130	1.3	3.9	38	32	55	38	1200	2500	96
Ukraine	1.6	440	340–540	190	5.1	1.5	1.5	43	42	–	–	–	1000	98
United Arab Emirates	–	–	–	–	–	–	–	–	–	–	–	–	–	–

...TABLE 4

	Estimated adult HIV prevalence rate (aged 15–49), 2007	Estimated number of people (all ages) living with HIV, 2007 (thousands)		Mother-to-child transmission — Estimated number of women (aged 15+) living with HIV, 2007 (thousands)	Paediatric infections — Estimated number of children (aged 0–14) living with HIV, 2007 (thousands)	Prevention among young people — HIV prevalence among young people (aged 15–24), 2007		Prevention among young people — % who have comprehensive knowledge of HIV, 2002–2007*		Prevention among young people — % who used condom at last higher-risk sex, 2002–2007*		Orphans — Children (aged 0–17) orphaned by AIDS, 2007 estimate (thousands)	Orphans — Children (aged 0–17) orphaned due to all causes, 2007 estimate (thousands)	Orphan school attendance ratio 2002–2007*
		estimate	low estimate–high estimate			male	female	male	female	male	female			
United Kingdom	0.2	77	37–160	22	–	0.3	0.1	–	–	–	–	–	520	–
United Republic of Tanzania	6.2	1400	1300–1500	760	140	0.5	0.9	40	45	46	34	970	2600	102
United States	0.6	1200	690–1900	230	–	0.7	0.3	–	–	–	–	–	2800	–
Uruguay	0.6	10	5.9–19	2.8	–	0.6	0.3	–	–	–	–	–	46	–
Uzbekistan	0.1	16	8.1–45	4.6	<0.2	0.1	0.1	–	31	–	61	–	690	–
Vanuatu	–	–	–	–	–	–	–	–	–	–	–	–	–	–
Venezuela (Bolivarian Republic of)	–	–	–	–	–	–	–	–	–	–	–	–	430	–
Viet Nam	0.5	290	180–470	76	–	0.6	0.3	–	44	68	–	–	1500	–
Yemen	–	–	–	–	–	–	–	–	–	–	–	–	–	–
Zambia	15.2	1100	1000–1200	560	95	3.6	11.3	37	34	48	38	600	1100	103y
Zimbabwe	15.3	1300	1200–1400	680	120	2.9	7.7	46	44	68	42	1000	1300	95

SUMMARY INDICATORS

Sub-Saharan Africa	5.0	22000	20500–23600	12000	1800	1.1	3.2	30	24	44	29	11600	47500	83
Eastern and Southern Africa	7.8	16400	15300–17600	8970	1300	1.5	4.5	38	31	47	30	8700	24900	92
West and Central Africa	2.6	5600	4800–6300	3000	480	0.7	1.9	23	19	42	29	3000	22700	76
Middle East and North Africa	0.3	480	370–620	220	28	0.1	0.2	–	–	–	–	–	5900	–
South Asia	0.3	2600	2000–3400	930	110	0.3	0.2	36	18	38	22	–	37400	73
East Asia and Pacific	0.2	2400	1900–3000	750	41	0.2	0.1	7**	18**	–	–	–	30100	–
Latin America and Caribbean	0.6	1900	1700–2400	660	55	0.5	0.4	–	–	–	–	–	9400	–
CEE/CIS	0.8	1500	1100–1900	460	11	0.8	0.5	–	–	–	–	–	7600	–
Industrialized countries§	0.3	2000	1400–2900	460	5.8	0.4	0.2	–	–	–	–	–	7200	–
Developing countries§	0.9	29500	27300–32100	14600	2000	0.4	0.7	30**	19**	–	–	–	130000	77
Least developed countries§	2.2	10000	9500–11000	5300	900	0.6	1.4	32	23	45	29	–	40400	86
World	0.8	33000	30000–36000	15500	2000	0.4	0.6	–	–	–	–	15000	145000	–

§ Also includes territories within each country category or regional group. Countries and territories in each country category or regional group are listed on page 152.

DEFINITIONS OF THE INDICATORS

Estimated adult HIV prevalence rate – Percentage of adults (aged 15–49) living with HIV as of 2007.

Estimated number of people (all ages) living with HIV – Estimated number of people (all ages) living with HIV as of 2007.

Estimated number of women (aged 15+) living with HIV – Estimated number of women (aged 15+) living with HIV as of 2007.

Estimated number of children (aged 0–14) living with HIV – Estimated number of children (aged 0–14) living with HIV as of 2007.

HIV prevalence among young people – Percentage of young men and women (aged 15–24) living with HIV as of 2007.

Comprehensive knowledge of HIV – Percentage of young men and women (aged 15–24) who correctly identify the two major ways of preventing the sexual transmission of HIV (using condoms and limiting sex to one faithful, uninfected partner), who reject the two most common local misconceptions about HIV transmission and who know that a healthy-looking person can be HIV-infected.

Condom use at last higher-risk sex – Percentage of young men and women (aged 15–24) who say they used a condom the last time they had sex with a non-marital, non-cohabiting partner, of those who have had sex with such a partner during the past 12 months.

Children orphaned by AIDS – Estimated number of children (aged 0–17) who have lost one or both parents to AIDS as of 2007.

Children orphaned due to all causes – Estimated number of children (aged 0–17) who have lost one or both parents due to any cause as of 2007.

Orphan school attendance ratio – Percentage of children (aged 10–14) who have lost both biological parents and who are currently attending school as a percentage of non-orphaned children of the same age who live with at least one parent and who are attending school.

MAIN DATA SOURCES

Estimated adult HIV prevalence rate – Joint United Nations Programme on HIV/AIDS (UNAIDS), *Report on the Global AIDS Epidemic*, 2008.

Estimated number of people (all ages) living with HIV – UNAIDS, *Report on the Global AIDS Epidemic*, 2008.

Estimated number of women (aged 15+) living with HIV – UNAIDS, *Report on the Global AIDS Epidemic*, 2008.

Estimated number of children (aged 0–14) living with HIV – UNAIDS, *Report on the Global AIDS Epidemic*, 2008.

HIV prevalence among young people – UNAIDS, *Report on the Global AIDS Epidemic*, 2008.

Comprehensive knowledge of HIV – AIDS Indicator Surveys (AIS), Behavioural Surveillance Surveys (BSS), Demographic and Health Surveys (DHS), Multiple Indicator Cluster Surveys (MICS), Reproductive Health Surveys (RHS) and other national household surveys, 2002–2007; 'HIV/AIDS Survey Indicators Database', <www.measuredhs.com/hivdata>.

Condom use at last higher-risk sex – AIS, BSS, DHS, RHS and other national household surveys, 2002–2007; 'HIV/AIDS Survey Indicators Database', <www.measuredhs.com/hivdata>.

Children orphaned by AIDS – UNAIDS, *Report on the Global AIDS Epidemic*, 2008.

Children orphaned due to all causes – UNAIDS unpublished estimates.

Orphan school attendance ratio – AIS, DHS, MICS and other national household surveys, 2002–2007; 'HIV/AIDS Survey Indicators Database', <www.measuredhs.com/hivdata>.

NOTES
- – Data not available.
- x Data refer to years or periods other than those specified in the column heading, differ from the standard definition or refer to only part of a country. Such data are not included in the calculation of regional and global averages.
- y Data refer to years or periods other than those specified in the column heading, differ from the standard definition or refer to only part of a country. Such data are included in the calculation of regional and global averages.
- p Proportion of orphans (aged 10–14) attending school is based on small denominators (typically 25–49 unweighted cases).
- * Data refer to the most recent year available during the period specified in the column heading.
- ** Excludes China.

TABLE 5. EDUCATION

Countries and territories	Youth (15–24 years) literacy rate 2000–2007*		Number per 100 population 2006		Primary school enrolment ratio 2000–2007*				Primary school attendance ratio 2000–2007* net		Survival rate to last primary grade (%) 2000–2007*		Secondary school enrolment ratio 2000–2007*				Secondary school attendance ratio 2000–2007* net	
					gross		net						gross		net			
	male	female	phones	Internet users	male	female	male	female	male	female	admin. data	survey data	male	female	male	female	male	female
Afghanistan	49	18	8	2	126	75	74	46	66	40	–	90	28	9	–	–	18	6
Albania	99	100	60	15	106	105	94	93	92	92	90	100	78	75	74	72	79	77
Algeria	94	91	63	7	114	106	96	94	97	96	91	–	80	86	65	68	57	65
Andorra	–	–	97	56	90	90	83	83	–	–	–	–	83	87	73	75	–	–
Angola	84	63	14	1	69x	59x	–	–	58	59	–	83	19	16	–	–	22	20
Antigua and Barbuda	–	–	134	64	–	–	–	–	–	–	–	–	–	–	–	–	–	–
Argentina	99	99	81	21	113	112	99	98	–	–	87	–	80	89	75	82	–	–
Armenia	100	100	–	6	96	100	80	84	99	98	99	100	88	91	84	88	93	95
Australia	–	–	97	52	105	105	96	97	–	–	–	–	154	146	87	88	–	–
Austria	–	–	113	51	102	101	97	98	–	–	99	–	104	100	–	–	–	–
Azerbaijan	100	100	39	10	98	95	86	83	74	72	97	99	85	81	79	76	82	80
Bahamas	–	–	77	34	98	98	87	89	–	–	81	–	91	91	83	85	–	–
Bahrain	100	100	123	28	120	119	98	98	86	87	99	99	100	104	91	96	77	85
Bangladesh	71	73	13	0	101	105	87	91	79	84	65	94	43	45	40	42	36	41
Barbados	–	–	88	93	104	102	97	96	–	–	97	–	100	104	88	89	–	–
Belarus	100	100	61	56	97	95	90	89	93	94	99	100	95	97	87	89	95	97
Belgium	–	–	93	47	102	102	97	98	–	–	94	–	112	108	89	85	–	–
Belize	–	89	44	11	125	121	97	97	95	95	92	–	77	81	64	70	58	60
Benin	63	41	12	1	105	87	87	73	72	62	65	89	41	23	23	11	40	27
Bhutan	83	73	10	4	103	101	79	79	74	67	84	–	51	46	38	39	–	–
Bolivia	99	98	31	6	109	109	95	95	78	77	82	41	84	81	72	70	57	56
Bosnia and Herzegovina	100	100	48	24	–	–	–	–	92	89	–	100	–	–	–	–	89	89
Botswana	93	95	47	5	108	106	83	85	83	86	75	–	75	78	52	60	36	44
Brazil	97	99	53	23	141	133	94	95	95x	95x	81	88	101	111	75	83	42x	50x
Brunei Darussalam	100	100	79	42	107	106	94	94	–	–	98	–	96	100	88	92	–	–
Bulgaria	98	97	108	47	101	100	93	92	–	–	95	–	108	104	90	88	–	–
Burkina Faso	47	33	7	1	66	54	52	42	49	44	64	90	17	12	14	10	17	15
Burundi	77	70	3	1	108	98	76	73	72	70	78	74	16	12	–	–	8	6
Cambodia	90	83	12	0	127	118	91	89	84	86	49	92	43	34	33	28	29	26
Cameroon	72	59	19	2	117	98	–	–	86	81	59	95	27	21	–	–	45	42
Canada	–	–	58	77	100	99	99	100	–	–	–	–	119	116	–	–	–	–
Cape Verde	97	98	21	6	108	103	88	87	97x	96x	89	–	75	86	56	63	–	–
Central African Republic	70	47	3	0	72	49	53	38	64	54	39	65	–	–	13	9	16	10
Chad	56	23	5	1	90	61	71	50	41	31	26	94	23	8	16	5	13	7
Chile	99	99	76	25	107	102	–	–	–	–	98	–	90	92	–	–	–	–
China	99	99	35	10	112	111	99	99	–	–	–	–	75	76	–	–	–	–
Colombia	98	98	64	14	117	115	89	88	90	92	82	89	78	87	62	69	64	72
Comoros	92	87	5	3	91	80	75	71	31	31	72	19	40	30	15	15	10	11
Congo	99	98	19	2	113	102	58	52	86	87	55	93	47	39	–	–	39	40
Cook Islands	–	–	–	27	79	80	73	75	–	–	–	–	71	74	62	68	–	–
Costa Rica	98	99	33	28	112	111	91	93	87	89	91	–	83	89	58	64	59	65
Côte d'Ivoire	–	40	22	2	79	62	61	49	66	57	86	90	32	18	25	14	32	22
Croatia	100	100	96	37	99	99	91	90	–	–	100	–	90	93	86	88	–	–
Cuba	100	100	1	2	102	100	96	97	–	–	97	–	93	94	86	88	–	–
Cyprus	100	100	103	42	103	102	99	99	–	–	99	–	96	97	93	95	–	–
Czech Republic	–	–	122	35	100	100	91	94	–	–	100	–	96	97	–	–	–	–
Democratic People's Republic of Korea	–	–	–	–	–	–	–	–	–	–	–	–	–	–	–	–	–	–
Democratic Republic of the Congo	78	63	7	0	68	54	–	–	55	49	–	49	28	16	–	–	18	15
Denmark	–	–	107	58	99	99	95	96	–	–	92	–	118	121	88	90	–	–
Djibouti	–	48	5	1	49	40	42	34	80	78	–	–	27	18	26	17	50	42
Dominica	–	–	–	37	85	87	75	80	–	–	88	–	107	105	77	85	–	–
Dominican Republic	95	97	51	16	101	96	77	79	84	88	61	81	63	75	47	57	27	39
Ecuador	96	97	63	12	117	117	96	97	–	–	76	–	67	68	57	58	–	–
Egypt	90	82	24	8	108	102	98	94	96	94	97	98	91	85	82	78	72	67
El Salvador	95	96	55	10	116	112	94	94	–	–	67	–	63	66	53	56	–	–
Equatorial Guinea	95	95	27	2	125	119	91	83	61	60	33	–	41	23	–	–	23	22
Eritrea	85	70	1	2	69	56	50	43	69	64	74	–	39	23	30	20	23	21
Estonia	100	100	125	55	100	98	95	94	–	–	96	–	99	101	90	92	–	–
Ethiopia	62	39	1	0	97	85	74	69	45	45	58	84	37	24	29	19	30	23
Fiji	–	–	–	9	101	99	91	91	–	–	81	–	80	88	76	83	–	–
Finland	–	–	108	56	98	98	97	97	–	–	99	–	109	114	96	96	–	–

...TABLE 5

| | Youth (15–24 years) literacy rate 2000–2007* | | Number per 100 population 2006 | | Primary school enrolment ratio 2000–2007* | | | | Primary school attendance ratio 2000–2007* net | | Survival rate to last primary grade (%) 2000–2007* | | Secondary school enrolment ratio 2000–2007* | | | | Secondary school attendance ratio 2000–2007* net | |
| | | | | | gross | | net | | | | | | gross | | net | | | |
	male	female	phones	Internet users	male	female	male	female	male	female	admin. data	survey data	male	female	male	female	male	female
France	–	–	85	50	110	109	98	99	–	–	98x	–	114	114	98	100	–	–
Gabon	98	96	64	6	153	152	88	88	94	94	56	–	53	46	–	–	34	36
Gambia	63	41	26	5	71	77	59	64	60	62	–	95	47	43	40	37	39	34
Georgia	–	99	38	7	94	97	88	91	94	95	100	–	83	86	77	81	89	88
Germany	–	–	104	47	103	103	98	98	–	–	99	–	102	100	–	–	–	–
Ghana	80	76	23	3	98	97	73	71	75	75	60	98	52	46	47	43	45	45
Greece	99	99	99	18	102	102	100	99	–	–	98	–	104	102	92	93	–	–
Grenada	–	–	45	21	94	91	84	83	–	–	83	–	99	102	78	80	–	–
Guatemala	88	83	56	10	118	109	96	92	80x	76x	63	–	56	51	40	37	23x	24x
Guinea	59	34	–	1	96	81	77	66	55	48	76	96	45	24	35	20	27	17
Guinea-Bissau	94	87	10	2	84	56	53	37	54	53	–	81	23	13	11	6	8	7
Guyana	–	–	–	23	125	124	–	–	96	96	59	96	106	104	–	–	66	73
Haiti	76	87	14	8	–	–	–	–	48	52	–	85	–	–	–	–	18	21
Holy See	–	–	0	0	–	–	–	–	–	–	–	–	–	–	–	–	–	–
Honduras	88	93	30	5	119	118	96	97	77	80	81	–	66	86	–	–	29	36
Hungary	98	99	99	35	98	96	89	88	–	–	98	–	96	95	90	90	–	–
Iceland	–	–	109	65	98	97	98	97	–	–	99	–	108	111	89	91	–	–
India	87	77	15	11	114	109	90	87	85	81	73	95	59	49	–	–	59	49
Indonesia	99	99	28	5	116	112	97	94	94	95	80	–	64	64	59	59	54	56
Iran (Islamic Republic of)	98	97	24	26	104	132	91	100	94	91	88	–	83	78	79	75	–	–
Iraq	89	81	32	0	109	90	95	82	91	80	70	83	54	36	45	32	46	34
Ireland	–	–	113	34	104	103	95	95	–	–	–	–	108	116	85	90	–	–
Israel	–	–	123	28	109	111	96	98	–	–	100	–	93	92	88	89	–	–
Italy	100	100	135	53	104	103	99	98	–	–	100	–	101	100	93	94	–	–
Jamaica	91	98	94	49	95	95	90	90	97	98	87	–	86	89	77	80	88	92
Japan	–	–	79	68	100	100	100	100	–	–	–	–	101	102	99	99	–	–
Jordan	99	99	74	14	96	98	89	91	99	99	96	–	88	90	81	83	85	89
Kazakhstan	100	100	53	9	105	106	90	90	99	98	100	100	93	92	86	86	97	97
Kenya	80	81	21	8	107	104	75	76	79	79	84	90	52	49	43	42	12	13
Kiribati	–	–	–	2	112	114	96	98	–	–	81	–	82	94	65	72	–	–
Kuwait	100	100	91	29	97	96	84	83	–	–	96	–	87	91	75	79	–	–
Kyrgyzstan	100	100	24	12	97	96	86	85	91	93	99	99	86	87	80	81	90	92
Lao People's Democratic Republic	85	80	17	1	123	109	86	81	81	77	62	93	49	38	38	32	40	33
Latvia	100	100	95	47	96	93	89	92	–	–	98	–	98	99	–	–	–	–
Lebanon	–	–	31	26	96	93	82	82	97	97	87	93	78	85	70	77	61	68
Lesotho	75	91	20	3	115	114	71	74	82	88	62	84	33	42	19	29	16	27
Liberia	68	76	8	0	96	87	40	39	–	–	–	–	37	27	22	13	–	–
Libyan Arab Jamahiriya	100	98	66	4	113	108	–	–	–	–	–	–	86	101	–	–	–	–
Liechtenstein	–	–	82	64	106	107	87	89	–	–	–	–	120	104	62	69	–	–
Lithuania	100	100	138	32	95	94	90	89	–	–	97	–	99	99	92	93	–	–
Luxembourg	–	–	117	72	102	103	96	98	–	–	88	–	94	98	82	86	–	–
Madagascar	73	68	5	1	142	137	96	96	74	77	36	93	24	23	17	18	17	21
Malawi	84	82	5	0	117	121	88	94	86	88	36	71	32	27	25	23	27	26
Malaysia	98	98	75	54	101	100	100	100	–	–	99	–	66	72	66	72	–	–
Maldives	98	98	88	9	118	114	97	97	–	–	–	–	80	86	65	70	–	–
Mali	36	23	11	1	90	71	68	54	45	33	73	90	35	21	–	–	15	11
Malta	96	99	86	34	101	99	92	91	–	–	99	–	99	100	84	90	–	–
Marshall Islands	–	–	–	–	94	92	67	66	–	–	–	–	66	67	43	47	–	–
Mauritania	70	63	34	1	99	104	78	82	56	59	45	–	27	23	16	15	21	17
Mauritius	95	97	62	25	102	102	94	96	–	–	99	–	89	88	81	82	–	–
Mexico	98	98	53	19	114	111	98	97	97	97	92	–	86	88	71	70	–	–
Micronesia (Federated States of)	–	–	19	14	109	111	–	–	–	–	–	–	80	86	–	–	–	–
Moldova	100	100	32	17	97	96	88	88	84	85	97	100	87	91	80	83	82	85
Monaco	–	–	52	56	–	–	–	–	–	–	–	–	–	–	–	–	–	–
Mongolia	94	97	29	12	99	102	90	93	96	98	91	97	84	95	77	87	85	91
Montenegro	–	93	107	44	–	–	–	–	98	97	–	97	–	–	–	–	90	92
Morocco	84	67	52	20	112	100	91	85	91	87	74	–	53	45	37	32	39	36
Mozambique	58	48	12	1	113	97	79	73	63	57	40	68	18	13	4	4	8	7
Myanmar	97	96	0	0	114	115	99	100	83	84	72	100	49	49	46	46	51	48
Namibia	91	94	30	4	107	107	74	79	91	91	77	90	53	61	30	40	40	53
Nauru	–	–	–	–	78	80	–	–	–	–	25	–	42	50	–	–	–	–

STATISTICAL TABLES

TABLE 5. EDUCATION

	Youth (15–24 years) literacy rate 2000–2007*		Number per 100 population 2006		Primary school enrolment ratio 2000–2007*				Primary school attendance ratio 2000–2007* net		Survival rate to last primary grade (%) 2000–2007*		Secondary school enrolment ratio 2000–2007*				Secondary school attendance ratio 2000–2007* net	
					gross		net						gross		net			
	male	female	phones	Internet users	male	female	male	female	male	female	admin. data	survey data	male	female	male	female	male	female
Nepal	85	73	4	1	129	123	91	87	86	82	81	95	46	41	–	–	46	38
Netherlands	–	–	106	86	108	105	99	97	–	–	98	–	119	117	88	89	–	–
New Zealand	–	–	94	79	102	102	99	99	–	–	–	–	117	123	91	93	–	–
Nicaragua	85	92	33	3	117	115	90	90	77	84	50	56	62	70	40	47	35	47
Niger	53	26	3	0	58	43	56	40	44	31	53	88	14	9	12	7	13	9
Nigeria	89	85	24	6	105	87	68	59	66	58	63	96	36	29	28	23	38	33
Niue	–	–	–	–	107	102	–	–	–	–	–	–	96	102	91x	96x	–	–
Norway	–	–	108	82	98	98	98	98	–	–	100	–	113	113	96	97	–	–
Occupied Palestinian Territory	99	99	22	7	82	83	76	76	91	92	98	–	91	97	87	92	–	–
Oman	99	98	70	11	82	83	73	75	–	–	99	–	90	87	78	77	–	–
Pakistan	80	60	22	8	94	74	74	57	60	51	70	–	34	26	33	26	23	18
Palau	–	–	0	0	108	101	98	95	–	–	–	–	96	105	–	–	–	–
Panama	97	96	66	15	113	110	99	98	–	–	85	–	67	73	61	68	–	–
Papua New Guinea	63	65	–	2	60	50	–	–	–	–	–	–	–	–	–	–	–	–
Paraguay	96	97	51	4	113	110	94	95	95	96	84	–	66	67	56	59	81	80
Peru	99	97	31	23	116	117	96	97	94	94	85	94	93	96	72	72	70	70
Philippines	94	95	51	6	110	109	91	93	88	89	70	90	79	88	55	66	55	70
Poland	100	99	95	37	98	97	96	96	–	–	98	–	100	99	93	94	–	–
Portugal	100	100	116	30	118	112	98	98	–	–	–	–	94	102	78	86	–	–
Qatar	97	98	110	35	105	104	93	94	–	–	89	–	103	100	91	90	–	–
Republic of Korea	–	–	84	71	107	103	100	93	–	–	99	–	100	95	99	93	–	–
Romania	97	98	80	52	105	104	93	93	–	–	94	–	86	86	74	73	–	–
Russian Federation	100	100	106	18	96	96	91	91	–	–	99	–	85	83	–	–	–	–
Rwanda	79	77	3	1	138	142	76	81	84	87	31	76	14	13	–	–	5	5
Saint Kitts and Nevis	–	–	–	32	86	103	64	78	–	–	78	–	110	100	70	61	–	–
Saint Lucia	–	–	–	62	122	114	99	97	–	–	96	–	80	95	65	80	–	–
Saint Vincent and the Grenadines	–	–	74	29	94	100	93	88	–	–	64	–	67	83	57	71	–	–
Samoa	99	100	25	4	100	100	90	91	–	–	96x	–	76	86	62	71	–	–
San Marino	–	–	64	57	–	–	–	–	–	–	–	–	–	–	–	–	–	–
Sao Tome and Principe	95	96	12	14	128	127	97	98	94	95	61	83	44	47	31	34	39	41
Saudi Arabia	98	96	78	19	–	–	–	–	–	–	–	–	–	–	–	–	–	–
Senegal	59	44	25	5	81	79	71	70	58	59	54	93	27	21	23	18	20	16
Serbia	–	96	63	13	97	97	95	95	98	98	–	100	87	89	–	–	90	93
Seychelles	99	99	87	36	126	125	99	100	–	–	99	–	105	119	94	100	–	–
Sierra Leone	64	44	–	0	155	139	–	–	69	69	–	91	38	26	27	19	21	17
Singapore	100	100	109	59	–	–	–	–	–	–	–	–	–	–	–	–	–	–
Slovakia	–	–	91	42	101	99	92	92	–	–	97	–	94	95	–	–	–	–
Slovenia	100	100	93	64	101	100	96	95	–	–	99	–	96	95	90	91	–	–
Solomon Islands	–	–	–	2	102	98	62	62	–	–	–	–	33	27	29	25	–	–
Somalia	–	24	6	1	–	–	–	–	24	20	–	85	–	–	–	–	8	4
South Africa	95	96	83	8	108	103	88	88	80x	83x	77	–	92	98	59	66	41x	48x
Spain	100	100	106	43	106	104	100	99	–	–	100	–	115	122	92	96	–	–
Sri Lanka	97	98	26	2	108	108	98	97	–	–	100	–	86	88	–	–	–	–
Sudan	85	71	12	9	71	61	45	37	56	52	74	56	35	33	–	–	17	22
Suriname	96	95	71	8	121	121	95	98	94	93	–	80	66	90	57	79	55	66
Swaziland	87	90	24	4	110	102	78	79	83	86	71	80	47	47	29	35	31	41
Sweden	–	–	106	77	96	95	95	95	–	–	–	–	104	103	99	99	–	–
Switzerland	–	–	99	58	98	97	89	89	–	–	–	–	95	90	84	80	–	–
Syrian Arab Republic	95	92	24	8	129	123	97	92	97	96	92	–	72	68	64	61	64	65
Tajikistan	100	100	–	–	103	98	99	95	89	88	99	100	90	75	87	74	89	74
Thailand	98	98	63	13	108	108	95	94	98	98	–	–	75	82	68	75	77	84
The former Yugoslav Republic of Macedonia	99	99	70	13	98	98	92	92	97	93	98	–	85	83	82	80	79	78
Timor-Leste	–	–	5	0	103	95	70	67	76	74	–	–	53	54	–	–	–	–
Togo	84	64	11	5	110	95	86	75	82	76	68	84	54	27	30	14	45	32
Tonga	100	100	29	3	116	110	98	94	–	–	91	–	92	96	54	68	–	–
Trinidad and Tobago	100	100	69	22	96	94	85	85	98	98	84	97	75	78	64	67	84	90
Tunisia	97	94	72	13	110	107	96	97	95	93	94	–	81	89	61	68	–	–
Turkey	98	94	71	18	96	92	93	89	91	87	94	95	86	71	74	64	52	43
Turkmenistan	100	100	4	1	–	–	–	–	99	99	–	100	–	–	–	–	84	84

...TABLE 5

	Youth (15–24 years) literacy rate 2000–2007*		Number per 100 population 2006		Primary school enrolment ratio 2000–2007*				Primary school attendance ratio 2000–2007* net		Survival rate to last primary grade (%) 2000–2007*		Secondary school enrolment ratio 2000–2007*				Secondary school attendance ratio 2000–2007* net	
					gross		net						gross		net			
	male	female	phones	Internet users	male	female	male	female	male	female	admin. data	survey data	male	female	male	female	male	female
Tuvalu	–	–	15	19	106	105	–	–	–	–	63	–	87	81	–	–	–	–
Uganda	88	84	7	5	116	117	–	–	83	82	25	72	20	16	16	14	16	15
Ukraine	100	100	107	20	102	102	90	90	96	98	98	100	94	93	83	84	90	93
United Arab Emirates	99	97	119	37	104	103	88	88	–	–	99	–	89	91	78	80	–	–
United Kingdom	–	–	117	63	105	106	98	99	–	–	–	–	97	99	91	94	–	–
United Republic of Tanzania	79	76	15	1	113	111	98	97	71	75	83	91	7x	6x	22	20	8	8
United States	–	–	80	70	98	99	91	93	–	–	96	–	94	94	88	88	–	–
Uruguay	98	99	67	24	117	113	100	100	–	–	92	–	94	109	–	–	–	–
Uzbekistan	99	99	9	4	97	94	–	–	100	100	99	100	103	102	–	–	91	90
Vanuatu	92	92	–	–	110	106	88	86	–	–	69x	–	43	37	41	35	–	–
Venezuela (Bolivarian Republic of)	96	98	69	15	106	103	91	91	91	93	90	82	73	82	62	71	30	43
Viet Nam	95	94	18	17	109	103	–	–	94	94	92	98	68	62	–	–	77	78
Yemen	93	67	14	1	100	74	85	65	68x	41x	60	–	61	30	49	26	35x	13x
Zambia	73x	66x	14	4	118	116	90	94	55	58	76	80	33	27	31	25	17	19
Zimbabwe	98	99	6	9	102	101	87	88	91	93	62	79	42	39	38	36	46	43

SUMMARY INDICATORS

	male	female	phones	Internet users	male	female	male	female	male	female	admin. data	survey data	male	female	male	female	male	female
Sub-Saharan Africa	77	68	18	3	101	90	75	70	64	61	61	84	36	29	28	24	26	22
Eastern and Southern Africa	78	69	19	3	110	104	83	81	66	66	60	82	39	34	30	27	20	18
West and Central Africa	77	66	18	3	93	77	67	58	63	56	62	86	33	24	26	20	31	26
Middle East and North Africa	93	85	37	13	102	97	86	81	88	85	83	–	73	67	67	62	54	52
South Asia	84	74	15	9	111	104	88	83	81	77	72	94	54	45	–	–	51	43
East Asia and Pacific	98	98	36	12	111	110	98	97	92**	92**	80**	–	73	73	60**	62**	60**	63**
Latin America and Caribbean	97	97	54	19	120	116	94	95	90	91	84	–	87	94	69	74	–	–
CEE/CIS	99	99	81	20	98	96	92	90	93	91	96	97	89	85	79	75	79	76
Industrialized countries§	–	–	93	59	101	101	95	96	–	–	97	–	102	101	91	92	–	–
Developing countries§	90	84	30	11	109	103	89	86	80**	77**	74**	90	62	58	51**	49**	48**	43**
Least developed countries§	75	65	9	1	101	91	79	74	65	63	60	82	35	29	30	26	26	24
World	90	85	42	18	108	103	90	87	80**	77**	76**	90	67	63	58**	57**	48**	44**

§ Also includes territories within each country category or regional group. Countries and territories in each country category or regional group are listed on page 152.

DEFINITIONS OF THE INDICATORS

Youth literacy rate – Number of literate persons aged 15–24, expressed as a percentage of the total population in that age group.

Primary school gross enrolment ratio – Number of children enrolled in primary school, regardless of age, expressed as a percentage of the total number of children of official primary school age.

Secondary school gross enrolment ratio – Number of children enrolled in secondary school, regardless of age, expressed as a percentage of the total number of children of official secondary school age.

Primary school net enrolment ratio – Number of children enrolled in primary school who are of official primary school age, expressed as a percentage of the total number of children of official primary school age.

Secondary school net enrolment ratio – Number of children enrolled in secondary school who are of official secondary school age, expressed as a percentage of the total number of children of official secondary school age.

Primary school net attendance ratio – Number of children attending primary or secondary school who are of official primary school age, expressed as a percentage of the total number of children of official primary school age.

Secondary school net attendance ratio – Number of children attending secondary or tertiary school who are of official secondary school age, expressed as a percentage of the total number of children of official secondary school age.

Survival rate to the last grade of primary school – Percentage of children entering the first grade of primary school who eventually reach the last grade of primary school.

MAIN DATA SOURCES

Youth literacy – UNESCO Institute for Statistics (UIS).
Phone and Internet use – International Telecommunications Union, Geneva.
Primary and secondary school enrolment – UIS.
Primary and secondary school attendance – Demographic and Health Surveys (DHS) and Multiple Indicator Cluster Surveys (MICS).
Survival rate to the last grade of primary school – Administrative data: UIS, survey data: DHS and MICS.

NOTES
– Data not available.
x Data refer to years or periods other than those specified in the column heading, differ from the standard definition or refer to only part of a country. Such data are not included in the calculation of regional and global averages.
* Data refer to the most recent year available during the period specified in the column heading.
** Excludes China.

TABLE 6. DEMOGRAPHIC INDICATORS

Countries and territories	Population (thousands) 2007		Population annual growth rate (%)		Crude death rate			Crude birth rate			Life expectancy			Total fertility rate 2007	% of population urbanized 2007	Average annual growth rate of urban population (%)	
	under 18	under 5	1970–1990	1990–2007	1970	1990	2007	1970	1990	2007	1970	1990	2007			1970–1990	1990–2007
Afghanistan	14526	5002	0.3	4.5	29	23	20	52	52	48	35	41	44	7.1	24	2.9	6.4
Albania	986	250	2.2	-0.2	8	6	6	33	24	16	67	72	76	2.1	47	2.9	1.4
Algeria	11780	3271	3.0	1.7	16	7	5	49	32	21	53	67	72	2.4	65	4.4	3.2
Andorra	14	4	3.9	2.0	–	–	–	–	–	–	–	–	–	–	91	3.8	2.0
Angola	9022	3162	2.7	2.8	27	24	21	52	53	48	37	40	42	6.5	55	7.3	5.4
Antigua and Barbuda	28	8	-0.6	1.9	–	–	–	–	–	–	–	–	–	–	38	-0.3	2.5
Argentina	12279	3364	1.5	1.1	9	8	8	23	22	18	66	71	75	2.3	90	2.0	1.5
Armenia	760	167	1.7	-1.0	5	8	10	23	21	12	70	68	72	1.4	64	2.3	-1.4
Australia	4802	1272	1.4	1.2	9	7	7	20	15	12	71	77	81	1.8	89	1.4	1.5
Austria	1573	393	0.2	0.5	13	11	9	15	12	9	70	76	80	1.4	66	0.2	0.5
Azerbaijan	2536	564	1.7	0.9	7	7	7	29	27	16	65	66	67	1.8	52	2.0	0.7
Bahamas	106	28	2.0	1.5	7	6	6	31	24	17	66	70	73	2.0	91	3.1	2.2
Bahrain	227	65	4.0	2.5	9	4	3	40	29	17	62	72	76	2.3	97	4.3	3.2
Bangladesh	64486	18900	2.4	2.0	20	12	8	45	35	25	44	54	64	2.9	26	7.2	3.8
Barbados	66	17	0.6	0.5	9	8	7	22	16	11	69	75	77	1.5	54	1.0	1.7
Belarus	1870	454	0.6	-0.3	7	11	15	16	14	9	71	71	69	1.2	73	2.7	0.2
Belgium	2128	558	0.2	0.3	12	11	10	14	12	10	71	76	79	1.6	97	0.3	0.4
Belize	124	36	2.1	2.6	8	5	4	40	35	25	66	72	76	3.0	49	1.7	2.9
Benin	4553	1525	3.0	3.3	22	15	11	47	47	40	46	53	56	5.5	41	6.7	4.5
Bhutan	248	60	3.0	1.1	23	14	7	47	38	19	41	52	66	2.2	12	6.1	4.2
Bolivia	4167	1245	2.3	2.1	20	11	8	46	36	28	46	59	65	3.5	65	4.0	3.2
Bosnia and Herzegovina	825	189	0.9	-0.5	7	7	9	23	15	9	66	72	75	1.2	47	2.8	0.5
Botswana	783	218	3.3	1.9	13	7	15	45	35	25	55	64	50	2.9	59	11.8	4.1
Brazil	62565	18110	2.2	1.5	10	7	6	35	24	19	59	66	72	2.3	85	3.7	2.4
Brunei Darussalam	132	41	3.4	2.5	7	3	3	36	28	22	67	74	77	2.3	74	3.7	3.4
Bulgaria	1298	341	0.2	-0.8	9	12	15	16	12	9	71	71	73	1.3	71	1.4	-0.5
Burkina Faso	7778	2670	2.4	3.0	24	17	15	51	49	44	42	50	52	6.0	19	6.8	5.2
Burundi	4383	1541	2.4	2.4	20	19	16	44	48	47	44	46	49	6.8	11	7.3	5.8
Cambodia	6247	1708	1.7	2.3	20	12	9	42	44	26	44	55	59	3.2	21	2.0	5.7
Cameroon	8908	2866	2.9	2.4	19	13	15	45	42	35	46	55	50	4.4	56	6.4	4.6
Canada	6909	1720	1.2	1.0	7	7	7	17	14	10	73	77	81	1.5	80	1.3	1.4
Cape Verde	242	74	1.4	2.4	12	8	5	40	39	29	56	65	72	3.4	59	5.5	4.3
Central African Republic	2137	674	2.4	2.2	22	16	18	42	42	36	42	50	44	4.6	38	3.9	2.5
Chad	5690	1989	2.5	3.3	21	16	15	46	48	46	45	52	51	6.2	26	5.5	5.0
Chile	4848	1234	1.6	1.4	10	6	5	29	23	15	62	73	79	1.9	88	2.1	1.8
China	341820	84062	1.6	0.9	8	7	7	33	21	13	62	68	73	1.7	42	3.9	3.6
Colombia	16196	4388	2.2	1.6	9	6	6	38	27	19	61	68	73	2.2	73	3.2	2.2
Comoros	403	130	3.3	2.7	18	11	7	50	41	34	48	56	65	4.4	38	5.1	4.8
Congo	1825	595	3.0	2.6	14	11	12	44	39	35	54	57	55	4.5	61	4.7	3.5
Cook Islands	5	1	-0.9	-1.7	–	–	–	–	–	–	–	–	–	–	73	-0.5	-0.3
Costa Rica	1482	394	2.6	2.2	7	4	4	33	27	18	67	75	79	2.1	63	4.0	3.7
Côte d'Ivoire	9271	2872	4.4	2.4	18	13	16	51	45	36	49	54	48	4.5	46	6.1	3.5
Croatia	846	204	0.4	0.0	10	11	12	15	12	9	69	72	76	1.3	57	1.9	0.4
Cuba	2571	632	1.0	0.4	7	7	8	29	17	11	70	74	78	1.5	75	2.0	0.5
Cyprus	200	50	0.5	1.3	10	8	7	19	19	12	71	76	79	1.6	70	3.0	1.7
Czech Republic	1822	469	0.2	-0.1	12	12	11	16	12	9	70	72	76	1.2	73	2.1	-0.2
Democratic People's Republic of Korea	6656	1562	1.7	1.0	7	6	10	35	21	13	62	71	67	1.9	62	2.1	1.4
Democratic Republic of the Congo	33784	12268	3.1	2.9	20	18	18	48	49	50	45	47	46	6.7	33	2.6	4.3
Denmark	1210	318	0.2	0.3	10	12	10	16	12	11	73	75	78	1.8	86	0.5	0.4
Djibouti	369	107	6.2	2.3	21	14	11	49	42	29	43	51	55	4.0	87	7.3	3.3
Dominica	22	6	0.3	-0.1	–	–	–	–	–	–	–	–	–	–	73	2.1	0.3
Dominican Republic	3788	1113	2.3	1.7	11	6	6	42	29	24	58	67	72	2.8	68	3.9	3.1
Ecuador	5060	1403	2.7	1.5	12	6	5	42	29	21	58	68	75	2.6	64	4.4	2.5
Egypt	29422	8719	2.2	1.8	17	9	6	41	32	24	50	62	71	2.9	43	2.4	1.9
El Salvador	2696	772	1.8	1.7	12	7	6	44	30	23	57	65	72	2.7	60	2.9	3.1
Equatorial Guinea	247	82	0.8	2.4	25	19	15	41	42	39	40	47	51	5.4	39	2.0	3.3
Eritrea	2402	837	2.7	2.5	21	16	9	47	41	40	43	48	58	5.1	20	3.8	4.2
Estonia	254	68	0.7	-0.9	11	13	14	15	14	11	71	69	71	1.5	69	1.1	-1.2
Ethiopia	42124	13651	2.7	2.9	21	18	13	49	47	38	43	47	53	5.3	16	4.6	4.7

...TABLE 6

	Population (thousands) 2007		Population annual growth rate (%)		Crude death rate			Crude birth rate			Life expectancy			Total fertility rate 2007	% of population urbanized 2007	Average annual growth rate of urban population (%)	
	under 18	under 5	1970–1990	1990–2007	1970	1990	2007	1970	1990	2007	1970	1990	2007			1970–1990	1990–2007
Fiji	320	88	1.6	0.9	8	6	7	34	29	21	60	67	69	2.8	52	2.5	2.3
Finland	1093	287	0.4	0.3	10	10	10	14	13	11	70	75	79	1.8	61	1.4	0.3
France	13573	3828	0.6	0.5	11	9	9	17	13	12	72	77	81	1.9	77	0.8	0.8
Gabon	555	159	2.8	2.2	20	11	12	34	36	26	47	61	57	3.1	85	6.6	3.6
Gambia	803	264	3.5	3.4	28	15	10	50	43	35	37	51	59	4.8	56	6.8	5.9
Georgia	1006	233	0.7	-1.3	9	9	12	19	16	11	67	71	71	1.4	52	1.5	-1.7
Germany	14286	3499	0.1	0.2	12	11	11	14	11	8	71	75	79	1.4	75	0.1	0.4
Ghana	10553	3216	2.7	2.4	16	11	9	45	40	30	49	57	60	3.9	49	3.9	4.5
Greece	1906	514	0.7	0.5	8	9	10	17	10	9	72	77	79	1.3	59	1.3	0.6
Grenada	42	10	0.1	0.6	9	10	8	28	28	18	64	66	69	2.3	31	0.1	0.3
Guatemala	6588	2093	2.5	2.4	15	9	6	44	39	34	52	62	70	4.2	48	3.2	3.5
Guinea	4656	1566	2.3	2.6	27	19	12	50	47	40	38	47	56	5.5	34	5.1	3.9
Guinea-Bissau	918	333	2.8	3.0	29	23	19	49	50	50	36	42	46	7.1	30	5.9	3.5
Guyana	267	70	0.1	0.1	11	9	8	38	25	17	60	62	66	2.3	28	0.2	-0.2
Haiti	4211	1250	2.1	1.8	18	13	9	39	37	28	47	54	61	3.6	40	4.1	3.8
Holy See	–	–	–	–	–	–	–	–	–	–	–	–	–	–	–	–	–
Honduras	3257	948	3.0	2.2	15	7	6	47	38	28	52	66	70	3.3	47	4.6	3.4
Hungary	1903	471	0.0	-0.2	11	14	13	15	12	9	69	69	73	1.3	67	0.5	-0.1
Iceland	78	21	1.1	1.0	7	7	6	21	17	14	74	78	82	2.0	93	1.4	1.2
India	446646	126808	2.2	1.8	16	10	8	38	32	23	49	59	64	2.8	29	3.5	2.8
Indonesia	76805	21630	2.1	1.4	17	9	6	41	26	19	48	61	70	2.2	50	5.0	4.6
Iran (Islamic Republic of)	24229	6472	3.4	1.3	14	7	5	43	35	20	54	64	71	2.0	68	4.9	2.6
Iraq	13847	4217	3.0	2.6	12	8	9	46	39	32	56	63	59	4.3	67	4.1	2.5
Ireland	1063	323	0.9	1.2	11	9	7	22	15	16	71	75	79	2.0	61	1.3	1.7
Israel	2262	683	2.2	2.5	7	6	5	27	22	20	71	76	81	2.8	92	2.6	2.8
Italy	9882	2734	0.3	0.2	10	10	10	17	10	9	72	77	81	1.4	68	0.4	0.3
Jamaica	1007	273	1.2	0.8	8	7	7	35	25	20	68	72	72	2.5	54	2.1	1.4
Japan	21206	5549	0.8	0.2	7	7	9	19	10	8	72	79	83	1.3	66	1.7	0.5
Jordan	2500	731	3.5	3.5	16	6	4	52	36	26	54	67	72	3.1	83	4.8	4.6
Kazakhstan	4558	1316	1.2	-0.4	9	9	10	26	23	19	62	67	67	2.3	58	1.7	-0.3
Kenya	18593	6359	3.7	2.8	15	10	12	51	42	39	52	60	53	5.0	21	6.5	3.9
Kiribati	35	10	2.5	1.6	–	–	–	–	–	–	–	–	–	–	50	4.0	4.1
Kuwait	785	242	5.3	1.7	6	2	2	48	24	18	66	75	78	2.2	98	6.0	1.8
Kyrgyzstan	1945	514	2.0	1.1	11	8	8	31	31	22	60	66	66	2.5	36	2.0	0.9
Lao People's Democratic Republic	2681	720	2.3	2.1	19	13	7	44	43	27	46	54	64	3.2	21	4.7	4.3
Latvia	411	103	0.6	-0.9	11	13	14	14	14	9	70	69	73	1.3	68	1.3	-1.1
Lebanon	1365	362	1.0	1.9	9	7	7	33	26	18	65	69	72	2.2	87	2.7	2.3
Lesotho	953	271	2.2	1.3	17	11	19	43	36	29	49	59	42	3.4	19	5.7	2.1
Liberia	2017	725	2.2	3.3	22	21	18	49	50	50	42	43	45	6.8	60	4.9	5.2
Libyan Arab Jamahiriya	2183	688	3.9	2.0	16	5	4	49	26	24	51	68	74	2.8	85	6.7	2.7
Liechtenstein	7	2	1.5	1.1	–	–	–	–	–	–	–	–	–	–	22	1.6	1.6
Lithuania	688	150	0.8	-0.5	9	11	12	17	15	9	71	71	73	1.3	66	2.4	-0.7
Luxembourg	102	27	0.6	1.2	12	11	9	13	13	11	70	75	79	1.7	83	1.0	1.4
Madagascar	9829	3190	2.8	2.9	21	15	10	47	44	37	44	51	59	4.8	27	5.3	4.0
Malawi	7479	2461	3.7	2.3	24	18	15	56	50	41	41	49	48	5.6	18	7.0	5.2
Malaysia	9663	2756	2.6	2.3	9	5	4	37	30	21	61	70	74	2.6	69	4.5	4.5
Maldives	121	31	2.9	2.0	17	9	6	40	40	23	50	60	68	2.6	31	6.8	3.2
Mali	6721	2321	2.3	2.8	26	20	15	52	52	48	39	47	54	6.5	32	4.7	4.9
Malta	84	20	0.9	0.7	9	8	8	17	15	10	70	76	79	1.4	96	0.9	1.1
Marshall Islands	22	6	4.2	1.3	–	–	–	–	–	–	–	–	–	–	67	4.3	1.6
Mauritania	1443	462	2.6	2.8	18	11	8	45	40	33	47	57	64	4.4	41	7.6	3.1
Mauritius	358	94	1.2	1.0	7	6	7	28	20	15	62	69	73	1.9	42	1.4	0.9
Mexico	37772	10342	2.4	1.4	10	5	5	44	28	20	61	70	76	2.2	77	3.4	1.8
Micronesia (Federated States of)	50	14	2.2	0.8	9	7	6	41	34	26	62	66	68	3.8	22	2.4	0.0
Moldova	932	211	1.0	-0.9	10	10	12	18	19	11	65	68	69	1.4	47	2.9	-0.9
Monaco	6	2	1.2	0.5	–	–	–	–	–	–	–	–	–	–	100	1.2	0.5
Mongolia	898	232	2.8	1.0	14	9	7	42	33	19	53	61	67	1.9	57	4.0	1.1
Montenegro	142	38	0.6	0.1	3	5	10	10	11	14	69	75	74	1.8	–	–	–
Morocco	11075	3005	2.4	1.4	17	8	6	47	30	20	52	64	71	2.4	60	4.1	2.8

TABLE 6. DEMOGRAPHIC INDICATORS

	Population (thousands) 2007		Population annual growth rate (%)		Crude death rate			Crude birth rate			Life expectancy			Total fertility rate 2007	% of population urbanized 2007	Average annual growth rate of urban population (%)	
	under 18	under 5	1970–1990	1990–2007	1970	1990	2007	1970	1990	2007	1970	1990	2007			1970–1990	1990–2007
Mozambique	10909	3700	1.8	2.7	25	20	20	48	43	40	39	43	42	5.2	36	8.3	6.2
Myanmar	15617	4132	2.1	1.1	15	11	10	40	27	18	51	59	62	2.1	32	2.5	2.8
Namibia	939	248	3.0	2.2	15	9	13	43	42	26	53	62	52	3.2	36	4.1	4.1
Nauru	4	1	1.7	0.6	–	–	–	–	–	–	–	–	–	–	100	1.7	0.6
Nepal	12606	3651	2.3	2.3	21	13	8	42	39	28	43	54	64	3.3	17	6.3	6.4
Netherlands	3576	969	0.7	0.6	8	9	9	17	13	11	74	77	80	1.7	81	1.2	1.6
New Zealand	1064	285	1.0	1.2	9	8	7	22	17	14	71	75	80	2.0	86	1.2	1.4
Nicaragua	2441	673	2.7	1.8	13	7	5	47	37	25	54	64	73	2.8	60	3.3	2.6
Niger	7724	2797	3.1	3.5	26	22	14	58	56	49	40	46	57	7.2	17	5.9	4.4
Nigeria	75065	24823	2.8	2.6	22	18	17	47	47	40	42	47	47	5.4	50	5.3	5.0
Niue	1	0	–	–	–	–	–	–	–	–	–	–	–	–	37	–	–
Norway	1092	284	0.4	0.6	10	11	9	17	14	12	74	77	80	1.8	78	0.9	1.1
Occupied Palestinian Territory	2095	685	3.4	3.7	19	7	4	49	46	36	54	68	73	5.2	72	4.5	4.2
Oman	1013	271	4.5	2.0	17	4	3	50	38	22	49	70	76	3.0	72	9.3	2.7
Pakistan	70609	19333	3.2	2.2	16	11	7	43	42	27	51	60	65	3.5	36	4.2	3.3
Palau	8	2	1.4	1.8	–	–	–	–	–	–	–	–	–	–	68	2.2	1.8
Panama	1181	344	2.4	1.9	8	5	5	38	26	21	65	72	75	2.6	73	3.0	3.9
Papua New Guinea	2941	894	2.4	2.5	19	11	10	42	37	30	43	54	57	3.8	14	3.9	2.9
Paraguay	2537	734	2.7	2.2	7	6	6	37	33	25	65	68	72	3.1	60	4.0	3.6
Peru	10273	2817	2.5	1.5	14	7	6	42	30	21	53	65	71	2.5	73	3.4	1.9
Philippines	36804	11095	2.6	2.1	11	7	5	40	33	26	57	65	72	3.3	64	4.5	4.0
Poland	7471	1767	0.8	0.0	8	10	10	17	15	9	70	71	76	1.2	62	1.6	0.1
Portugal	1996	558	0.7	0.4	11	10	11	21	12	11	67	74	78	1.5	59	1.8	1.7
Qatar	208	65	7.2	3.5	13	3	2	34	23	16	60	69	76	2.7	96	7.4	3.9
Republic of Korea	10418	2319	1.5	0.7	9	6	6	31	16	9	60	71	79	1.2	81	4.5	1.3
Romania	4154	1051	0.7	-0.5	9	11	12	21	14	10	68	69	72	1.3	54	2.2	-0.5
Russian Federation	27044	7302	0.7	-0.2	9	12	16	14	14	11	69	68	65	1.3	73	1.5	-0.3
Rwanda	4921	1685	3.3	1.7	20	33	17	53	49	44	44	33	46	5.9	21	5.9	10.3
Saint Kitts and Nevis	17	5	-0.5	1.3	–	–	–	–	–	–	–	–	–	–	32	-0.4	0.8
Saint Lucia	54	15	1.4	1.1	8	7	7	41	25	19	64	71	74	2.2	28	2.4	0.8
Saint Vincent and the Grenadines	42	12	0.9	0.6	11	7	7	40	25	20	61	69	71	2.2	47	3.0	1.5
Samoa	88	24	0.6	0.9	10	7	5	39	34	25	55	65	71	4.0	23	0.8	1.4
San Marino	6	2	1.2	1.5	–	–	–	–	–	–	–	–	–	–	89	3.1	1.4
Sao Tome and Principe	76	23	2.3	1.8	13	10	8	47	38	33	55	62	65	3.9	60	4.2	3.9
Saudi Arabia	9781	2921	5.2	2.5	18	5	4	48	36	25	52	68	73	3.4	81	7.5	3.0
Senegal	5998	1942	2.9	2.6	21	12	9	48	43	35	45	57	63	4.7	42	4.2	3.3
Serbia	2204	610	0.8	0.2	9	10	12	18	15	13	68	71	74	1.8	–	–	–
Seychelles	44	15	1.6	1.1	–	–	–	–	–	–	–	–	–	–	50	4.8	1.2
Sierra Leone	2889	1019	2.1	2.1	29	26	22	47	48	46	35	39	42	6.5	42	4.8	4.4
Singapore	994	200	1.9	2.3	5	5	5	23	18	8	69	75	80	1.3	100	1.9	2.4
Slovakia	1087	260	0.7	0.1	10	10	10	19	15	10	70	72	75	1.2	56	2.3	0.1
Slovenia	343	89	0.7	0.2	10	10	10	17	11	9	69	73	78	1.3	51	2.3	0.4
Solomon Islands	229	71	3.3	2.7	10	12	7	46	40	31	54	57	63	3.9	18	5.5	4.4
Somalia	4389	1539	3.1	1.5	24	22	17	51	46	43	40	42	48	6.1	36	4.5	2.8
South Africa	18385	5235	2.4	1.7	14	8	17	38	29	23	53	62	50	2.7	60	2.9	2.7
Spain	7742	2321	0.7	0.8	9	8	9	20	10	11	72	77	81	1.4	77	1.4	0.9
Sri Lanka	5504	1464	1.6	0.7	8	7	7	31	21	15	65	70	72	1.9	15	1.0	-0.1
Sudan	17961	5528	2.9	2.3	20	14	10	47	41	32	44	53	58	4.3	43	5.3	5.4
Suriname	158	44	0.4	0.8	8	6	7	37	24	20	63	68	70	2.4	75	2.4	1.4
Swaziland	534	147	3.2	1.6	18	10	21	50	41	29	48	59	40	3.5	25	7.5	2.2
Sweden	1912	505	0.3	0.4	10	11	10	14	14	11	74	78	81	1.8	84	0.4	0.5
Switzerland	1488	358	0.5	0.5	9	9	8	16	12	9	73	78	82	1.4	76	1.6	1.2
Syrian Arab Republic	8424	2544	3.5	2.6	13	5	3	47	37	27	55	68	74	3.1	51	4.1	3.1
Tajikistan	3081	857	2.9	1.4	10	8	6	40	39	27	60	63	67	3.4	24	2.2	-0.1
Thailand	16430	4518	1.9	1.0	10	7	9	37	19	15	59	67	70	1.8	33	3.6	1.7
The former Yugoslav Republic of Macedonia	476	115	1.0	0.4	8	8	9	24	17	11	66	71	74	1.4	70	2.0	1.6
Timor-Leste	590	199	1.0	2.6	22	19	9	46	43	42	40	46	61	6.6	27	3.4	4.5
Togo	3260	1061	3.1	3.0	18	12	10	48	44	37	48	58	58	4.9	42	4.9	5.2
Tonga	44	12	-0.2	0.3	6	6	6	37	30	25	65	70	73	3.8	24	0.4	0.8

THE STATE OF THE WORLD'S CHILDREN 2009

...TABLE 6

	Population (thousands) 2007		Population annual growth rate (%)		Crude death rate			Crude birth rate			Life expectancy			Total fertility rate 2007	% of population urbanized 2007	Average annual growth rate of urban population (%)	
	under 18	under 5	1970–1990	1990–2007	1970	1990	2007	1970	1990	2007	1970	1990	2007			1970–1990	1990–2007
Trinidad and Tobago	357	94	1.2	0.5	7	7	8	27	21	15	66	70	70	1.6	13	-0.5	3.1
Tunisia	3178	830	2.4	1.3	14	6	6	39	27	17	54	69	74	1.9	66	3.8	2.1
Turkey	24623	6646	2.3	1.6	12	8	6	39	26	18	56	65	72	2.1	68	4.5	2.6
Turkmenistan	1845	494	2.6	1.8	11	8	8	37	35	22	58	63	63	2.5	47	2.3	2.1
Tuvalu	4	1	1.3	0.7	–	–	–	–	–	–	–	–	–	–	57	4.6	2.8
Uganda	17349	6028	3.2	3.2	16	15	14	49	50	47	50	51	51	6.5	13	5.7	4.4
Ukraine	8389	2025	0.4	-0.6	9	13	16	15	13	9	71	70	68	1.2	68	1.4	-0.5
United Arab Emirates	1006	327	10.6	5.0	11	3	1	36	27	16	61	73	79	2.3	77	10.5	5.1
United Kingdom	13100	3503	0.1	0.4	12	11	10	16	14	12	72	76	79	1.8	90	0.8	0.5
United Republic of Tanzania	20630	7050	3.1	2.7	18	15	13	48	44	40	47	51	52	5.2	25	7.5	4.6
United States	75992	20957	1.0	1.0	9	9	8	16	16	14	71	75	78	2.1	81	1.1	1.6
Uruguay	938	252	0.5	0.4	10	10	9	21	18	15	69	72	76	2.1	92	0.9	0.7
Uzbekistan	10593	2879	2.7	1.7	10	7	7	36	35	23	63	67	67	2.5	37	3.1	1.2
Vanuatu	103	31	2.8	2.4	14	7	5	43	37	29	53	64	70	3.8	24	4.9	4.2
Venezuela (Bolivarian Republic of)	10089	2896	3.0	2.0	7	5	5	37	29	22	65	71	74	2.6	94	3.8	2.8
Viet Nam	30263	8109	2.2	1.6	18	8	5	41	31	19	49	65	74	2.2	27	2.7	3.6
Yemen	11729	3740	3.3	3.5	27	13	8	56	51	38	38	54	62	5.5	28	5.5	5.6
Zambia	6270	2030	3.2	2.3	17	16	19	49	44	40	49	49	42	5.2	35	4.5	1.7
Zimbabwe	6175	1706	3.5	1.4	13	8	19	48	37	28	55	63	43	3.2	37	6.1	3.0
SUMMARY INDICATORS																	
Sub-Saharan Africa	383988	127624	2.9	2.6	20	16	15	48	45	39	45	50	50	5.2	36	4.7	4.3
Eastern and Southern Africa	186875	61296	2.9	2.5	19	15	15	47	43	38	46	51	50	4.9	29	4.7	3.9
West and Central Africa	197113	66328	2.9	2.7	22	17	16	48	47	41	43	49	50	5.5	43	4.8	4.6
Middle East and North Africa	153178	44789	3.0	2.0	16	8	6	45	35	25	51	63	69	3.0	58	4.4	2.9
South Asia	614747	175250	2.3	1.9	17	11	8	39	33	24	49	59	64	3.0	29	3.8	3.0
East Asia and Pacific	559872	144441	1.8	1.0	10	7	7	35	22	15	59	67	72	1.9	44	3.9	3.5
Latin America and Caribbean	197226	55622	2.2	1.5	10	7	6	37	27	20	60	68	73	2.4	78	3.3	2.2
CEE/CIS	100110	26458	1.0	0.2	9	11	12	20	18	14	67	68	68	1.7	62	2.0	0.3
Industrialized countries§	204334	54922	0.7	0.6	10	9	9	17	13	11	71	76	79	1.7	76	1.0	0.9
Developing countries§	1962419	562128	2.2	1.6	13	9	8	38	29	22	55	63	67	2.8	44	3.8	3.1
Least developed countries§	383853	124237	2.5	2.5	21	16	12	47	42	36	44	51	55	4.7	28	4.9	4.4
World	2213456	629106	1.8	1.4	12	9	9	32	26	20	59	65	68	2.6	49	2.7	2.3

§ Also includes territories within each country category or regional group. Countries and territories in each country category or regional group are listed on page 152.

DEFINITIONS OF THE INDICATORS

Life expectancy at birth – Number of years newborn children would live if subject to the mortality risks prevailing for the cross section of population at the time of their birth.

Crude death rate – Annual number of deaths per 1,000 population.

Crude birth rate – Annual number of births per 1,000 population.

Total fertility rate – Number of children who would be born per woman if she lived to the end of her childbearing years and bore children at each age in accordance with prevailing age-specific fertility rates.

Urban population – Percentage of population living in urban areas as defined according to the national definition used in the most recent population census.

MAIN DATA SOURCES

Child population – United Nations Population Division.

Crude death and birth rates – United Nations Population Division.

Life expectancy – United Nations Population Division.

Fertility – United Nations Population Division.

Urban population – United Nations Population Division.

NOTES — Data not available.

TABLE 7. ECONOMIC INDICATORS

Countries and territories	GNI per capita (US$) 2007	GDP per capita average annual growth rate (%)		Average annual rate of inflation (%) 1990–2007	% of population below international poverty line of US$1.25 per day 2005	% of central government expenditure (1997–2006*) allocated to:			ODA inflow in millions US$ 2006	ODA inflow as a % of recipient GNI 2006	Debt service as a % of exports of goods and services	
		1970–1990	1990–2007			health	education	defence			1990	2006
Afghanistan	250x	–	–	–	–	–	–	–	3000	37	–	–
Albania	3290	-0.7x	5.2	18	1	4	4	2	321	3	4x	3
Algeria	3620	1.6	1.4	13	7	17	4	24	209	0	62	–
Andorra	d	–	–	–	–	–	–	–	–	–	–	–
Angola	2560	0.4x	2.9	319	54	34x	6x	15x	171	1	7	13
Antigua and Barbuda	11520	8.3x	1.7	2	–	–	–	–	3	0	–	–
Argentina	6050	-0.7	1.5	6	5	3	5	5	114	0	30	13
Armenia	2640	–	5.8	69	11	–	–	–	213	4	–	6
Australia	35960	1.5	2.4	2	–	6	15	10	–	–	–	–
Austria	42700	2.4	1.8	2	–	2	14	10	–	–	–	–
Azerbaijan	2550	–	2.8	71	0	12	1	4	206	1	–	1
Bahamas	15730x	1.8	0.4x	3x	–	3	16	20	–	–	–	–
Bahrain	19350	-1.3x	2.4x	2x	–	14	8	15	57x	1x	–	–
Bangladesh	470	0.6	3.1	4	50y	10	7	17	1223	2	17	3
Barbados	d	1.5	1.3x	3x	–	–	–	–	-1	0	–	–
Belarus	4220	–	3.4	162	0	4	3	4	73	0	–	2
Belgium	40710	2.2	1.8	2	–	3	16	3	–	–	–	–
Belize	3800	2.9	2.4	1	–	5x	8x	20x	8	1	5	16
Benin	570	0	1.3	6	47	17x	6x	31x	375	8	7	6x
Bhutan	1770	6.8x	5.2	7	26	–	9	13	94	10	–	–
Bolivia	1260	-1.1	1.3	7	20	5	10	22	581	6	31	8
Bosnia and Herzegovina	3580	–	10.8x	5x	0	–	–	–	494	4	–	7
Botswana	5840	8.2	4.2	8	31	8x	5x	26x	65	1	4	1
Brazil	5910	2.3	1.2	72	8y	3	6	6	82	0	19	36
Brunei Darussalam	26930x	-2.2x	-0.3x	4x	–	–	–	–	–	–	–	–
Bulgaria	4590	3.4x	2.3	51	0	6	11	5	–	–	19	10
Burkina Faso	430	1.3	2.5	3	57	14x	7x	17x	871	14	6	–
Burundi	110	1.1	-2.7	12	81	23	2	15	415	52	41	40
Cambodia	540	–	6.2x	3x	40	–	–	–	529	8	0x	1
Cameroon	1050	3.3	0.6	4	33	10	3	12	1684	9	18	15x
Canada	39420	2	2.2	2	–	6	9	3	–	–	–	–
Cape Verde	2430	–	3.3	4	21	–	–	–	138	13	5	4
Central African Republic	380	-1.3	-0.8	3	62	–	–	–	134	9	8	–
Chad	540	-1	2.4	7	62	–	8x	8x	284	6	2	–
Chile	8350	1.5	3.7	6	1	7	15	17	83	0	20	19
China	2360	6.6	8.9	5	16y	12	0	2	1245	0	10	2
Colombia	3250	2	1	14	15	13	9	20	988	1	39	31
Comoros	680	0.1x	-0.4	4	46	–	–	–	30	7	2	–
Congo	1540	3.2	-0.2	8	54	10	4	4	254	7	32	2x
Cook Islands	–	–	–	–	–	–	–	–	32	0	–	–
Costa Rica	5560	0.7	2.5	13	2	0	21	22	24	0	21	4
Côte d'Ivoire	910	-1.9	-0.7	6	23	4x	4x	21x	251	2	26	0
Croatia	10460	–	3	33	0	4	13	8	200	0	–	33
Cuba	c	–	3.6x	4x	–	–	23x	10x	78	0	–	–
Cyprus	24940	5.9x	2.2	4	–	4	6	12	–	–	–	–
Czech Republic	14450	–	2.4	7	0	4	16	10	–	–	–	–
Democratic People's Republic of Korea	a	–	–	–	–	–	–	–	55	0	–	–
Democratic Republic of the Congo	140	-2.4	-4.3	335	59	18	0	0	2056	27	–	–
Denmark	54910	2	1.9	2	–	5	1	12	–	–	–	–
Djibouti	1090	–	-2.1	3	19	–	–	–	117	14	4x	6
Dominica	4250	4.7x	2.4	1	–	–	–	–	19	7	4	13x
Dominican Republic	3550	2.1	3.8	11	5	4	10	13	53	0	7	8
Ecuador	3080	1.3	1.2	5	10	13x	11x	18x	189	0	27	23
Egypt	1580	4.3	2.5	7	2	9	3	15	873	1	18	5
El Salvador	2850	-1.8	1.8	4	14	3	14	14	157	1	14	12
Equatorial Guinea	12860	–	21.1	13	–	–	–	–	27	1	2	–
Eritrea	230	–	-0.3x	12x	–	–	–	–	129	15	–	–
Estonia	13200	1.5x	5.2	24	0	5	16	7	–	–	–	–
Ethiopia	220	–	2.2	5	39	17	1	5	1947	15	33	7
Fiji	3800	0.6x	1.5x	4x	–	6x	9x	18x	56	2	12	1
Finland	44400	2.8	2.8	2	–	4	3	10	–	–	–	–

142 THE STATE OF THE WORLD'S CHILDREN 2009

...TABLE 7

	GNI per capita (US$) 2007	GDP per capita average annual growth rate (%)		Average annual rate of inflation (%) 1990–2007	% of population below international poverty line of US$1.25 per day 2005	% of central government expenditure (1997–2006*) allocated to:			ODA inflow in millions US$ 2006	ODA inflow as a % of recipient GNI 2006	Debt service as a % of exports of goods and services	
		1970–1990	1990–2007			health	education	defence			1990	2006
France	38500	2.2	1.6	1	–	6x	16x	7x	–	–	–	–
Gabon	6670	0.3	-0.7	6	5	–	–	–	31	0	4	5x
Gambia	320	0.9	0.2	8	34	4x	7x	12x	74	15	18	11
Georgia	2120	3.2	1.8	102	13	23	7	11	361	5	–	7
Germany	38860	2.3x	1.4	1	–	4	19	1	–	–	–	–
Ghana	590	-2.1	2.1	24	30	5x	7x	22x	1176	10	21	4
Greece	29630	1.3	2.7	6	–	8	7	11	–	–	–	–
Grenada	4670	4.9	2.5	2	–	–	10x	17x	27	6	2	5x
Guatemala	2440	0.2	1.4	7	12	11x	11x	17x	487	1	11	4
Guinea	400	0.3x	1.3	8	70	29x	3x	11x	164	4	18	17x
Guinea-Bissau	200	-0.2	-2.6	16	49	4x	1x	3x	82	27	21	35x
Guyana	1300	-1.5	3.1	8	8	–	–	–	173	20	20x	3
Haiti	560	-0.3	-2.1	18	55	–	–	–	581	14	4	3
Holy See	–	–	–	–	–	–	–	–	–	–	–	–
Honduras	1600	0.8	1.5	15	22	7x	10x	19x	587	7	30	5
Hungary	11570	3	3.3	13	0	3	6	5	–	–	30	32
Iceland	54100	3.2	2.4	4	–	0	27	11	–	–	–	–
India	950	2.1	4.5	6	42y	14	2	4	1379	0	25	7
Indonesia	1650	4.7	2.3	15	21y	7	1	4	1405	0	31	9
Iran (Islamic Republic of)	3470	-2.3	2.5	23	1	14	6	7	121	0	1	–
Iraq	2170x	–	–	–	–	–	–	–	8661	0	–	–
Ireland	48140	2.8	5.8	4	–	3	16	14	–	–	–	–
Israel	21900	1.9	1.7	6	–	19	12	15	–	–	–	–
Italy	33540	2.8	1.2	3	–	3	3	10	–	–	–	–
Jamaica	3710	-1.3	0.8	15	0	2	7	15	37	0	20	11
Japan	37670	3	0.9	-1	–	4x	2x	6x	–	–	–	–
Jordan	2850	2.5x	2	2	0	19	10	16	580	4	18	5
Kazakhstan	5060	–	3.2	75	3	6	5	6	172	0	–	33
Kenya	680	1.2	0	11	20	6	7	26	943	5	26	6
Kiribati	1170	-5.3	1.8	2	–	–	–	–	-45	-36	–	–
Kuwait	31640	-6.8x	1.1x	4x	–	14	6	12	–	–	–	–
Kyrgyzstan	590	–	-0.5	46	22	7	12	11	311	12	–	4
Lao People's Democratic Republic	580	–	4.2	25	44	–	–	–	364	13	8	–
Latvia	9930	3.4	4.7	21	0	5	12	6	–	–	0x	29
Lebanon	5770	–	2.5	8	–	11	2	7	707	3	–	19
Lesotho	1000	3.1	1.8	8	43	5	6	25	72	4	4	4
Liberia	150	-4.2	1.9	42	84	9x	5x	11x	269	57	–	0
Libyan Arab Jamahiriya	9010	-4.9x	–	–	–	–	–	–	37	0	–	–
Liechtenstein	d	–	–	–	–	–	–	–	–	–	–	–
Lithuania	9920	–	3	29	0	5	12	7	–	–	–	21
Luxembourg	75880	2.7	3.2	2	–	1	13	10	–	–	–	–
Madagascar	320	-2.4	-0.4	14	68	5	8	13	754	14	32	5x
Malawi	250	-0.1	0.3	30	74	5x	7x	12x	669	30	23	–
Malaysia	6540	4	3.2	4	1	11	6	23	240	0	12	4
Maldives	3200	–	5.5x	1x	–	5	8	14	39	4	4	5
Mali	500	-0.3	2.2	5	51	8x	2x	9x	825	13	8	4
Malta	15310	6.5	2.7x	3	–	2	14	13	11x	0x	–	–
Marshall Islands	3070	–	-2	5	–	–	–	–	55	28	–	–
Mauritania	840	-0.9	0.6	8	21	–	4x	23x	188	8	24	–
Mauritius	5450	5.1x	3.7	6	–	1	9	15	19	0	6	6
Mexico	8340	1.6	1.6	14	1	3	5	25	247	0	16	19
Micronesia (Federated States of)	2470	–	-0.2	2	–	–	–	–	109	41	–	–
Moldova	1260	1.8x	-1.3	52	8	1	13	9	228	6	–	10
Monaco	d	–	–	–	–	–	–	–	–	–	–	–
Mongolia	1290	–	2.2	30	22	9	6	9	203	9	17x	2
Montenegro	5180	–	3.4x	–	–	–	–	–	1586	68	–	–
Morocco	2250	2	2	3	3	13	3	18	1046	2	18	12
Mozambique	320	-1x	4.1	20	75	35x	5x	10x	1611	23	21	2
Myanmar	220x	1.5	6.8x	24x	–	23	3	13	147	0	17	1
Namibia	3360	-2.3x	1.8	9	49	7x	10x	22x	145	2	–	–
Nauru	–	–	–	–	–	–	–	–	17	0	–	–

STATISTICAL TABLES 143

TABLE 7. ECONOMIC INDICATORS

	GNI per capita (US$) 2007	GDP per capita average annual growth rate (%) 1970–1990	GDP per capita average annual growth rate (%) 1990–2007	Average annual rate of inflation (%) 1990–2007	% of population below international poverty line of US$1.25 per day 2005	% of central government expenditure (1997–2006*) allocated to: health	% of central government expenditure (1997–2006*) allocated to: education	% of central government expenditure (1997–2006*) allocated to: defence	ODA inflow in millions US$ 2006	ODA inflow as a % of recipient GNI 2006	Debt service as a % of exports of goods and services 1990	Debt service as a % of exports of goods and services 2006
Nepal	340	1.2	1.9	7	55	11	5	18	514	6	12	5
Netherlands	45820	1.5	2.1	2	–	4	10	11	–	–	–	–
New Zealand	28780	0.8	2	2	–	3	16	19	–	–	–	–
Nicaragua	980	-3.7	1.9	21	16	6x	13x	15x	733	14	2	4
Niger	280	-2.2	-0.6	4	66	–	–	–	401	11	12	5x
Nigeria	930	-1.4	1.2	23	64	3x	1x	3x	11434	12	22	16x
Niue	–	–	–	–	–	–	–	–	9	0	–	–
Norway	76450	3.2	2.6	4	–	5	16	6	–	–	–	–
Occupied Palestinian Territory	1230	–	-2.9x	4x	–	–	–	–	1449	33	–	–
Oman	11120	3.3	2.2x	2x	–	33	7	15	35	0	12	1
Pakistan	870	3	1.6	10	23	18	1	2	2147	2	16	8
Palau	8210	–	–	3x	–	–	–	–	37	23	–	–
Panama	5510	0.3	2.6	2	9	–	18	16	30	0	3	25
Papua New Guinea	850	-0.7	-0.6	8	36	4	7	22	279	6	37	9x
Paraguay	1670	2.8	-0.3	11	9	11x	7x	22x	56	1	12	6
Peru	3450	-0.6	2.7	13	8	–	13	7	468	1	6	12
Philippines	1620	0.8	1.7	7	23	5	2	19	562	0	23	18
Poland	9840	–	4.4	13	0	4	11	12	–	–	4	24
Portugal	18950	2.6	1.9	4	–	3	16	16	–	–	–	–
Qatar	12000x	–	–	–	–	–	–	–	–	–	–	–
Republic of Korea	19690	6.2	4.4	4	–	10	0	14	–	–	–	–
Romania	6150	0.9x	2.3	57	1	5	14	5	–	–	0	16
Russian Federation	7560	–	1.2	71	0	12	8	4	–	–	–	13
Rwanda	320	1.1	1.1	9	77	–	5x	26x	585	25	9	9
Saint Kitts and Nevis	9630	6.3x	2.8	3	–	–	–	–	5	1	3	22x
Saint Lucia	5530	5.3x	1.3	2	21	–	–	–	18	2	2	6x
Saint Vincent and the Grenadines	4210	3.3	3	2	–	–	12	16	5	1	3	11x
Samoa	2430	–	2.6	6	–	–	–	–	47	11	5	6
San Marino	45130	–	–	–	–	–	18	9	–	–	–	–
Sao Tome and Principe	870	–	–	–	–	–	–	–	22	17	28	37
Saudi Arabia	15440	-1.5	0.3	4	–	36x	6x	14x	25	0	–	–
Senegal	820	-0.7	1.1	4	34	7	3	14	825	9	14	10x
Serbia	4730	–	2.6x	–	–	–	–	–	96	0	–	–
Seychelles	8960	2.9	1.4	3	–	3	9	8	14	2	7	18
Sierra Leone	260	-0.4	-0.4	19	53	10x	10x	13x	364	27	8	8
Singapore	32470	5.6	3.8	1	–	31	6	22	–	–	–	–
Slovakia	11730	–	3.3	8	0	5	19	4	–	–	–	–
Slovenia	20960	–	3.5	15	0	3	15	13	53x	0x	–	–
Solomon Islands	730	3.4	-1.6	7	–	–	–	–	205	62	10	2
Somalia	140x	-0.9	–	–	–	38x	1x	2x	392	0	25x	–
South Africa	5760	0.1	1	8	26	–	–	–	718	0	–	6
Spain	29450	1.9	2.4	4	–	4	15	2	–	–	–	–
Sri Lanka	1540	3	3.9	9	14	18	6	10	796	3	10	7
Sudan	960	0.1	3.6	38	–	28	1	8	2058	7	4	4
Suriname	4730	-2.4x	1.8	54	16	–	–	–	64	4	–	–
Swaziland	2580	3.1	-0.3	12	63	8	8	20	35	1	6	2
Sweden	46060	1.8	2.2	2	–	5	3	6	–	–	–	–
Switzerland	59880	1.2	0.7	1	–	5	0	5	–	–	–	–
Syrian Arab Republic	1760	2	1.5	7	–	24	2	9	27	0	20	1
Tajikistan	460	–	-2.2	99	21	9	2	4	240	9	–	5
Thailand	3400	5	2.9	3	0	6	9	20	-216	0	14	9
The former Yugoslav Republic of Macedonia	3460	–	0.5	30	0	–	–	–	200	3	–	15
Timor-Leste	1510	–	–	–	53	–	–	–	210	24	–	–
Togo	360	-0.6	-0.2	4	39	11x	5x	20x	79	4	8	0x
Tonga	2320	–	2	4	–	–	7x	13x	21	10	2	3
Trinidad and Tobago	14100	0.5	5.1	5	4	2	9	17	13	0	–	–
Tunisia	3200	2.5	3.4	4	3	5	5	20	432	1	22	13
Turkey	8020	1.9	2.2	52	3	8	3	10	570	0	27	25
Turkmenistan	b	–	-6.8x	408x	25	–	–	–	26	0	–	–
Tuvalu	–	–	–	–	–	–	–	–	15	0	–	–
Uganda	340	–	3.1	8	52	26x	2x	15x	1551	17	47	5

...TABLE 7

	GNI per capita (US$) 2007	GDP per capita average annual growth rate (%)		Average annual rate of inflation (%) 1990–2007	% of population below international poverty line of US$1.25 per day 2005	% of central government expenditure (1997–2006*) allocated to:			ODA inflow in millions US$ 2006	ODA inflow as a % of recipient GNI 2006	Debt service as a % of exports of goods and services	
		1970–1990	1990–2007			health	education	defence			1990	2006
Ukraine	2550	–	-0.7	93	0	3	3	6	484	1	–	16
United Arab Emirates	26210x	-4.8x	-0.3x	3x	–	30	7	17	–	–	–	–
United Kingdom	42740	2	2.4	3	–	7	15	4	–	–	–	–
United Republic of Tanzania	400	–	1.8	15	88	16x	6x	8x	1825	14	25	3
United States	46040	2.2	2	2	–	20	25	3	–	–	–	–
Uruguay	6380	0.9	1.5	18	0	4	7	8	21	0	31	43
Uzbekistan	730	–	1.2	106	46	–	–	–	149	1	–	–
Vanuatu	1840	1.1x	-0.4	3	–	–	–	–	49	13	2	1
Venezuela (Bolivarian Republic of)	7320	-1.6	-0.2	35	18	5	8	21	58	0	22	13
Viet Nam	790	–	6	10	21	–	4	14	1846	3	–	2
Yemen	870	–	1.6	17	18	19	4	22	284	2	4	2
Zambia	800	-2.3	0.1	34	64	4	13	14	1425	19	13	3
Zimbabwe	340	-0.4	-2.1x	62x	–	7	8	24	280	6	19	–

SUMMARY INDICATORS

	GNI per capita (US$) 2007	1970–1990	1990–2007	Inflation 1990–2007	Poverty 2005	health	education	defence	ODA 2006	ODA % GNI 2006	Debt 1990	Debt 2006
Sub-Saharan Africa	965	-0.1	1.3	35	51	–	–	–	35799	6	17	7
Eastern and Southern Africa	1245	–	1.4	40	49	–	–	–	13793	3	14	7
West and Central Africa	698	-0.6	1.3	26	53	–	–	–	22006	11	19	–
Middle East and North Africa	3666	-0.1	1.6	11	4	15	5	14	16660	1	21	8
South Asia	889	2.1	4.1	6	40	14	2	5	9191	1	21	7
East Asia and Pacific	2742	5.7	6.8	5	17	11	1	7	7477	0	16	4
Latin America and Caribbean	5628	1.4	1.5	35	8	4	7	14	5989	0	20	21
CEE/CIS	5686	–	1.6	67	4	9	7	6	5928	0	–	17
Industrialized countries§	38579	2.3	1.9	2	–	12	18	4	–	–	–	–
Developing countries§	2405	2.4	4	18	25	10	3	9	77364	1	19	10
Least developed countries§	491	-0.2	2.5	60	54	14	5	14	28181	9	12	6
World	7952	2.3	2.4	8	–	11	14	6	81045	0	18	11

§ Also includes territories within each country category or regional group. Countries and territories in each country category or regional group are listed on page 152.

DEFINITIONS OF THE INDICATORS

GNI per capita – Gross national income (GNI) is the sum of value added by all resident producers plus any product taxes (less subsidies) not included in the valuation of output plus net receipts of primary income (compensation of employees and property income) from abroad. GNI per capita is gross national income divided by midyear population. GNI per capita in US dollars is converted using the World Bank Atlas method.

GDP per capita – Gross domestic product (GDP) is the sum of value added by all resident producers plus any product taxes (less subsidies) not included in the valuation of output. GDP per capita is gross domestic product divided by midyear population. Growth is calculated from constant price GDP data in local currency.

% of population below international poverty line of US$1.25 per day – Percentage of population living on less than US$1.25 per day at 2005 prices, adjusted for purchasing power parity. The new poverty threshold reflects revisions to purchasing power parity exchange rates based on the results of the 2005 International Comparison Program. The revisions reveal that the cost of living is higher across the developing world than previously estimated. As a result of these revisions, poverty rates for individual countries cannot be compared with poverty rates reported in previous editions. More detailed information on the definition, methodology and sources of the data presented is available at <www.worldbank.org>.

ODA – Net official development assistance.

Debt service – Sum of interest payments and repayments of principal on external public and publicly guaranteed long-term debts.

MAIN DATA SOURCES

GNI per capita – World Bank.

GDP per capita – World Bank.

Rate of inflation – World Bank.

% of population below international poverty line of US$1.25 per day – World Bank.

Expenditure on health, education and defence – International Monetary Fund (IMF).

ODA – Organisation for Economic Co-operation and Development (OECD).

Debt service – World Bank.

NOTES

a: low income ($935 or less).
b: lower-middle income ($936 to $3,705).
c: upper-middle income ($3,706 to $11,455).
d: high income ($11,456 or more).

– Data not available.
x Data refer to years or periods other than those specified in the column heading, differ from the standard definition or refer to only part of a country. Such data are not included in the calculation of regional and global averages.
y Data refer to years or periods other than those specified in the column heading, differ from the standard definition or refer to only part of a country. Such data are included in the calculation of regional and global averages.
* Data refer to the most recent year available during the period specified in the column heading.

TABLE 8. WOMEN

Countries and territories	Life expectancy: females as a % of males 2007	Adult literacy rate: females as a % of males 2000–2007*	Enrolment and attendance ratios: females as a % of males				Contraceptive prevalence (%) 2000–2007*	Antenatal care coverage (%) 2000–2007*		Delivery care coverage (%) 2000–2007*		Maternal mortality ratio[†]		
			Net primary school 2000–2007*		Net secondary school 2000–2007*			At least once	At least four times	Skilled attendant at birth	Institutional delivery	2000–2007* reported	2005 Adjusted	Lifetime risk of maternal death. 1 in:
			enrolled	attending	enrolled	attending								
Afghanistan	100	29	63	60	–	33	10	16	–	14	13	1600	1800	8
Albania	109	99	99	100	98	97	60	97	–	100	98	20	92	490
Algeria	104	79	98	99	106	112	61	89	–	95	95	120x	180	220
Andorra	–	–	101	–	103	–	–	–	–	–	–	–	–	–
Angola	108	65	–	102	–	90	6	80	–	47	46	–	1400	12
Antigua and Barbuda	–	–	–	–	–	–	53	100	–	100	–	0	–	–
Argentina	111	100	99	–	110	–	–	99	89y	99	99	48	77	530
Armenia	110	100	105	99	104	102	53	93	71	98	97	27	76	980
Australia	106	–	101	–	102	–	–	100x	–	100x	–	–	4	13300
Austria	107	–	101	–	–	–	51x	100x	–	100x	–	–	4	21500
Azerbaijan	112	99	97	98	96	98	51	77	45	88	78	29	82	670
Bahamas	108	–	103	–	102	–	–	98	–	99	–	–	16	2700
Bahrain	104	96	100	100	105	111	62x	97x	–	98x	98x	46x	32	1300
Bangladesh	103	82	104	106	104	114	56	51	21	18	15	320	570	51
Barbados	107	–	99	–	101	–	55x	100	–	100	–	0x	16	4400
Belarus	119	100	98	101	102	102	73	99	–	100	100	12	18	4800
Belgium	108	–	100	–	96	–	78x	–	–	–	–	–	8	7800
Belize	108	–	101	100	108	103	34	94	76x	96	88	42	52	560
Benin	104	53	84	87	50	66	17	84	61	74	78	400	840	20
Bhutan	105	63	100	91	101	–	35y	88	–	56	55	260	440	55
Bolivia	107	90	101	99	98	98	58	79	58	67	57	230	290	89
Bosnia and Herzegovina	107	95	–	97	–	100	36	99	–	100	100	9	3	29000
Botswana	100	100	103	103	114	122	48	97	–	94	80x	330x	380	130
Brazil	111	101	102	100x	111	119x	77x	97	87	88x	97	53	110	370
Brunei Darussalam	106	96	100	–	105	–	–	100x	–	99x	–	0x	13	2900
Bulgaria	110	99	99	–	98	–	86x	–	–	99	–	7	11	7400
Burkina Faso	106	59	82	90	72	91	17	85	18	54	51	480x	700	22
Burundi	106	78	97	97	–	79	9	92	–	34	29	620	1100	16
Cambodia	109	79	98	102	85	90	40	69	27	44	22	470	540	48
Cameroon	102	78	–	94	–	93	29	82	60	63	61	670	1000	24
Canada	106	–	100	–	–	–	75x	–	–	98	–	–	7	11000
Cape Verde	109	88	99	100x	113	–	61	98	64x	78	78	15	210	120
Central African Republic	106	52	72	84	71	64	19	69	40x	53	51	540	980	25
Chad	105	31	70	76	33	51	3	39	18	14	13	1100	1500	11
Chile	108	100	–	–	–	–	58y	95x	–	100	100	20	16	3200
China	105	93	100	–	–	–	85	90	–	98	88	41	45	1300
Colombia	111	100	100	102	111	111	78	94	83	96	92	73	130	290
Comoros	107	87	95	100	101	103	26	75	52x	62	43x	380	400	52
Congo	105	89	90	101	–	104	21	86	75	83	82	780	740	22
Cook Islands	–	–	103	–	110	–	44	–	–	98	–	6x	–	–
Costa Rica	106	101	102	102	110	110	96	92	–	99	94	36	30	1400
Côte d'Ivoire	104	63	80	87	57	69	13	85	45	57	54	540	810	27
Croatia	110	98	99	–	102	–	–	–	–	100	–	10	7	10500
Cuba	105	100	101	–	103	–	77	100	–	100	–	21	45	1400
Cyprus	107	98	100	–	102	–	–	–	–	–	–	0x	10	6400
Czech Republic	108	–	103	–	–	–	69x	99x	97x	100	–	8	4	18100
Democratic People's Republic of Korea	106	–	–	–	–	–	62x	–	–	97	–	110x	370	140
Democratic Republic of the Congo	106	67	–	89	–	81	31	85	–	74	70	1300	1100	13
Denmark	106	–	101	–	103	–	–	–	–	–	–	10x	3	17800
Djibouti	105	–	82	97	66	84	18	92	7	61	74	74x	650	35
Dominica	–	–	106	–	110	–	50x	100	–	99	–	0	–	–
Dominican Republic	109	101	103	104	122	145	73	99	95	98	98	160	150	230
Ecuador	108	98	101	–	102	–	73	84	58	99x	74	110	210	170
Egypt	107	73	96	97	94	93	59	70	59	74	65	84	130	230
El Salvador	109	94	100	–	105	–	67	86	71	92	69	71	170	190
Equatorial Guinea	105	86	90	98	–	95	–	86	–	65	–	–	680	28
Eritrea	109	–	87	93	67	92	8	70	41	28	26	1000x	450	44
Estonia	117	100	99	–	102	–	70	–	–	100	–	7	25	2900
Ethiopia	105	46	92	101	65	77	15	28	12	6	5	670	720	27
Fiji	107	–	100	–	110	–	44	–	–	99	–	34	210	160
Finland	108	–	100	–	100	–	–	100x	–	100x	100	6x	7	8500
France	109	–	100	–	102	–	75x	99x	–	99x	–	10x	8	6900
Gabon	101	91	99	100	–	106	33	94	63	86	85	520	520	53

...TABLE 8

Countries and territories	Life expectancy: females as a % of males 2007	Adult literacy rate: females as a % of males 2000–2007*	Enrolment and attendance ratios: females as a % of males				Contraceptive prevalence (%) 2000–2007*	Antenatal care coverage (%) 2000–2007*		Delivery care coverage (%) 2000–2007*		Maternal mortality ratio†		
			Net primary school 2000–2007*		Net secondary school 2000–2007*								2005	
			enrolled	attending	enrolled	attending		At least once	At least four times	Skilled attendant at birth	Institutional delivery	2000–2007* reported	Adjusted	Lifetime risk of maternal death. 1 in:
Gambia	103	–	109	103	94	87	18	98	–	57	55	730	690	32
Georgia	112	–	103	101	105	98	47	94	75	98	96	23	66	1100
Germany	107	–	100	–	–	–	75x	–	–	–	–	8x	4	19200
Ghana	101	81	97	100	91	99	17	92	69	50	49	210x	560	45
Greece	106	98	100	–	101	–	–	–	–	–	–	1x	3	25900
Grenada	105	–	99	–	102	–	54y	100	–	100	–	0	–	–
Guatemala	111	86	96	94x	92	103x	43	84	–	41	42	130	290	71
Guinea	106	42	86	87	57	66	9	82	49	38	31	980	910	19
Guinea-Bissau	107	72	71	97	55	88	10	78	–	39	36	410	1100	13
Guyana	109	–	–	100	–	110	34	81	–	83	83	120	470	90
Haiti	106	106	–	107	–	117	32	85	54	26	25	630	670	44
Holy See	–	–	–	–	–	–	–	–	–	–	–	–	–	–
Honduras	110	102	102	104	–	123	65	92	81	67	67	110x	280	93
Hungary	112	100	99	–	100	–	77x	–	–	100	–	8	6	13300
Iceland	104	–	99	–	102	–	–	–	–	–	–	–	4	12700
India	105	71	96	96	–	83	56	74	37	47	39	300	450	70
Indonesia	106	93	97	101	100	104	61	93	81	72	40	310	420	97
Iran (Islamic Republic of)	105	88	110	97	94	–	79	77x	94y	97	96	25	140	300
Iraq	107	76	86	88	70	75	50	84	–	89	63	84	300	72
Ireland	106	–	101	–	106	–	–	–	–	100	100	6x	1	47600
Israel	105	–	101	–	100	–	–	–	–	–	–	5x	4	7800
Italy	108	99	99	–	101	–	60x	–	–	–	–	7x	3	26600
Jamaica	108	113	100	100	105	105	69	91	87x	97	94	95	170	240
Japan	109	–	100	–	100	–	56	–	–	100x	–	8x	6	11600
Jordan	105	93	102	100	103	104	57	99	94	99	99	41x	62	450
Kazakhstan	118	100	100	99	100	100	51	100	70x	100	100	70	140	360
Kenya	104	90	102	100	97	114	39	88	52	42	40	410	560	39
Kiribati	–	–	101	–	111	–	21x	88x	–	85x	–	56	–	–
Kuwait	105	97	99	–	105	–	50x	95x	–	98x	98x	5x	4	9600
Kyrgyzstan	113	100	99	103	102	103	48	97	81x	98	97	100	150	240
Lao People's Democratic Republic	104	83	94	95	86	84	38	27	–	19	–	410	660	33
Latvia	116	100	103	–	–	–	48x	–	–	100	–	9	10	8500
Lebanon	106	–	99	99	110	113	58	96	–	98x	–	100x	150	290
Lesotho	99	123	104	108	154	171	37	90	70	55	52	760x	960	45
Liberia	104	85	97	–	58	–	11	85	–	51	37	580x	1200	12
Libyan Arab Jamahiriya	107	83	–	–	–	–	45x	81x	–	94x	–	77x	97	350
Liechtenstein	–	–	103	–	111	–	–	–	–	–	–	–	–	–
Lithuania	116	100	99	–	101	–	47x	–	–	100	–	13	11	7800
Luxembourg	108	–	101	–	105	–	–	–	–	100	–	0x	12	5000
Madagascar	106	85	100	104	104	125	27	80	40	51	32	470	510	38
Malawi	101	82	106	102	93	96	42	92	57	54	54	810	1100	18
Malaysia	107	95	100	–	110	–	55x	79	–	98	98	28	62	560
Maldives	102	100	100	–	109	–	39	81	–	84	–	140	120	200
Mali	109	51	79	74	–	68	8	70	35	45	45	460	970	15
Malta	105	104	99	–	107	–	–	–	–	98x	–	–	8	8300
Marshall Islands	–	–	99	–	108	–	34	–	–	95x	–	74	–	–
Mauritania	106	76	105	105	90	82	8	64	16	57	49	750	820	22
Mauritius	110	94	102	–	102	–	76	–	–	98	98	22	15	3300
Mexico	107	96	99	100	99	–	71	86x	–	93	86	62	60	670
Micronesia (Federated States of)	102	–	–	–	–	–	45x	–	–	88	–	270x	–	–
Moldova	111	99	100	102	104	103	68	98	89	100	99	16	22	3700
Monaco	–	–	–	–	–	–	–	–	–	–	–	–	–	–
Mongolia	110	101	102	102	113	106	66	99	–	99	99	90	46	840
Montenegro	106	–	–	–	99	–	101	39	97	–	99	100	23	–	–
Morocco	106	63	94	95	84	93	63	68	31	63	61	230	240	150
Mozambique	102	58	93	90	91	80	17	85	53	48	48	410	520	45
Myanmar	111	92	101	102	100	94	34	76	–	57	16	320	380	110
Namibia	101	99	106	101	132	132	55	95	70	81	81	270	210	170
Nauru	–	–	–	–	–	–	–	–	–	–	–	–	–	–

STATISTICAL TABLES 147

TABLE 8. WOMEN

Countries and territories	Life expectancy: females as a % of males 2007	Adult literacy rate: females as a % of males 2000–2007*	Enrolment and attendance ratios: females as a % of males				Contraceptive prevalence (%) 2000–2007*	Antenatal care coverage (%) 2000–2007*		Delivery care coverage (%) 2000–2007*		Maternal mortality ratio†		
			Net primary school 2000–2007*		Net secondary school 2000–2007*			At least once	At least four times	Skilled attendant at birth	Institutional delivery	2000–2007* reported	2005 Adjusted	Lifetime risk of maternal death, 1 in:
			enrolled	attending	enrolled	attending								
Nepal	102	62	96	95	–	83	48	44	29	19	18	280	830	31
Netherlands	106	–	99	–	101	–	79x	–	–	100x	–	–	6	10200
New Zealand	105	–	100	–	103	–	75x	95x	–	100x	–	15x	9	5900
Nicaragua	109	102	100	108	116	132	72	90	78	74	66	87	170	150
Niger	97	37	71	70	63	65	11	46	15	33	17	650	1800	7
Nigeria	102	80	86	88	84	87	13	58	47	35	33	–	1100	18
Niue	–	–	–	–	105x	–	–	–	–	100	–	–	–	–
Norway	106	–	101	–	101	–	–	–	–	–	–	6x	7	7700
Occupied Palestinian Territory	104	92	100	101	106	–	50	99	–	99	97	–	–	–
Oman	104	87	102	–	99	–	32	100	83y	98	98	13	64	420
Pakistan	101	59	78	85	77	78	30	61	28	39	34	530x	320	74
Palau	–	–	96	–	–	–	17	–	–	100	–	0x	–	–
Panama	107	99	99	–	111	–	–	72x	–	91	92	66	130	270
Papua New Guinea	111	86	–	–	–	–	26x	78x	–	41	–	370x	470	55
Paraguay	106	99	101	100	106	99	73	94	79	77	74	120	150	170
Peru	107	90	102	101	100	100	71	91	87	71	72	190	240	140
Philippines	106	101	102	102	121	127	51	88	70	60	38	160	230	140
Poland	112	99	101	–	102	–	49x	–	–	100	–	3	8	10600
Portugal	108	97	99	–	110	–	–	–	–	100	–	8x	11	6400
Qatar	102	100	101	–	98	–	43x	–	–	99x	98x	10x	12	2700
Republic of Korea	110	–	93	–	94	–	81x	–	–	100x	–	20x	14	6100
Romania	110	99	100	–	98	–	70	94	76	98	98	15	24	3200
Russian Federation	123	100	100	–	–	–	–	–	–	100	–	24	28	2700
Rwanda	107	84	107	103	–	88	17	94	13	39	28	750	1300	16
Saint Kitts and Nevis	–	–	122	–	87	–	54y	100	–	100	–	0	–	–
Saint Lucia	105	–	98	–	124	–	47x	99	–	100	–	0	–	–
Saint Vincent and the Grenadines	106	–	96	–	124	–	48y	95	–	100	–	0	–	–
Samoa	109	99	100	–	114	–	43x	–	–	100x	–	29	–	–
San Marino	–	–	–	–	–	–	–	–	–	–	–	–	–	–
Sao Tome and Principe	106	89	101	101	111	105	30	97	–	81	78	150	–	–
Saudi Arabia	106	89	–	–	–	–	32x	90x	–	91x	91x	–	18	1400
Senegal	107	61	98	102	76	78	12	87	40	52	62	400	980	21
Serbia	106	–	100	100	–	103	41	98	–	99	99	13	–	–
Seychelles	–	101	101	–	106	–	–	–	–	–	–	57	–	–
Sierra Leone	108	54	–	101	71	79	5	81	–	43	19	1800	2100	8
Singapore	105	94	–	–	–	–	62x	–	–	100x	–	6x	14	6200
Slovakia	111	–	101	–	–	–	74x	–	–	100	–	4	6	13800
Slovenia	110	100	100	–	101	–	74x	98x	–	100	–	17	6	14200
Solomon Islands	103	–	99	–	87	–	7	–	–	85x	–	140x	220	100
Somalia	105	–	–	82	–	51	15	26	6	33	9	1000	1400	12
South Africa	103	98	100	104x	112	117x	60	92	73x	92	–	170	400	110
Spain	108	98	99	–	103	–	81x	–	–	–	–	6x	4	16400
Sri Lanka	111	96	100	–	–	–	68	99	–	99	98	43	58	850
Sudan	105	73	83	93	–	133	7	60	–	87	–	550x	450	53
Suriname	110	95	103	99	138	121	46	90	–	90	88	150	72	530
Swaziland	100	97	101	103	121	132	51	85	79	69	74	590	390	120
Sweden	106	–	100	–	100	–	–	–	–	–	–	5x	3	17400
Switzerland	107	–	99	–	95	–	82x	–	–	–	–	5x	5	13800
Syrian Arab Republic	105	85	95	100	95	101	58	84	–	93	70	65	130	210
Tajikistan	108	100	96	99	84	83	38	77	–	83	62	97	170	160
Thailand	113	97	99	100	111	109	77	98	–	97	97	12	110	500
The former Yugoslav Republic of Macedonia	107	97	100	96	98	99	–	94	–	99	99	4	10	6500
Timor-Leste	103	–	96	98	–	–	20	61	30	18	10	–	380	35
Togo	106	56	87	93	48	70	17	84	46x	62	63	480x	510	38
Tonga	103	100	97	–	125	–	33	–	–	95	–	78	–	–
Trinidad and Tobago	106	99	100	100	104	107	43	96	–	98	97	45x	45	1400
Tunisia	106	80	101	98	110	–	66	92	–	90	89	69x	100	500
Turkey	107	84	96	96	86	83	71	81	54	83	78	29	44	880
Turkmenistan	114	100	–	100	–	100	48	99	83	100	98	14	130	290

148 THE STATE OF THE WORLD'S CHILDREN 2009

...TABLE 8

Countries and territories	Life expectancy: females as a % of males 2007	Adult literacy rate: females as a % of males 2000–2007*	Enrolment and attendance ratios: females as a % of males				Contraceptive prevalence (%) 2000–2007*	Antenatal care coverage (%) 2000–2007*		Delivery care coverage (%) 2000–2007*		Maternal mortality ratio†		
			Net primary school 2000–2007*		Net secondary school 2000–2007*			At least once	At least four times	Skilled attendant at birth	Institutional delivery	2000–2007* reported	2005 Adjusted	Lifetime risk of maternal death, 1 in:
			enrolled	attending	enrolled	attending								
Tuvalu	–	–	–	–	–	–	32	–	–	100	–	–	–	–
Uganda	103	80	–	99	90	94	24	94	47	42	41	440	550	25
Ukraine	119	100	100	102	101	102	67	99	–	99	99	17	18	5200
United Arab Emirates	106	98	100	–	102	–	28x	97x	–	99x	99x	3x	37	1000
United Kingdom	106	–	101	–	104	–	84	–	–	99x	–	7x	8	8200
United Republic of Tanzania	104	83	99	106	90	108	26	78	62	43	47	580	950	24
United States	107	–	102	–	100	–	76x	–	–	99x	–	8x	11	4800
Uruguay	110	101	100	–	–	–	84	94x	97	100x	–	35	20	2100
Uzbekistan	110	98	–	100	–	98	65	99	79x	100	97	28	24	1400
Vanuatu	106	95	99	–	87	–	28	–	–	88x	–	68x	–	–
Venezuela (Bolivarian Republic of)	108	99	100	102	114	147	77x	94	–	95	95	61	57	610
Viet Nam	105	93x	–	100	–	102	76	91	29	88	64	160	150	280
Yemen	105	53	76	60x	53	37x	28	41	11x	36	24	370	430	39
Zambia	101	78x	104	105	80	112	34	93	72	43	44	730	830	27
Zimbabwe	97	94	101	102	96	93	60	94	71	69	68	560	880	43

SUMMARY INDICATORS

Sub-Saharan Africa	104	75	93	95	84	87	23	72	42	45	40	–	920	22
Eastern and Southern Africa	104	79	98	101	90	92	30	72	40	40	33	–	760	29
West and Central Africa	103	72	86	89	77	84	17	71	44	49	46	–	1100	17
Middle East and North Africa	105	78	94	96	92	97	56	72	–	81	71	–	210	140
South Asia	104	71	94	95	–	85	53	68	34	41	35	–	500	59
East Asia and Pacific	106	93	99	101**	103**	105**	78	89	66**	87	73	–	150	350
Latin America and Caribbean	109	99	100	101	107	–	69	94	83	85	86	–	130	280
CEE/CIS	115	97	98	98	95	96	64	90	–	94	89	–	46	1300
Industrialized countries§	108	–	101	–	101	–	72	–	–	–	–	–	8	8000
Developing countries§	105	86	96	96**	97**	91**	60	77	46**	61	54	–	450	76
Least developed countries§	104	72	94	97	86	94	29	64	32	39	32	–	870	24
World	106	88	97	96**	98**	91**	62	77	47**	62	54	–	400	92

§ Also includes territories within each country category or regional group. Countries and territories in each country category or regional group are listed on page 152.

DEFINITIONS OF THE INDICATORS

Life expectancy at birth – Number of years newborn children would live if subject to the mortality risks prevailing for the cross section of population at the time of their birth.
Adult literacy rate – Number of literate persons aged 15 and above, expressed as a percentage of the total population in that age group.
Enrolment and attendance ratios: females as a % of males – Girls' net enrolment and attendance ratios divided by those of boys, as a percentage.
Primary or secondary school net enrolment ratio – Number of children enrolled in primary or secondary school who are of official primary or secondary school age, expressed as a percentage of the total number of children of official primary or secondary school age.
Primary school net attendance ratio – Number of children attending primary or secondary school who are of official primary school age, expressed as a percentage of the total number of children of official primary school age.
Secondary school net attendance ratio – Number of children attending secondary or tertiary school who are of official secondary school age, expressed as a percentage of the total number of children of official secondary school age.
Contraceptive prevalence – Percentage of women in union aged 15–49 currently using contraception.
Antenatal care coverage – Percentage of women 15–49 years old attended at least once during pregnancy by skilled health personnel (doctors, nurses or midwives) and the percentage attended by any provider at least four times.
Skilled attendant at birth – Percentage of births attended by skilled health personnel (doctors, nurses or midwives).
Institutional delivery – Proportion of women 15–49 years old who gave birth during the two years preceding the survey and delivered in a health facility.
Maternal mortality ratio – Annual number of deaths of women from pregnancy-related causes per 100,000 live births. The 'reported' column shows country-reported figures that are not adjusted for under-reporting and misclassification.
Lifetime risk of maternal death – Lifetime risk of maternal death takes into account both the probability of becoming pregnant and the probability of dying as a result of that pregnancy accumulated across a woman's reproductive years.

MAIN DATA SOURCES

Life expectancy – United Nations Population Division.
Adult literacy – UNESCO Institute for Statistics (UIS).
Primary and secondary school enrolment – UIS.
Primary and secondary school attendance – Demographic and Health Surveys (DHS) and Multiple Indicator Cluster Surveys (MICS).
Contraceptive prevalence – DHS, MICS, United Nations Population Division and UNICEF.
Antenatal care coverage – DHS, MICS and other national household surveys.
Skilled attendant at birth – DHS, MICS, WHO and UNICEF.
Institutional delivery – DHS, MICS, WHO and UNICEF.
Maternal mortality – WHO and UNICEF.
Lifetime risk – WHO and UNICEF.

† The maternal mortality data in the column headed 'reported' are those reported by national authorities. Periodically, UNICEF, WHO, UNFPA and the World Bank evaluate these data and make adjustments to account for the well-documented problems of under-reporting and misclassification of maternal deaths and to develop estimates for countries with no data. The column with 'adjusted' estimates for the year 2005 reflects the most recent of these reviews.

NOTES
– Data not available.
x Data refer to years or periods other than those specified in the column heading, differ from the standard definition or refer to only part of a country. Such data are not included in the calculation of regional and global averages.
y Data refer to years or periods other than those specified in the column heading, differ from the standard definition or refer to only part of a country. Such data are included in the calculation of regional and global averages.
* Data refer to the most recent year available during the period specified in the column heading.
** Excludes China.

TABLE 9. CHILD PROTECTION

Countries and territories	Child labour (5–14 years) 1999–2007* total	male	female	Child marriage 1998–2007* total	urban	rural	Birth registration 2000–2007* total	urban	rural	Female genital mutilation/cutting 2002–2007* women[a] (15–49 years) total	urban	rural	daughters[b] total	Attitude towards domestic violence 2001–2007* total	Child disability◊ 1999–2007* total	Child discipline 2005–2007* total
Afghanistan	30	28	33	43	–	–	6	12	4	–	–	–	–	–	–	–
Albania	12	14	9	8	7	8	98	97	98	–	–	–	–	30	16	49
Algeria	5	6	4	2	2	2	99	99	99	–	–	–	–	68	1y	86
Angola	24	22	25	–	–	–	29	34	19	–	–	–	–	–	–	–
Argentina	7y	8y	5y	–	–	–	91y	–	–	–	–	–	–	–	–	–
Armenia	4y	–	–	10	7	16	96	97	95	–	–	–	–	22	12y	–
Azerbaijan	7y	8y	5y	12	–	–	94	96	92	–	–	–	–	49	–	75
Bahrain	5	6	3	–	–	–	–	–	–	–	–	–	–	–	–	–
Bangladesh	13	18	8	64	58	69	10	13	9	–	–	–	–	–	21	–
Belarus	5	6	4	7	6	10	–	–	–	–	–	–	–	–	–	83
Belize	40	39	42	–	–	–	94	92	97	–	–	–	–	12	44	68
Benin	46	47	45	34	19	47	60	68	56	13	9	15	2	47	–	–
Bhutan	19y	16y	22y	–	–	–	–	–	–	–	–	–	–	–	–	–
Bolivia	22	22	22	26	22	37	74	76	72	–	–	–	–	–	–	–
Bosnia and Herzegovina	5	7	4	6	2	7	100	99	100	–	–	–	–	5	10	36
Botswana	–	–	–	10x	13x	9x	58	66	52	–	–	–	–	–	–	–
Brazil	6y	7y	4y	24x	22x	30x	89y	–	–	–	–	–	–	–	–	–
Burkina Faso	47y	46y	48y	48	29	61	64	86	58	73	76	71	25	71	–	83
Burundi	19	19	19	18	14	18	60	62	60	–	–	–	–	–	–	–
Cambodia	45y	45y	45y	23	18	25	66	71	66	–	–	–	–	55	–	–
Cameroon	31	31	30	36	23	57	70	86	58	1	1	2	1	56	33	92
Cape Verde	3y	4y	3y	–	–	–	–	–	–	–	–	–	–	–	1y	–
Central African Republic	47	44	49	61	57	64	49	72	36	26	21	29	7	–	48	88
Chad	53	54	51	72	65	73	9	36	3	45	47	44	21	–	3y	–
Chile	3	3	2	–	–	–	95y	–	–	–	–	–	–	–	–	–
China	–	–	–	–	–	–	–	–	–	–	–	–	–	–	2y	–
Colombia	5	6	4	23	19	38	90	97	77	–	–	–	–	–	3y	–
Comoros	27	26	28	30x	23x	33x	83	87	83	–	–	–	–	–	–	–
Congo	25	24	25	31	24	40	81y	88y	75y	–	–	–	–	76	–	–
Costa Rica	5	6	3	–	–	–	–	–	–	–	–	–	–	–	–	–
Côte d'Ivoire	35	36	34	35	27	43	55	79	41	36	34	39	9	65	–	90
Cuba	–	–	–	–	–	–	100	100	100	–	–	–	–	–	–	–
Democratic People's Republic of Korea	–	–	–	–	–	–	99	99	99	–	–	–	–	–	–	–
Democratic Republic of the Congo	32	29	34	–	–	–	34	30	36	–	–	–	–	–	–	–
Djibouti	8	8	8	5	5	13	89	90	82	93	93	96	49	–	–	70
Dominican Republic	10	12	7	40	38	47	78	82	70	–	–	–	–	9	5y	83
Ecuador	12	12	13	22	–	–	85	85	85	–	–	–	–	–	–	–
Egypt	7	8	5	17	9	22	99	99	99	96	92	98	28y	50	8y	92
El Salvador	6y	9y	4y	27	–	–	–	–	–	–	–	–	–	–	–	–
Equatorial Guinea	28	28	28	–	–	–	32	43	24	–	–	–	–	–	–	–
Eritrea	–	–	–	47	31	60	–	–	–	89	86	91	63	–	–	–
Ethiopia	53	59	46	49	27	55	7	29	5	74	69	76	38	81	–	–
Gabon	–	–	–	34	30	49	89	90	87	–	–	–	–	–	–	–
Gambia	25	20	29	36	24	45	55	57	54	78	72	83	64	74	–	84
Georgia	18	20	17	17	12	23	92	97	87	–	–	–	–	7	30	66
Ghana	34	34	34	22	15	28	51	69	42	4	2	6	1	47	21	89
Guatemala	29	25	32	34	25	44	–	–	–	–	–	–	–	–	2y	–
Guinea	25	26	24	63	45	75	43	78	33	96	94	96	57	86	–	–
Guinea-Bissau	39	41	37	24	14	32	39	53	33	45	39	48	35	52	–	80
Guyana	19	21	17	20	15	22	93	96	92	–	–	–	–	18	–	74
Haiti	21	22	19	30	27	33	81	87	78	–	–	–	–	29	–	–
Honduras	16	16	15	39	33	46	94	95	93	–	–	–	–	16	–	–
India	12	12	12	47	29	56	41	59	35	–	–	–	–	54	–	–
Indonesia	4y	5y	4y	24	15	33	55	69	43	–	–	–	–	25	–	–
Iraq	11	12	9	17	16	19	95	95	96	–	–	–	–	59	21	84
Jamaica	6	7	5	9	7	11	89	88	89	–	–	–	–	6	24	87
Jordan	–	–	–	10	–	–	–	–	–	–	–	–	–	90	–	–
Kazakhstan	2	2	2	7	6	9	99	99	99	–	–	–	–	10	–	52
Kenya	26	27	25	25	19	27	48y	64y	44y	32	21	36	21	68	–	–
Kyrgyzstan	4	4	3	10	7	14	94	96	93	–	–	–	–	38	–	51
Lao People's Democratic Republic	25	24	26	–	–	–	59	71	56	–	–	–	–	–	–	–
Lebanon	7	8	6	11	–	–	–	–	–	–	–	–	–	–	–	–
Lesotho	23	25	21	23	13	26	26	39	24	–	–	–	–	–	–	–
Liberia	–	–	–	40	–	–	–	–	–	–	–	–	–	–	–	–
Madagascar	32	36	28	39	29	42	75	87	72	–	–	–	–	28	–	–
Malawi	29	28	29	50	38	53	–	–	–	–	–	–	–	28	–	–
Maldives	–	–	–	–	–	–	73	–	–	–	–	–	–	70	–	–
Mali	34	35	33	71	60	77	53	75	45	85	81	87	69	75	–	–
Mauritania	4y	5y	3y	35	27	44	56	75	42	72	60	84	66	–	30	–
Mexico	16y	15y	16y	28x	31x	21x	–	–	–	–	–	–	–	–	–	–
Moldova	32	32	33	19	16	22	98	98	98	–	–	–	–	21	–	–
Mongolia	18	19	17	9	7	12	98	98	99	–	–	–	–	20	26	79
Montenegro	10	12	8	5	5	5	98	98	99	–	–	–	–	11	14	61
Morocco	11y	13y	9y	16	12	21	85	92	80	–	–	–	–	–	–	–
Mozambique	–	–	–	56	41	66	–	–	–	–	–	–	–	–	–	–
Myanmar	–	–	–	–	–	–	65y	88y	59y	–	–	–	–	–	–	–
Namibia	13y	15y	12y	9	–	–	67	83	59	–	–	–	–	35	–	–
Nepal	31y	30y	33y	51	41	54	35	42	34	–	–	–	–	23	–	–
Nicaragua	15	18	11	43	36	55	81	90	73	–	–	–	–	17	–	–
Niger	43	43	43	75	42	84	32	71	25	2	2	2	1	70	–	–
Nigeria	13y	–	–	43	27	52	33y	52y	25y	19	28	14	10	65	–	–
Occupied Palestinian Territory	–	–	–	19	–	–	96y	97y	96y	–	–	–	–	–	–	95
Pakistan	–	–	–	32x	21x	37x	–	–	–	–	–	–	–	–	–	–
Panama	3	5	2	–	–	–	–	–	–	–	–	–	–	–	–	–
Paraguay	15	17	12	24x	18x	32x	–	–	–	–	–	–	–	–	–	–

150 THE STATE OF THE WORLD'S CHILDREN 2009

...TABLE 9

Countries and territories	Child labour (5–14 years) 1999–2007* total	male	female	Child marriage 1998–2007* total	urban	rural	Birth registration 2000–2007* total	urban	rural	Female genital mutilation/cutting 2002–2007* women[a] (15–49 years) total	urban	rural	daughters[b] total	Attitude towards domestic violence 2001–2007* total	Child disability◊ 1999–2007* total	Child discipline 2005–2007* total
Peru	19	20	19	18	13	31	93	95	90	–	–	–	–	–	–	–
Philippines	12	13	11	14	10	22	83	87	78	–	–	–	–	24	–	–
Portugal	3y	4y	3y	–	–	–	–	–	–	–	–	–	–	–	–	–
Romania	1	1	1	–	–	–	–	–	–	–	–	–	–	–	–	–
Rwanda	35	36	35	13	9	14	82	79	83	–	–	–	–	48	2y	–
Sao Tome and Principe	8	8	7	33	31	37	69	70	67	–	–	–	–	32	29	–
Senegal	22	24	21	39	23	55	55	75	44	28	22	34	20	65	–	–
Serbia	4	5	4	6	4	8	99	99	99	–	–	–	–	6	14	73
Sierra Leone	48	49	48	56	34	66	48	62	44	94	86	97	35	85	34	92
Somalia	49	45	54	45	35	52	3	6	2	98	97	98	46	76y	–	–
South Africa	–	–	–	8	5	12	78y	–	–	–	–	–	–	–	–	–
Sri Lanka	8	9	7	12y	–	–	–	–	–	–	–	–	–	–	–	–
Sudan	13	14	12	34	24	40	33	53	22	89	88	90	43y	–	–	–
Suriname	–	–	–	19	14	33	97	98	95	–	–	–	–	13	39	84
Swaziland	9	9	9	5	1	6	30	38	28	–	–	–	–	38	–	–
Syrian Arab Republic	4	5	3	13	15	12	95	96	95	–	–	–	–	–	–	87
Tajikistan	10	9	11	13	13	13	88	85	90	–	–	–	–	74y	–	74
Thailand	8	8	8	20	12	23	99	100	99	–	–	–	–	–	15	–
The former Yugoslav Republic of Macedonia	6	7	5	4	3	4	94	95	93	–	–	–	–	21	21	69
Timor-Leste	4	4	4	–	–	–	53y	–	–	–	–	–	–	–	–	–
Togo	29	29	30	24	15	36	78	93	69	6	4	7	1	53	–	90
Trinidad and Tobago	1	1	1	8	–	–	96	–	–	–	–	–	–	8	–	75
Tunisia	–	–	–	10x	7x	14x	–	–	–	–	–	–	–	–	–	–
Turkey	5	4	6	18	17	22	84	87	79	–	–	–	–	39	–	–
Turkmenistan	–	–	–	7	9	6	96	96	95	–	–	–	–	38y	–	–
Uganda	36	37	36	46	27	52	21	24	21	1	0	1	–	70	11y	–
Ukraine	7	8	7	6	6	10	100	100	100	–	–	–	–	5	–	70
United Republic of Tanzania	36	37	34	41	23	49	8	22	4	15	7	18	4	60	–	–
Uruguay	8y	8y	8y	–	–	–	–	–	–	–	–	–	–	–	–	–
Uzbekistan	2	2	2	7	9	7	100	100	100	–	–	–	–	70	3	–
Venezuela (Bolivarian Republic of)	8	9	6	–	–	–	92	–	–	–	–	–	–	–	–	–
Viet Nam	16	15	16	10	3	13	88	94	86	–	–	–	–	64	4y	93
Yemen	11y	11y	12y	32	28	35	22	38	16	23x	26x	22x	20x	–	29	94
Zambia	12y	11y	12y	42	32	49	10	16	6	1	1	1	–	85	–	–
Zimbabwe	13y	12y	14y	34	20	44	74	83	71	–	–	–	–	48	–	–

SUMMARY INDICATORS

	total	male	female	total	urban	rural	total	urban	rural	total	urban	rural	total	total	total	total
Sub-Saharan Africa	35n	36n	34n	40	25	48	37	52	30	34	30	37	19	65	–	–
Eastern and Southern Africa	36	38	33	36	20	43	32	41	24	43	36	46	28	65	–	–
West and Central Africa	35n	34n	35n	44	28	55	41	57	35	28	28	29	14	64	–	–
Middle East and North Africa	9	10	8	18	12	23	75	86	67	–	–	–	–	–	–	89
South Asia	13	13	12	49	32	58	36	52	30	–	–	–	–	53	–	–
East Asia and Pacific	10**	11**	10**	19**	12**	25**	72**	81**	67**	–	–	–	–	34**	3	–
Latin America and Caribbean	11	11	10	–	–	–	89	92	82	–	–	–	–	–	–	–
CEE/CIS	5	5	5	11	11	13	92	93	92	–	–	–	–	32	–	–
Industrialized countries§	–	–	–	–	–	–	–	–	–	–	–	–	–	–	–	–
Developing countries§	16***	17***	15***	36**	22**	46**	50**	65**	39**	–	–	–	–	51**	–	–
Least developed countries§	30	31	28	49	37	55	29	42	25	–	–	–	–	–	–	–
World	–	–	–	–	–	–	–	–	–	–	–	–	–	–	–	–

§ Also includes territories within each country category or regional group. Countries and territories in each country category or regional group are listed on page 152.

DEFINITIONS OF THE INDICATORS

Child labour – Percentage of children 5–14 years old involved in child labour at the moment of the survey. A child is considered to be involved in child labour under the following conditions: (a) children 5–11 years old who, during the week preceding the survey, did at least one hour of economic activity or at least 28 hours of domestic work, or (b) children 12–14 years old who, during the week preceding the survey, did at least 14 hours of economic activity or at least 28 hours of domestic work.

Child labour background variables – Sex of the child; urban or rural place of residence; poorest 20 per cent or richest 20 per cent of the population constructed from household assets (a more detailed description of the household wealth estimation procedure can be found at <www.childinfo.org>); mother's education, reflecting mothers with and without some level of education.

Child marriage – Percentage of women 20–24 years old who were married or in union before they were 18 years old.

Birth registration – Percentage of children less than five years old who were registered at the moment of the survey. The numerator of this indicator includes children whose birth certificate was seen by the interviewer or whose mother or caretaker says the birth has been registered. MICS data refer to children alive at the time of the survey.

Female genital mutilation/cutting – (a) Women – the percentage of women 15–49 years old who have been mutilated/cut. (b) Daughters – the percentage of women 15–49 years old with at least one mutilated/cut daughter. Female genital mutilation/cutting is the cutting or alteration of the female genitalia for social reasons.

Attitudes towards domestic violence – Percentage of women 15–49 years old who consider a husband to be justified in hitting or beating his wife for at least one of the specified reasons. Women were asked whether a husband is justified in hitting or beating his wife under a series of circumstances, i.e., if his wife burns the food, argues with him, goes out without telling him, neglects the children or refuses sexual relations.

Child disability – Percentage of children 2–9 years old with at least one reported disability (i.e., cognitive, motor, seizure, vision, hearing or speech).

Child discipline – Percentage of children 2–14 years old who experience any psychological or physical punishment.

MAIN DATA SOURCES

Child labour – Multiple Indicator Cluster Surveys (MICS) and Demographic and Health Surveys (DHS).

Child marriage – MICS, DHS and other national surveys.

Birth registration – MICS, DHS, other national surveys and vital registration systems.

Female genital mutilation/cutting – MICS, DHS and other national surveys.

Attitudes towards domestic violence – MICS, DHS and other national surveys.

Child disability – MICS, DHS and other national surveys.

Child discipline – MICS, DHS and other national surveys.

NOTES
- – Data not available.
- x Data refer to years or periods other than those specified in the column heading, differ from the standard definition or refer to only part of a country. Such data are not included in the calculation of regional and global averages.
- y Data refer to years or periods other than those specified in the column heading, differ from the standard definition or refer to only part of a country. Such data are included in the calculation of regional and global averages.
- n Excludes Nigeria.
- ◊ A fuller explanation of the methodology and the recent changes in calculating these estimates can be found in the *General note on the data*, page 114.
- * Data refer to the most recent year available during the period specified in the column heading.
- ** Excludes China.
- *** Excludes China and Nigeria.

Summary indicators

Averages given at the end of each table are calculated using data from the countries and territories as grouped below.

Sub-Saharan Africa

Angola; Benin; Botswana; Burkina Faso; Burundi; Cameroon; Cape Verde; Central African Republic; Chad; Comoros; Congo; Côte d'Ivoire; Democratic Republic of the Congo; Equatorial Guinea; Eritrea; Ethiopia; Gabon; Gambia; Ghana; Guinea; Guinea-Bissau; Kenya; Lesotho; Liberia; Madagascar; Malawi; Mali; Mauritania; Mauritius; Mozambique; Namibia; Niger; Nigeria; Rwanda; Sao Tome and Principe; Senegal; Seychelles; Sierra Leone; Somalia; South Africa; Swaziland; Togo; Uganda; United Republic of Tanzania; Zambia; Zimbabwe

Middle East and North Africa

Algeria; Bahrain; Djibouti; Egypt; Iran (Islamic Republic of); Iraq; Jordan; Kuwait; Lebanon; Libyan Arab Jamahiriya; Morocco; Occupied Palestinian Territory; Oman; Qatar; Saudi Arabia; Sudan; Syrian Arab Republic; Tunisia; United Arab Emirates; Yemen

South Asia

Afghanistan; Bangladesh; Bhutan; India; Maldives; Nepal; Pakistan; Sri Lanka

East Asia and Pacific

Brunei Darussalam; Cambodia; China; Cook Islands; Democratic People's Republic of Korea; Fiji; Indonesia; Kiribati; Lao People's Democratic Republic; Malaysia; Marshall Islands; Micronesia (Federated States of); Mongolia; Myanmar; Nauru; Niue; Palau; Papua New Guinea; Philippines; Republic of Korea; Samoa; Singapore; Solomon Islands; Thailand; Timor-Leste; Tonga; Tuvalu; Vanuatu; Viet Nam

Latin America and Caribbean

Antigua and Barbuda; Argentina; Bahamas; Barbados; Belize; Bolivia; Brazil; Chile; Colombia; Costa Rica; Cuba; Dominica; Dominican Republic; Ecuador; El Salvador; Grenada; Guatemala; Guyana; Haiti; Honduras; Jamaica; Mexico; Nicaragua; Panama; Paraguay; Peru; Saint Kitts and Nevis; Saint Lucia; Saint Vincent and the Grenadines; Suriname; Trinidad and Tobago; Uruguay; Venezuela (Bolivarian Republic of)

CEE/CIS

Albania; Armenia; Azerbaijan; Belarus; Bosnia and Herzegovina; Bulgaria; Croatia; Georgia; Kazakhstan; Kyrgyzstan; Moldova, Republic of; Montenegro; Romania; Russian Federation; Serbia; Tajikistan; The former Yugoslav Republic of Macedonia; Turkey; Turkmenistan; Ukraine; Uzbekistan

Industrialized countries/territories

Andorra; Australia; Austria; Belgium; Canada; Cyprus; Czech Republic; Denmark; Estonia; Finland; France; Germany; Greece; Holy See; Hungary; Iceland; Ireland; Israel; Italy; Japan; Latvia; Liechtenstein; Lithuania; Luxembourg; Malta; Monaco; Netherlands; New Zealand; Norway; Poland; Portugal; San Marino; Slovakia; Slovenia; Spain; Sweden; Switzerland; United Kingdom; United States

Developing countries/territories

Afghanistan; Algeria; Angola; Antigua and Barbuda; Argentina; Armenia; Azerbaijan; Bahamas; Bahrain; Bangladesh; Barbados; Belize; Benin; Bhutan; Bolivia; Botswana; Brazil; Brunei Darussalam; Burkina Faso; Burundi; Cambodia; Cameroon; Cape Verde; Central African Republic; Chad; Chile; China; Colombia; Comoros; Congo; Cook Islands; Costa Rica; Côte d'Ivoire; Cuba; Cyprus; Democratic Republic of the Congo; Democratic People's Republic of Korea; Djibouti; Dominica; Dominican Republic; Ecuador; Egypt; El Salvador; Equatorial Guinea; Eritrea; Ethiopia; Fiji; Gabon; Gambia; Georgia; Ghana; Grenada; Guatemala; Guinea; Guinea-Bissau; Guyana; Haiti; Honduras; India; Indonesia; Iran (Islamic Republic of); Iraq; Israel; Jamaica; Jordan; Kazakhstan; Kenya; Kiribati; Kuwait; Kyrgyzstan; Lao People's Democratic Republic; Lebanon; Lesotho; Liberia; Libyan Arab Jamahiriya; Madagascar; Malawi; Malaysia; Maldives; Mali; Marshall Islands; Mauritania; Mauritius; Mexico; Micronesia (Federated States of); Mongolia; Morocco; Mozambique; Myanmar; Namibia; Nauru; Nepal; Nicaragua; Niger; Nigeria; Niue; Occupied Palestinian Territory; Oman; Pakistan; Palau; Panama; Papua New Guinea; Paraguay; Peru; Philippines; Qatar; Republic of Korea; Rwanda; Saint Kitts and Nevis; Saint Lucia; Saint Vincent and the Grenadines; Samoa; Sao Tome and Principe; Saudi Arabia; Senegal; Seychelles; Sierra Leone; Singapore; Solomon Islands; Somalia; South Africa; Sri Lanka; Sudan; Suriname; Swaziland; Syrian Arab Republic; Tajikistan; Thailand; Timor-Leste; Togo; Tonga; Trinidad and Tobago; Tunisia; Turkey; Turkmenistan; Tuvalu; Uganda; United Arab Emirates; United Republic of Tanzania; Uruguay; Uzbekistan; Vanuatu; Venezuela (Bolivarian Republic of); Viet Nam; Yemen; Zambia; Zimbabwe

Least developed countries/territories

Afghanistan; Angola; Bangladesh; Benin; Bhutan; Burkina Faso; Burundi; Cambodia; Cape Verde; Central African Republic; Chad; Comoros; Democratic Republic of the Congo; Djibouti; Equatorial Guinea; Eritrea; Ethiopia; Gambia; Guinea; Guinea-Bissau; Haiti; Kiribati; Lao People's Democratic Republic; Lesotho; Liberia; Madagascar; Malawi; Maldives; Mali; Mauritania; Mozambique; Myanmar; Nepal; Niger; Rwanda; Samoa; Sao Tome and Principe; Senegal; Sierra Leone; Solomon Islands; Somalia; Sudan; Timor-Leste; Togo; Tuvalu; Uganda; United Republic of Tanzania; Vanuatu; Yemen; Zambia

Measuring human development
An introduction to Table 10

If development is to be measured by a comprehensive and inclusive assessment, then the need arises for a method of measuring human as well as economic progress. From UNICEF's point of view, there is a need for an agreed method of measuring the level of child well-being and its rate of change.

The under-five mortality rate (U5MR) is used in Table 10 (*pages 150–153*) as the principal indicator of such progress. In 2007, the number of children dying before their fifth birthday fell to 9.2 million. In comparison, in 1960, approximately 20 million children were dying every year – highlighting an important long-term decline in the global number of under-five deaths.

The U5MR has several advantages. First, it measures an end result of the development process rather than an 'input', such as school enrolment level, per capita calorie availability or the number of doctors per thousand population – all of which are means to an end.

Second, the U5MR is known to be the result of a wide variety of inputs: antibiotics to treat pneumonia; insecticide-treated mosquito nets to prevent malaria; the nutritional health and the health knowledge of mothers; the level of immunization and oral rehydration therapy use; the availability of maternal and child health services, including prenatal care; income and food availability in the family; the availability of safe drinking water and basic sanitation; and the overall safety of the child's environment.

Third, the U5MR is less susceptible to the fallacy of the average than, for example, per capita gross national income (GNI). This is because the natural scale does not allow the children of the rich to be one thousand times as likely to survive, even if the human-made scale does permit them to have one thousand times as much income. In other words, it is much more difficult for a wealthy minority to affect a nation's U5MR, and it therefore presents a more accurate, if far from perfect, picture of the health status of the majority of children and of society as a whole.

The speed of progress in reducing the U5MR can be measured by calculating its average annual rate of reduction (AARR). Unlike the comparison of absolute changes, the AARR reflects the fact that the lower limits to U5MR are approached only with increasing difficulty. As lower levels of under-five mortality are reached, for example, the same absolute reduction obviously represents a greater percentage reduction. The AARR therefore shows a higher rate of progress for a 10-point reduction, for example, if that reduction happens at a lower level of under-five mortality. A fall in the U5MR of 10 points from 100 to 90 represents a reduction of 10 per cent, whereas the same 10-point fall from 20 to 10 represents a reduction of 50 per cent. (A negative value for the percentage reduction indicates an increase in the U5MR over the period specified.)

When used in conjunction with gross domestic product (GDP) growth rates, the U5MR and its rate of reduction can therefore give a picture of the progress being made by any country, territory or region, and over any period of time, towards the satisfaction of some of the most essential of human needs.

As Table 10 shows, there is no fixed relationship between the annual reduction rate of the U5MR and the annual rate of growth in per capita GDP. Such comparisons help to shed light on the relationship between economic advances and human development.

Finally, the table gives the total fertility rate for each country and territory and the corresponding average annual rate of reduction. It is clear that many of the nations that have achieved significant reductions in their U5MR have also achieved significant reductions in fertility.

TABLE 10. THE RATE OF PROGRESS

Countries and territories	Under-5 mortality rank	Under-5 mortality rate 1970	Under-5 mortality rate 1990	Under-5 mortality rate 2007	Average annual rate of reduction (%) 1970–1990	Average annual rate of reduction (%) 1990–2007	Reduction since 1990 (%)	GDP per capita average annual growth rate (%) 1970–1990	GDP per capita average annual growth rate (%) 1990–2007	Total fertility rate 1970	Total fertility rate 1990	Total fertility rate 2007	Average annual rate of reduction (%) 1970–1990	Average annual rate of reduction (%) 1990–2007
Afghanistan	2	320	260	257	1.0	0.1	1	–	–	7.7	8.0	7.1	-0.2	0.7
Albania	126	107	46	15	4.2	6.6	67	-0.7x	5.2	4.9	2.9	2.1	2.6	2.0
Algeria	75	220	69	37	5.8	3.7	46	1.6	1.4	7.4	4.7	2.4	2.3	4.0
Andorra	189	–	6	3	–	4.1	50	–	–	–	–	–	–	–
Angola	16	–	258	158	–	2.9	39	0.4x	2.9	7.3	7.2	6.5	0.1	0.6
Antigua and Barbuda	140	–	–	11	–	–	–	8.3x	1.7	–	–	–	–	–
Argentina	125	68	29	16	4.3	3.5	45	-0.7	1.5	3.1	3.0	2.3	0.1	1.7
Armenia	99	–	56	24	–	5.0	57	–	5.8	3.2	2.5	1.4	1.2	3.7
Australia	160	21	9	6	4.2	2.4	33	1.5	2.4	2.7	1.9	1.8	1.9	0.3
Austria	173	29	9	4	5.9	4.8	56	2.4	1.8	2.3	1.5	1.4	2.3	0.2
Azerbaijan	71	–	98	39	–	5.4	60	–	2.8	4.6	3.0	1.8	2.2	3.1
Bahamas	134	49	29	13	2.6	4.7	55	1.8	0.4x	3.6	2.6	2.0	1.6	1.5
Bahrain	145	82	19	10	7.3	3.8	47	-1.3x	2.4x	6.5	3.7	2.3	2.8	2.8
Bangladesh	58	238	151	61	2.3	5.3	60	0.6	3.1	6.4	4.4	2.9	1.9	2.5
Barbados	137	54	17	12	5.8	2.0	29	1.5	1.3x	3.1	1.7	1.5	3.1	0.6
Belarus	134	–	24	13	–	3.6	46	–	3.4	2.3	1.9	1.2	1.0	2.6
Belgium	166	24	10	5	4.4	4.1	50	2.2	1.8	2.2	1.6	1.6	1.7	-0.2
Belize	97	–	43	25	–	3.2	42	2.9	2.4	6.3	4.5	3.0	1.7	2.5
Benin	25	256	184	123	1.7	2.4	33	0	1.3	7.0	6.8	5.5	0.2	1.3
Bhutan	45	288	148	84	3.3	3.3	43	6.8x	5.2	6.7	5.9	2.2	0.6	5.7
Bolivia	61	243	125	57	3.3	4.6	54	-1.1	1.3	6.6	4.9	3.5	1.5	1.9
Bosnia and Herzegovina	132	82	22	14	6.6	2.7	36	–	10.8x	2.9	1.7	1.2	2.6	2.0
Botswana	69	144	57	40	4.6	2.1	30	8.2	4.2	6.6	4.7	2.9	1.7	2.8
Brazil	107	134	58	22	4.2	5.7	62	2.3	1.2	5.0	2.8	2.3	2.9	1.3
Brunei Darussalam	148	78	11	9	9.8	1.2	18	-2.2x	-0.3x	5.7	3.2	2.3	2.8	2.0
Bulgaria	137	33	18	12	3.0	2.4	33	3.4x	2.3	2.2	1.7	1.3	1.2	1.6
Burkina Faso	7	281	206	191	1.6	0.4	7	1.3	2.5	7.6	7.3	6.0	0.2	1.1
Burundi	10	219	189	180	0.7	0.3	5	1.1	-2.7	6.8	6.8	6.8	0.0	0.0
Cambodia	40	–	119	91	–	1.6	24	–	6.2x	5.9	5.8	3.2	0.1	3.5
Cameroon	18	215	139	148	2.2	-0.4	-6	3.3	0.6	6.2	5.9	4.4	0.2	1.8
Canada	160	22	8	6	5.1	1.7	25	2	2.2	2.2	1.7	1.5	1.5	0.5
Cape Verde	84	–	60	32	–	3.7	47	–	3.3	7.0	5.5	3.4	1.2	2.8
Central African Republic	12	232	171	172	1.5	0.0	-1	-1.3	-0.8	5.7	5.7	4.6	0.0	1.2
Chad	3	–	201	209	–	-0.2	-4	-1	2.4	6.5	6.7	6.2	-0.1	0.4
Chile	148	98	21	9	7.7	5.0	57	1.5	3.7	4.0	2.6	1.9	2.1	1.8
China	107	118	45	22	4.8	4.2	51	6.6	8.9	5.6	2.2	1.7	4.7	1.4
Colombia	112	105	35	20	5.5	3.3	43	2	1	5.6	3.0	2.2	3.1	1.8
Comoros	55	215	120	66	2.9	3.5	45	0.1x	-0.4	7.1	6.1	4.4	0.7	2.0
Congo	24	142	104	125	1.6	-1.1	-20	3.2	-0.2	6.3	5.4	4.5	0.8	1.0
Cook Islands	117	–	32	18	–	3.4	44	–	–	–	–	–	–	–
Costa Rica	140	83	18	11	7.6	2.9	39	0.7	2.5	5.0	3.2	2.1	2.3	2.4
Côte d'Ivoire	22	236	151	127	2.2	1.0	16	-1.9	-0.7	7.4	6.6	4.5	0.5	2.2
Croatia	160	42	13	6	5.9	4.5	54	–	3	2.0	1.7	1.3	0.9	1.3
Cuba	156	39	13	7	5.5	3.6	46	–	3.6x	4.0	1.8	1.5	4.2	0.9
Cyprus	166	31	11	5	5.2	4.6	55	5.9x	2.2	2.6	2.4	1.6	0.4	2.5
Czech Republic	173	24	12	4	3.5	6.5	67	–	2.4	2.0	1.8	1.2	0.5	2.3
Democratic People's Republic of Korea	62	70	55	55	1.2	0.0	0	–	–	4.0	2.4	1.9	2.6	1.5
Democratic Republic of the Congo	15	235	200	161	0.8	1.3	20	-2.4	-4.3	6.4	6.7	6.7	-0.3	0.0
Denmark	173	16	9	4	2.9	4.8	56	2	1.9	2.1	1.7	1.8	1.2	-0.5
Djibouti	22	–	175	127	–	1.9	27	–	-2.1	7.4	6.2	4.0	0.9	2.5
Dominica	140	60	18	11	6.0	2.9	39	4.7x	2.4	–	–	–	–	–
Dominican Republic	73	131	66	38	3.4	3.2	42	2.1	3.8	6.2	3.3	2.8	3.1	0.9
Ecuador	107	140	57	22	4.5	5.6	61	1.3	1.2	6.3	3.7	2.6	2.7	2.0
Egypt	77	236	93	36	4.7	5.6	61	4.3	2.5	6.2	4.4	2.9	1.7	2.4
El Salvador	99	162	60	24	5.0	5.4	60	-1.8	1.8	6.4	3.7	2.7	2.7	1.8
Equatorial Guinea	4	–	170	206	–	-1.1	-21	–	21.1	5.7	5.9	5.4	-0.2	0.5
Eritrea	50	237	147	70	2.4	4.4	52	–	-0.3x	6.6	6.2	5.1	0.3	1.2
Estonia	160	20	18	6	0.5	6.5	67	1.5x	5.2	2.1	1.9	1.5	0.4	1.6
Ethiopia	27	241	204	119	0.8	3.2	42	–	2.2	6.8	6.8	5.3	0.0	1.4
Fiji	117	–	22	18	–	1.2	18	0.6x	1.5x	4.5	3.4	2.8	1.5	1.2
Finland	173	16	7	4	4.1	3.3	43	2.8	2.8	1.9	1.7	1.8	0.3	-0.2

...TABLE 10

	Under-5 mortality rank	Under-5 mortality rate			Average annual rate of reduction (%)⊖		Reduction since 1990 (%)⊖	GDP per capita average annual growth rate (%)		Total fertility rate			Average annual rate of reduction (%)	
		1970	1990	2007	1970–1990	1990–2007		1970–1990	1990–2007	1970	1990	2007	1970–1990	1990–2007
France	173	18	9	4	3.5	4.8	56	2.2	1.6	2.5	1.8	1.9	1.7	-0.5
Gabon	40	–	92	91	–	0.1	1	0.3	-0.7	4.8	4.8	3.1	0.0	2.6
Gambia	34	311	153	109	3.5	2.0	29	0.9	0.2	6.7	6.0	4.8	0.5	1.4
Georgia	88	–	47	30	–	2.6	36	3.2	1.8	2.6	2.1	1.4	1.0	2.4
Germany	173	26	9	4	5.3	4.8	56	2.3x	1.4	2.0	1.4	1.4	1.9	0.0
Ghana	30	183	120	115	2.1	0.3	4	-2.1	2.1	6.7	5.8	3.9	0.7	2.3
Greece	173	32	11	4	5.3	6.0	64	1.3	2.7	2.4	1.4	1.3	2.5	0.5
Grenada	114	–	37	19	–	3.9	49	4.9	2.5	4.6	3.7	2.3	1.1	2.8
Guatemala	71	168	82	39	3.6	4.4	52	0.2	1.4	6.2	5.6	4.2	0.6	1.7
Guinea	17	326	231	150	1.7	2.5	35	0.3x	1.3	7.0	6.7	5.5	0.2	1.2
Guinea-Bissau	5	–	240	198	–	1.1	18	-0.2	-2.6	6.8	7.1	7.1	-0.2	0.0
Guyana	59	–	88	60	–	2.3	32	-1.5	3.1	5.6	2.6	2.3	3.8	0.6
Haiti	47	222	152	76	1.9	4.1	50	-0.3	-2.1	5.8	5.4	3.6	0.3	2.5
Holy See	–	–	–	–	–	–	–	–	–	–	–	–	–	–
Honduras	99	169	58	24	5.3	5.2	59	0.8	1.5	7.3	5.1	3.3	1.7	2.5
Hungary	156	40	17	7	4.3	5.2	59	3	3.3	2.0	1.8	1.3	0.6	2.0
Iceland	189	16	7	3	4.1	5.0	57	3.2	2.4	3.0	2.2	2.0	1.6	0.3
India	49	190	117	72	2.4	2.9	38	2.1	4.5	5.4	4.0	2.8	1.5	2.0
Indonesia	86	172	91	31	3.2	6.3	66	4.7	2.3	5.5	3.1	2.2	2.8	2.1
Iran (Islamic Republic of)	83	191	72	33	4.9	4.6	54	-2.3	2.5	6.6	5.0	2.0	1.3	5.3
Iraq	66	125	53	44	4.3	1.1	17	–	–	7.2	5.9	4.3	1.0	1.9
Ireland	173	23	9	4	4.7	4.8	56	2.8	5.8	3.9	2.1	2.0	3.1	0.4
Israel	166	29	12	5	4.4	5.1	58	1.9	1.7	3.8	3.0	2.8	1.2	0.4
Italy	173	33	10	4	6.0	5.4	60	2.8	1.2	2.4	1.3	1.4	3.1	-0.3
Jamaica	86	62	33	31	3.2	0.4	6	-1.3	0.8	5.5	2.9	2.5	3.1	1.1
Japan	173	17	6	4	5.2	2.4	33	3	0.9	2.1	1.6	1.3	1.3	1.3
Jordan	99	107	40	24	4.9	3.0	40	2.5x	2	7.9	5.5	3.1	1.8	3.3
Kazakhstan	84	88	60	32	1.9	3.7	47	–	3.2	3.5	2.8	2.3	1.1	1.3
Kenya	26	156	97	121	2.4	-1.3	-25	1.2	0	8.1	5.9	5.0	1.6	1.0
Kiribati	57	–	88	63	–	2.0	28	-5.3	1.8	–	–	–	–	–
Kuwait	140	59	15	11	6.8	1.8	27	-6.8x	1.1x	7.2	3.5	2.2	3.6	2.8
Kyrgyzstan	73	–	74	38	–	3.9	49	–	-0.5	4.9	3.9	2.5	1.2	2.7
Lao People's Democratic Republic	50	218	163	70	1.5	5.0	57	–	4.2	6.4	6.2	3.2	0.2	3.9
Latvia	148	20	17	9	0.8	3.7	47	3.4	4.7	1.9	1.9	1.3	0.0	2.3
Lebanon	91	54	37	29	1.9	1.4	22	–	2.5	5.1	3.1	2.2	2.4	2.1
Lesotho	45	171	102	84	2.6	1.1	18	3.1	1.8	5.8	4.9	3.4	0.8	2.2
Liberia	20	284	205	133	1.6	2.5	35	-4.2	1.9	6.9	6.9	6.8	0.0	0.1
Libyan Arab Jamahiriya	117	160	41	18	6.8	4.8	56	-4.9x	–	7.6	4.8	2.8	2.3	3.3
Liechtenstein	189	–	10	3	–	7.1	70	–	–	–	–	–	–	–
Lithuania	151	22	16	8	1.6	4.1	50	–	3	2.3	2.0	1.3	0.7	2.7
Luxembourg	189	23	9	3	4.7	6.5	67	2.7	3.2	2.0	1.6	1.7	1.1	-0.3
Madagascar	32	180	168	112	0.3	2.4	33	-2.4	-0.4	6.8	6.2	4.8	0.4	1.5
Malawi	33	334	209	111	2.3	3.7	47	-0.1	0.3	7.3	7.0	5.6	0.2	1.2
Malaysia	140	70	22	11	5.8	4.1	50	4	3.2	5.6	3.7	2.6	2.0	2.1
Maldives	88	–	111	30	–	7.7	73	–	5.5x	7.0	6.2	2.6	0.6	5.1
Mali	6	372	250	196	2.0	1.4	22	-0.3	2.2	7.5	7.4	6.5	0.0	0.8
Malta	166	28	11	5	4.7	4.6	55	6.5	2.7x	2.1	2.0	1.4	0.0	2.4
Marshall Islands	64	–	92	54	–	3.1	41	–	-2	–	–	–	–	–
Mauritania	27	233	130	119	2.9	0.5	8	-0.9	0.6	6.6	5.8	4.4	0.6	1.6
Mauritius	126	86	24	15	6.4	2.8	38	5.1x	3.7	3.7	2.2	1.9	2.5	1.1
Mexico	78	111	52	35	3.8	2.3	33	1.6	1.6	6.7	3.4	2.2	3.4	2.5
Micronesia (Federated States of)	69	–	58	40	–	2.2	31	–	-0.2	6.9	5.0	3.8	1.7	1.6
Moldova	117	65	37	18	2.8	4.2	51	1.8x	-1.3	2.6	2.4	1.4	0.3	3.2
Monaco	173	–	9	4	–	4.8	56	–	–	–	–	–	–	–
Mongolia	67	–	98	43	–	4.8	56	–	2.2	7.5	4.1	1.9	3.0	4.6
Montenegro	145	–	16	10	–	2.8	38	–	3.4x	2.4	2.0	1.8	0.9	0.6
Morocco	81	184	89	34	3.6	5.7	62	2	2	7.1	4.0	2.4	2.8	3.1
Mozambique	14	277	201	168	1.6	1.1	16	-1x	4.1	6.6	6.2	5.2	0.3	1.1
Myanmar	36	179	130	103	1.6	1.4	21	1.5	6.8x	6.1	3.4	2.1	2.8	3.0
Namibia	53	126	87	68	1.9	1.4	22	-2.3x	1.8	6.5	5.8	3.2	0.5	3.5
Nauru	88	–	–	30	–	–	–	–	–	–	–	–	–	–

STATISTICAL TABLES

TABLE 10. THE RATE OF PROGRESS

	Under-5 mortality rank	Under-5 mortality rate			Average annual rate of reduction (%)		Reduction since 1990 (%)	GDP per capita average annual growth rate (%)		Total fertility rate			Average annual rate of reduction (%)	
		1970	1990	2007	1970–1990	1990–2007		1970–1990	1990–2007	1970	1990	2007	1970–1990	1990–2007
Nepal	62	237	142	55	2.6	5.6	61	1.2	1.9	5.9	5.2	3.3	0.6	2.6
Netherlands	166	16	8	5	3.5	2.8	38	1.5	2.1	2.4	1.6	1.7	2.2	-0.6
New Zealand	160	21	11	6	3.2	3.6	45	0.8	2	3.1	2.1	2.0	2.0	0.2
Nicaragua	78	165	68	35	4.4	3.9	49	-3.7	1.9	6.9	4.8	2.8	1.9	3.2
Niger	11	318	304	176	0.2	3.2	42	-2.2	-0.6	8.1	7.9	7.2	0.1	0.5
Nigeria	8	265	230	189	0.7	1.2	18	-1.4	1.2	6.9	6.8	5.4	0.1	1.3
Niue	–	–	–	–	–	–	–	–	–	–	–	–	–	–
Norway	173	16	9	4	2.9	4.8	56	3.2	2.6	2.5	1.9	1.8	1.5	0.1
Occupied Palestinian Territory	95	–	38	27	–	2.0	29	–	-2.9x	7.9	6.4	5.2	1.0	1.3
Oman	137	200	32	12	9.2	5.8	63	3.3	2.2x	7.2	6.6	3.0	0.4	4.6
Pakistan	43	184	132	90	1.7	2.3	32	3	1.6	6.6	6.3	3.5	0.2	3.4
Palau	145	–	21	10	–	4.4	52	–	–	–	–	–	–	–
Panama	104	68	34	23	3.5	2.3	32	0.3	2.6	5.3	3.0	2.6	2.8	0.9
Papua New Guinea	56	156	94	65	2.5	2.2	31	-0.7	-0.6	6.2	4.8	3.8	1.2	1.3
Paraguay	91	75	41	29	3.0	2.0	29	2.8	-0.3	5.7	4.5	3.1	1.2	2.2
Peru	112	170	78	20	3.9	8.0	74	-0.6	2.7	6.3	3.9	2.5	2.4	2.6
Philippines	94	89	62	28	1.8	4.7	55	0.8	1.7	6.3	4.3	3.3	1.8	1.7
Poland	156	35	17	7	3.6	5.2	59	–	4.4	2.2	2.0	1.2	0.4	3.0
Portugal	173	66	15	4	7.4	7.8	73	2.6	1.9	2.8	1.5	1.5	3.0	0.3
Qatar	126	51	26	15	3.4	3.2	42	–	–	6.9	4.4	2.7	2.3	2.9
Republic of Korea	166	54	9	5	9.0	3.5	44	6.2	4.4	4.5	1.6	1.2	5.2	1.7
Romania	126	52	32	15	2.4	4.5	53	0.9x	2.3	2.9	1.9	1.3	2.0	2.3
Russian Federation	126	40	27	15	2.0	3.5	44	–	1.2	2.0	1.9	1.3	0.3	2.0
Rwanda	9	223	195	181	0.7	0.4	7	1.1	1.1	8.2	7.6	5.9	0.4	1.5
Saint Kitts and Nevis	117	–	36	18	–	4.1	50	6.3x	2.8	–	–	–	–	–
Saint Lucia	117	66	21	18	5.7	0.9	14	5.3x	1.3	6.1	3.3	2.2	3.0	2.5
Saint Vincent and the Grenadines	114	72	22	19	5.9	0.9	14	3.3	3	6.0	3.0	2.2	3.5	1.8
Samoa	95	101	50	27	3.5	3.6	46	–	2.6	6.1	4.8	4.0	1.2	1.0
San Marino	173	–	13	4	–	6.9	69	–	–	–	–	–	–	–
Sao Tome and Principe	38	104	101	99	0.1	0.1	2	–	–	6.5	5.4	3.9	0.9	1.9
Saudi Arabia	97	185	44	25	7.2	3.3	43	-1.5	0.3	7.3	5.8	3.4	1.1	3.2
Senegal	31	276	149	114	3.1	1.6	23	-0.7	1.1	7.0	6.6	4.7	0.3	1.9
Serbia	151	–	–	8	–	–	–	–	2.6x	2.4	2.1	1.8	0.6	1.0
Seychelles	134	59	19	13	5.7	2.2	32	2.9	1.4	–	–	–	–	–
Sierra Leone	1	371	290	262	1.2	0.6	10	-0.4	-0.4	6.5	6.5	6.5	0.0	0.0
Singapore	189	27	8	3	6.1	5.8	63	5.6	3.8	3.0	1.8	1.3	2.7	1.9
Slovakia	151	31	15	8	3.6	3.7	47	–	3.3	2.5	2.0	1.2	1.0	2.9
Slovenia	173	29	11	4	4.8	6.0	64	–	3.5	2.3	1.5	1.3	2.0	1.0
Solomon Islands	50	–	121	70	–	3.2	42	3.4	-1.6	6.9	5.9	3.9	0.8	2.4
Somalia	19	–	203	142	–	2.1	30	-0.9	–	7.3	6.8	6.1	0.3	0.6
South Africa	60	113	64	59	2.8	0.5	8	0.1	1	5.6	3.6	2.7	2.2	1.7
Spain	173	25	9	4	5.1	4.8	56	1.9	2.4	2.9	1.3	1.4	3.9	-0.2
Sri Lanka	110	100	32	21	5.7	2.5	34	3	3.9	4.4	2.5	1.9	2.7	1.7
Sudan	34	168	125	109	1.5	0.8	13	0.1	3.6	6.6	6.0	4.3	0.5	1.9
Suriname	91	–	51	29	–	3.3	43	-2.4x	1.8	5.7	2.7	2.4	3.6	0.7
Swaziland	40	199	96	91	3.6	0.3	5	3.1	-0.3	6.9	5.7	3.5	0.9	2.9
Sweden	189	13	7	3	3.1	5.0	57	1.8	2.2	2.0	2.0	1.8	0.1	0.7
Switzerland	166	18	8	5	4.1	2.8	38	1.2	0.7	2.0	1.5	1.4	1.4	0.5
Syrian Arab Republic	123	128	37	17	6.2	4.6	54	2	1.5	7.6	5.5	3.1	1.6	3.4
Tajikistan	54	138	117	67	0.8	3.3	43	–	-2.2	6.9	5.2	3.4	1.4	2.5
Thailand	156	103	31	7	6.0	8.8	77	5	2.9	5.5	2.1	1.8	4.8	0.8
The former Yugoslav Republic of Macedonia	123	119	38	17	5.7	4.7	55	–	0.5	3.2	1.9	1.4	2.4	1.8
Timor-Leste	39	–	184	97	–	3.8	47	–	–	6.3	5.3	6.6	0.8	-1.2
Togo	37	219	150	100	1.9	2.4	33	-0.6	-0.2	7.0	6.4	4.9	0.5	1.6
Tonga	104	50	32	23	2.2	1.9	28	–	2	5.9	4.6	3.8	1.3	1.2
Trinidad and Tobago	78	54	34	35	2.3	-0.2	-3	0.5	5.1	3.5	2.4	1.6	1.8	2.4
Tunisia	110	201	52	21	6.8	5.3	60	2.5	3.4	6.6	3.6	1.9	3.0	3.7
Turkey	104	201	82	23	4.5	7.5	72	1.9	2.2	5.5	3.0	2.1	3.0	2.1
Turkmenistan	65	–	99	50	–	4.0	49	–	-6.8x	6.3	4.3	2.5	1.9	3.2

...TABLE 10

	Under-5 mortality rank	Under-5 mortality rate			Average annual rate of reduction (%)ᶿ		Reduction since 1990 (%)ᶿ	GDP per capita average annual growth rate (%)		Total fertility rate			Average annual rate of reduction (%)	
		1970	1990	2007	1970–1990	1990–2007		1970–1990	1990–2007	1970	1990	2007	1970–1990	1990–2007
Tuvalu	75	–	53	37	–	2.1	30	–	–	–	–	–	–	–
Uganda	21	195	175	130	0.5	1.7	26	–	3.1	7.1	7.1	6.5	0.0	0.5
Ukraine	99	36	25	24	1.8	0.2	4	–	-0.7	2.1	1.9	1.2	0.6	2.6
United Arab Emirates	151	84	15	8	8.6	3.7	47	-4.8x	-0.3x	6.6	4.4	2.3	2.1	3.8
United Kingdom	160	21	9	6	4.2	2.4	33	2	2.4	2.3	1.8	1.8	1.2	0.0
United Republic of Tanzania	29	217	157	116	1.6	1.8	26	–	1.8	6.8	6.1	5.2	0.5	0.9
United States	151	23	11	8	3.7	1.9	27	2.2	2	2.2	2.0	2.1	0.6	-0.2
Uruguay	132	60	25	14	4.4	3.4	44	0.9	1.5	2.9	2.5	2.1	0.7	1.0
Uzbekistan	68	–	74	41	–	3.5	45	–	1.2	6.5	4.2	2.5	2.2	3.0
Vanuatu	81	155	62	34	4.6	3.5	45	1.1x	-0.4	6.3	4.9	3.8	1.2	1.6
Venezuela (Bolivarian Republic of)	114	62	32	19	3.3	3.1	41	-1.6	-0.2	5.4	3.4	2.6	2.2	1.7
Viet Nam	126	85	56	15	2.1	7.7	73	–	6	7.0	3.7	2.2	3.2	3.2
Yemen	48	309	127	73	4.4	3.3	43	–	1.6	8.6	8.1	5.5	0.3	2.2
Zambia	13	179	163	170	0.5	-0.2	-4	-2.3	0.1	7.4	6.5	5.2	0.7	1.2
Zimbabwe	43	131	95	90	1.6	0.3	5	-0.4	-2.1x	7.4	5.2	3.2	1.8	2.8

SUMMARY INDICATORS

		1970	1990	2007	1970–1990	1990–2007		1970–1990	1990–2007	1970	1990	2007	1970–1990	1990–2007
Sub-Saharan Africa		232	186	148	1.1	1.3	20	-0.1	1.3	6.8	6.3	5.2	0.4	1.1
Eastern and Southern Africa		202	165	123	1.0	1.7	25	–	1.4	6.8	6.0	4.9	0.6	1.2
West and Central Africa		260	206	169	1.2	1.2	18	-0.6	1.3	6.8	6.6	5.5	0.1	1.1
Middle East and North Africa		195	79	46	4.5	3.2	42	-0.1	1.6	6.8	5.0	3.0	1.5	3.0
South Asia		197	125	78	2.3	2.8	38	2.1	4.1	5.7	4.3	3.0	1.4	2.2
East Asia and Pacific		121	56	27	3.9	4.3	52	5.7	6.8	5.6	2.5	1.9	4.1	1.6
Latin America and Caribbean		122	55	26	4.0	4.4	53	1.4	1.5	5.3	3.2	2.4	2.5	1.8
CEE/CIS		91	53	25	2.7	4.4	53	–	1.6	2.8	2.3	1.7	0.9	1.9
Industrialized countries§		24	10	6	4.4	3.0	40	2.3	1.9	2.3	1.7	1.7	1.3	0.2
Developing countries§		162	103	74	2.3	1.9	28	2.4	4	5.8	3.6	2.8	2.3	1.6
Least developed countries§		241	179	130	1.5	1.9	27	-0.2	2.5	6.7	5.8	4.7	0.7	1.3
World		143	93	68	2.2	1.8	27	2.3	2.4	4.7	3.2	2.6	1.9	1.3

§ Also includes territories within each country category or regional group. Countries and territories in each country category or regional group are listed on page 152.

DEFINITIONS OF THE INDICATORS

Under-five mortality rate – Probability of dying between birth and exactly five years of age, expressed per 1,000 live births.

Reduction since 1990 (%) – Percentage reduction in the under-five mortality rate (U5MR) from 1990 to 2007. The United Nations Millennium Declaration in 2000 established a goal of a two-thirds (67 per cent) reduction in U5MR from 1990 to 2015. This indicator provides a current assessment of progress towards this goal.

GDP per capita – Gross domestic product (GDP) is the sum of value added by all resident producers plus any product taxes (less subsidies) not included in the valuation of output. GDP per capita is gross domestic product divided by midyear population. Growth is calculated from constant price GDP data in local currency.

Total fertility rate – Number of children who would be born per woman if she lived to the end of her childbearing years and bore children at each age in accordance with prevailing age-specific fertility rates.

MAIN DATA SOURCES

Under-five mortality rate – UNICEF, United Nations Population Division and United Nations Statistics Division.

GDP per capita – World Bank.

Fertility – United Nations Population Division.

NOTES

– Data not available.

x Data refer to years or periods other than those specified in the column heading, differ from the standard definition or refer to only part of a country. Such data are not included in the calculation of regional and global averages.

ᶿ A negative value indicates an increase in the under-five mortality rate since 1990.

Acronyms

ACSD	Accelerated Child Survival and Development	**MICS**	Multiple Indicator Cluster Surveys
AIDS	acquired immune deficiency syndrome	**OECD**	Organisation of Economic Co-operation and Development
EmOC	emergency obstetric care	**PMTCT**	prevention of mother-to-child transmission (of HIV)
FGM/C	female genital mutilation/cutting		
GDP	gross domestic product	**UN SG**	United Nations Secretary-General
HIV	human immunodeficiency virus	**UNAIDS**	Joint United Nations Programme on HIV/AIDS
HMN	Health Metrics Network	**UNESCO**	United Nations Educational, Scientific and Cultural Organization
IMCI	Integrated Management of Childhood Illness	**UNFPA**	United Nations Population Fund
IMNCH	Integrated Management of Newborn and Child Health	**UNICEF**	United Nations Children's Fund
MDG	Millennium Development Goal	**WHO**	World Health Organization